T0366712

# NESTED ECOLOGIES

THE WILLIAM & BETTYE NOWLIN SERIES
*in Art, History, and Culture of the Western Hemisphere*

# NESTED ECOLOGIES

## A Multilayered Ethnography of Functional Medicine

Rosalynn A. Vega

University of Texas Press

*Austin*

Requests for permission to reproduce material from this work should be sent to:
    Permissions
    University of Texas Press
    P.O. Box 7819
    Austin, TX 78713-7819
    utpress.utexas.edu/rp-form

♾ The paper used in this book meets the minimum requirements of ANSI/NISO
Z39.48-1992 (R1997) (Permanence of Paper).

Library of Congress Cataloging-in-Publication Data

Names: Vega, Rosalynn A., author.
Title: Nested ecologies : a multilayered ethnography of functional medicine /
Rosalynn A. Vega.
Description: First edition. | Austin : University of Texas Press, 2023. | Includes
bibliographical references and index.
Identifiers: LCCN 2022025718
    ISBN 978-1-4773-2685-5 (cloth)
    ISBN 978-1-4773-2686-2 (paperback)
    ISBN 978-1-4773-2687-9 (PDF)
    ISBN 978-1-4773-2688-6 (ePub)
Subjects: LCSH: Vega, Rosalynn A. | Functional medicine. | Chronically ill—Care. |
Medical anthropology. | Discrimination in medical care.
Classification: LCC R733 .V44 2023 | DDC 610—dc23/eng/20220628
LC record available at https://lccn.loc.gov/2022025718

doi:10.7560/326855

*For my daughter, Madelena*

# CONTENTS

# NESTED ECOLOGIES

# ∾ *Prelude* ∾

# ANTHROPOLOGY
# OF AND FOR HEALING

I come from a long line of Chinese women martyrs—my grandmother being the most loving and self-sacrificing of them all—so I received plenty of role modeling for silent suffering. As an example, when my grandmother fractured her spine in six places, she told no one for a whole day. When dinner was ready, we called her, but she didn't come—because she couldn't stand. I remember carrying her frail body in my arms (I'm a small woman, but she's even smaller) and placing her in the MRI machine. All the while, she was yelling how she didn't want to be X-rayed because the radiation could cause her to develop cancer in the future. She was about ninety at the time. I explained that the MRI was not an X-ray machine, but that didn't make any difference to her. "Lift me off of here immediately!" When I didn't mind her, she threatened me from inside the MRI tube. "As soon as I get out of here, I am going to whip you to death!" I retorted, "As soon as you are well enough to whip me to death, I will be so happy that I will allow you to!"

So, as I was saying, I come from a long line of Chinese women martyrs. My health issues were "nothing" in comparison to their suffering. Over time, I learned to adapt to different symptoms and limitations. I settled into a long-term state of "functional illness." By that, I mean I learned to cope with my illness, accept different limitations as part of who I am, and carry on with my daily responsibilities.

But I was not resilient. Even the common cold could knock me off my feet for weeks or months. I was using every strategy I had learned as a medical anthropologist and as someone who apprenticed to the curanderos and parteras (traditional medicine doctors and midwives) of Mexico, grew up with Traditional Chinese Medicine in her household, and studied in Brown University's Program in Liberal Medical Education. Still, I wasn't keeping my head above water.

Over time, I had been building up an extensive rap sheet of issues. Some of the problems began during childhood, like the digestive symptoms that started when I was around eight years old and were diagnosed as irritable bowel syndrome when I was fourteen. I started having pain in my neck and shoulders during my late teens and, about ten years later, was diagnosed with degenerative disc disease and arthritis. Some viruses I picked up in young adulthood while conducting research in rural Mexico for my first book. These included herpes simplex virus 1 and typhus. During that period, malnutrition took its toll on my body, paving the way for nutrient deficiencies resembling anemia. Other more recent diagnoses included autoimmunity, hypothyroidism, chronic fatigue syndrome, chronic Epstein-Barr viral infection, histamine intolerance, and estrogen dominance.

Other issues I had yet to find out. Among those diagnoses were mixed heavy metal poisoning, BPA poisoning, celiac disease, leaky gut, and microbial dysbiosis including a *Clostridium difficile* infection. Elevated LDL cholesterol leading to oxidized LDL cholesterol was also on the list, as were elevated Lp(a) (an independent risk factor of coronary heart disease), a mitochondrial disorder, exposure to mold, and multiple genetic single nucleotide polymorphisms (MTHFR C677T, slow COMT, a GSTM-1 deletion, etc.). "Genetic single nucleotide polymorphisms" means I have a limited ability to convert folic acid into bioavailable folate, metabolize estrogen and numerous neurotransmitters, and eliminate harmful toxins and viruses, among many other important functions.

At the time, like most patients, I didn't understand the interlinkages among all my health problems and was instead seeking to alleviate a range of seemingly unrelated symptoms. My esophagus was constantly stinging—the sensation was what I imagine it might feel like if one were to drink hard liquor nonstop. I was constantly itching everywhere, and I was allergic to everything, including the sun. For years, I had to wear long sleeves and pants, use a sun umbrella whenever I walked outside, and have an EpiPen with me at all times. I had hives on the inside of my eyelids, giving them a cobblestone texture. My hair was falling out in clumps. For the second time in my life, I was undergoing biopsies for cervical dysplasia—this time accompanied by a positive result for the human papillomavirus. I had migraines almost every day. Driving became difficult because I was often seeing double.

For months at a time, I could barely get out of bed, but I was determined to fulfill my professorial duties. On the days I was able to leave home, I grasped the lecture podium to keep from falling. When I was too weak to stand, I asked the departmental administrative assistant to set up a Skype session in my classroom so I could lecture to my students while lying down at home.[1] I feigned wellness for my students and colleagues, all the while fighting back nausea and gasping for air. During these Skype sessions, I propped myself up against the wall in bed, pulled my uncombed hair into a high bun, and did my very best to appear like I was seated somewhere—anywhere more professorial than where I actually was. As a woman of color, I am in the least represented demographic in my profession. I didn't want to give my students or colleagues any reason to focus on anything but the quality of my teaching and research. I was afraid that, were they to know the truth, they would define me by what felt like a steadily encroaching disability rather than by the scholarship of which I know I am capable.

I began seeking help from various doctors. Living on the US-Mexico border meant that a lot of the specialized attention I needed—for example, an immunologist who specializes in mast cell activation disorder—was totally inaccessible in the Rio Grande Valley. The Valley is home to mostly Hispanic residents, approximately a quarter of whom were identified in the Census Bureau's 2015 "ACS 1-Year Estimate" data set as "foreign-born persons." Some of the poorest counties in the United States are located in the Valley. While the region does have a booming health care industry (Gawande 2009), it is geared toward health problems relating to diabetes (Montoya 2011), obesity, and aging—issues that have taken on "epidemic" proportions in the Valley due to intersecting class and racialized inequalities.

In my case, I was "out of luck." When I sought help from my primary care doctor for my mast cells, he said, "I've never even heard of that! What kind of doctor works on that? Let me look it up on Google." I had to go farther to seek help, so I started scheduling regular visits in San Antonio, the nearest big city. This meant driving four or more hours away from the border, heading north in the direction of Austin. I could barely get out of bed, so there was no way I could manage the eight- to nine-hour round-trip drive on my own. My husband Rikin took sick leave to drive me to my doctor's appointments. As a federal public defender, Rikin represents the undocumented migrants who face criminal charges after entering the United States. It was difficult for him to leave his work so regularly, but he was committed to finding me the proper care and being my advocate for the short fifteen-minute visits we had with each doctor. Even though Rikin did all the driving, I would come back from those long days in the car, sometimes also having spent hours in the waiting room at the doctor's office, feeling totally beat. The situation was unsustainable.

Despite the great lengths Rikin and I went to seek help in San Antonio, I wasn't getting all the answers I needed to get better. During my initial visit with the primary care physician, the physician's assistant came into the consultation room after reviewing my intake form and told me that the doctor was refusing to see me until I whittled my list of health concerns down to three items. Confused, I asked the physician's assistant how it is possible, and why it is even useful, to isolate three issues, given that everything I listed on the intake form contributed to my overall state of illness. She responded that regular office visits are limited to fifteen minutes. In my case, the doctor was giving me an extended slot for my initial visit. But because my medical insurance will only pay for up to thirty minutes of the doctor's time, I would have to stick to three health issues and finish the appointment in under half an hour.

My experience with immunology in San Antonio was no better. The doctor prescribed three different types of antihistamines, to be taken in five pills throughout the day, to control my allergies to the sun, heat, and certain foods. The physician's assistant explained that eventually the treatment would become ineffective and I would have to switch to regular injections. I asked her if the injections were something I could do on my own at home. She explained that, since the solution had to be centrifuged, I would need to go to the clinic at least once a week for my injections. Her answer was unacceptable to me—I was not willing to spend my life tethered to a clinic or else risk anaphylactic shock. What the immunologist's office in San Antonio was offering me was not a cure—they simply wanted to throw more and more drugs at the problem. There had to be a better option. Even moving to a colder region seemed more feasible at that point.

I needed to take action. The medical doctors treating me didn't have the answers, so I needed to get the answers myself. While I had studied health sciences for several years in college (including a few credits at the medical school), had shadowed doctors from different specialties for a couple of years, and had been trained and certified in basic life support, I was far from being a medical doctor. However, in my final year of doctoral studies in medical anthropology and while on the job market for both academic and health care jobs, I crammed in a master's degree in epidemiology. The dean at the University of California, Berkeley raised the upper limit for credit hours so I could take fifty-two semester credits that year and graduate with both degrees. Thus, I had a decade of training in medical anthropology and epidemiology and six years of experience conducting ethnography. Armed with these tools, I set out to gain deep understanding into my own health issues.

My research into the epidemiological literature quickly revealed how seemingly discrete diagnoses and symptoms are all part of one disordered bodily system. Using the tools I had at hand—a black pen, a highlighter,

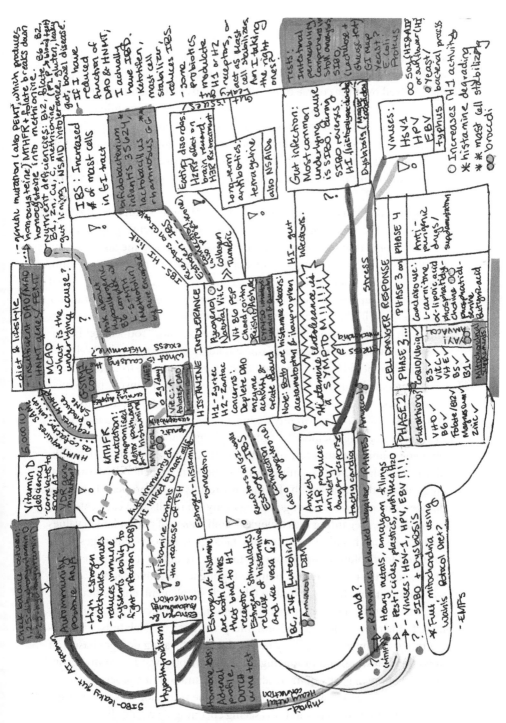

*Systems biology concept map.*

and the dry erase markers I use for teaching—I drew a concept map depicting how all of my health problems connect to one another in a network that evolved over the course of my life. The body's interconnectedness and the idea that underlying, systemic causes can manifest in different ways for different people were not strange concepts to me given that I regularly teach these concepts to my undergraduate students. However, I was now learning the underlying biological mechanisms undergirding these long-standing anthropological observations (see, for example, Foster 1976; Kleinman 1978).

I enlisted Rikin's help and support in creating a "Return to Wellness Workshop." We used our after-work hours to review emerging research and implement changes in our household that would help me take back my health. Some of these changes seemed a bit strange or unnecessary to him, especially since none involved medical intervention in the conventional sense, but he supported me nonetheless. At times, I doubted if I would ever get better, and in those moments, he reassured me. He looked into my eyes and, with tenderness and confidence in his voice, said, "You will get better. I know you will." I didn't feel the same confidence, but I thought, "Well, he's never lied to me, so it must be true." And I would continue to seek answers.

During my Return to Wellness Workshop sessions, I constantly updated a color-coded Microsoft Word table that included all the supplements I had at one point taken, was currently taking, or was considering for a later stage in my recovery. The document was organized into categories: general health, lipidology, immune support, neurotransmitter support, hormonal health, histamine balance, detox pathways/liver support, mitochondrial support, gut health, and thyroid health. To track my results and to properly titrate my dosages, I incorporated an ongoing log of my lab results into each category, as well as notes regarding the etiological significance of particular lab values for my personal health. Over time, the table grew to sixty-plus pages—180 rows and four columns—allowing me to compare different supplement formulas, identify my preferred brands, highlight contraindications, decide what time during the day is best to take each supplement, ensure that I was combining co-factors for proper absorption, and indicate plan notes for myself. The process of ordering and interpreting my own lab tests, identifying the best supplements for my unique biology, titrating dosages based on ongoing lab testing, and producing my own care plan was key to my recovery. I spent the majority of my health savings funds on this process.

However, the time we were dedicating to the workshop was not enough. We were finding answers and I was seeing encouraging results, but I needed more time to research my health issues so I could heal quicker. My goal was not to creep toward well-being, inch by inch, for the coming years. I wanted to feel better. I wanted to be normal again. I wanted to see straight. I wanted to have energy to do things. I wanted to travel without feeling like I had been run over by a train. And I wanted these things sooner rather than later.

I decided to make research regarding my health issues my full-time research project. I needed to dedicate all my remaining energy to the only thing that really mattered at that point—how to recover my health. I phased out my prior research projects, moving a handful of articles through the publication pipeline. At the same time, I started conceiving a new book project—a medical anthropology approach to reversing chronic disease. And thus began my ethnographic research into the world of functional medicine.

It turned out to be my training as a medical anthropologist that saved me. Without my commitment to the ethnographic research method, I would have never turned the corner in my journey toward wellness. Over the next fourteen months, I used ethnography to locate all the information I needed to heal myself of my chronic health issues. I addressed my nutrient deficiencies, reduced my toxic exposure, and upregulated my estrogen metabolism. At the same time, I successfully reversed my autoimmunity, chronic Epstein-Barr, chronic fatigue, leaky gut, hypothyroidism, histamine intolerance, seasonal allergies, cervical dysplasia, and irritable bowel syndrome.

This book is the story of how I used ethnography as the primary tool in my recovery, but it is also so much more. As I struggled to restore my own health, I faced glaring social inequalities and neoliberal interests that determine who stays ill and who gets well.

# INTRODUCTION

In this book, I use my healing journey to discuss issues that are much bigger and more important than one person's experiences. I am aware of how critical an issue chronic disease is for the tens of millions of Americans who either suffer from chronic disease or love someone who does. I describe paradigm shifts that are underway and open multiple possibilities for how to think about care, illness, and recovery.

I attribute my own recovery to functional medicine, a model that has been shown to produce better outcomes than conventional medicine in a 2019 study published in the *Journal of the American Medical Association* (see Beidelschies et al. 2019). Functional medicine is a personalized and holistic approach to treating chronic disease. It is both an alternative to and an outgrowth of conventional medicine. Many functional medicine doctors are conventionally trained. These doctors turned to functional medicine after becoming frustrated with a health care system that pharmaceuticalizes health problems instead of seeking to create lasting health. Thus, functional medicine presents a series of paradigm shifts to conventional medicine. One primary paradigm shift is the switch from the body-as-machine model to a systems biology approach. Functional medicine uses systems biology to identify root causes and, ultimately, promote healing and recovery. This involves exploring patients' biochemical individuality and may incorporate tools such as gut microbiome testing and genomic profiling.

The concept of "nested ecologies" illuminates how systems biology extends beyond the body to the surrounding environment, thus linking internal and external ecologies. At the same time, nested ecologies emphasize how contexts of social inequality frame health and disease. Thus, seen through the lens of nested ecologies, epigenetics is a molecular biological framework for assessing structural inequality, and the field of "sociogenomics" should be expanded to include the epigenetic effect of social inequality. When applied to the microbiome—the sum total of all microbiota living on or in the body—the lens of nested ecologies reconfigures humans as ecosystems and problematizes existing notions of what it means to be human.

How can we think of humans, teeming with trillions of bacteria, yeast, and fungi, as microbial? Given that the microbiome is shaped by physical and social environments, I argue that the constitution of individuals' microbiomes also reflects inequality in society (see also Benezra 2020). I also use nested ecologies as a heuristic when exploring how intersectional vulnerability shapes and determines individuals' exposomes, the sum total of environmental toxicants to which a person is exposed during their lifetime. In so doing, I highlight how existing food policies drive chronic disease among lower-income and minority communities.

Functional medicine has made healing possible for countless people, including hundreds of individuals I have encountered during my research for this book. However, like any approach, functional medicine is not flawless. I argue that despite functional medicine practitioners' well-intended attempts to cure chronic disease, they inadvertently reinscribe intersectional inequalities. Functional medicine interlocutors critique how the pharmaceuticalization of conventional medicine leads to the monetization of disease; however, they do not acknowledge how their delivery of personalized medicine reproduces socioeconomic and racialized privilege. Functional medicine's personalized approach relies heavily on informational biology such as genomic profiling. I signal how individuals' access to informational biology depends on their purchasing power as bioconsumers. This genomic approach uses "lifestyle medicine prescriptions" to produce better health outcomes while ignoring the effects of social inequality. Similarly, when treating the microbiome, functional medicine interlocutors tend to describe diet as a "choice," thus sidestepping important issues of access to nutritious food.

In the past, I have written primarily for scholars in my field. However, specific topics in this book—namely, epigenetics and the microbiome— have the potential to spark transdisciplinary cooperation and "a common way of speaking" among social and natural scientists (Nading 2017; Benezra 2017). Furthermore, my ethnographic examination of functional medicine, disease, and healing may be of interest to anyone whose life is affected by chronic disease. Thus, I aim to make my prose accessible to a wider audience, including undergraduate students at all levels and their families.

In so doing, I hope to fill a void between science writing and medical anthropology (see Benezra 2017). While science writers transform scientific information into publicly digestible bits, medical anthropologists critically reflect on the work of science and scientists. The reading public would clearly benefit from a critical yet digestible approach to science, yet science writers and medical anthropologists are rarely in conversation with one another. When examining how the microbiome is being presented to and understood by the public, Benezra asks, "Have academic anthropologists, sociologists of science, and science studies scholars jargoned and siloed themselves right out of usefulness when it comes to interacting with public readers?" (2017, 2). My challenge here is to write at the intersection of science writing and medical anthropology—that is, to bring medical anthropology to bear on functional medicine discourse using prose that is digestible and accessible to a wide range of readers.

## THE DATA COLLECTION PROCESS

Although my prose often resembles science writing, the research for this book reflects the ethnographic rigor of medical anthropology. My research spanned twenty-five months, between February 2019 and June 2021. My first pieces of ethnographic data emerged during an internet search on histamine intolerance. I was desperate to identify the underlying causes of my worsening allergic symptoms and to address those causes. My search led me to the web pages of Alison Vickery,[1] a functional diagnostic nutritionist and certified health coach, and Yasmina Ykelenstam, a health journalist and health coach. Both struggled with debilitating histamine intolerance before taking control of their conditions through nutrition and lifestyle approaches. Vickery's experience motivated her to seek further training on adverse drug interactions, functional immunology, mitochondrial disorders, the microbiome, detoxification, stress hormones, mold, small intestinal bacterial overgrowth (SIBO), methylation, and nutrigenomics. For her part, Ykelenstam funneled her experience working for *60 Minutes*, CNN, and the BBC into reading numerous studies and interviewing leading medical experts, best-selling authors, and healers of histamine intolerance, mast cell activation disorder, mastocytosis, and inflammatory diseases. Vickery provides online health coaching via video conferencing to people around the world. Meanwhile, Ykelenstam produces books, online courses, and webinars for purchase on her website.

Recognizing from their materials that I might have SIBO, I conducted an online search that led me to the website of Dr. Amy Myers, where I participated in a webinar on SIBO and purchased a kit for overcoming SIBO without the use of antibiotics. As an emergency medicine physician, Dr. Myers was a firsthand witness to the wonders of medical technology. However, in her own struggle with Graves' disease, she realized that conventional medicine had very little to offer when it came to healing her hyperthyroidism. In addition to starting a functional medicine clinic in Austin, Texas, she wrote two best-selling books, *The Autoimmune Solution* and *The Thyroid Connection*. Reading both was the initial step to reversing my autoimmunity and understanding my hypothyroidism.

Then, I stumbled upon HealthMeans (a.k.a. DrTalks), an online platform that hosts online summits and conferences on different functional medicine topics. I began listening to summit after summit, conference after conference, and this process exposed me to up-to-the-minute insights from dozens of functional medicine practitioners on a wide variety of health-related topics, many of which pertained to me. Registration for these online events often includes "free registration gifts" ranging from informational PDFs to study guides, eBooks, recipes, and master classes. Registrants' email addresses are added to the listservs of the different speakers in the online event. As a result of my participation in many different online events, I began receiving email newsletters from numerous functional medicine practitioners and their allies.

These emails often included links to practitioners' podcasts and blogs. The emails also offered free registration to the functional medicine practitioners' online webinars and eCourses. Thus, while the HealthMeans platform brought numerous functional medicine practitioners together for each online event, these webinars and eCourses were usually delivered by either a single functional medicine practitioner or a small group of functional medicine colleagues. Both formats were usually intended for other health professionals, especially those seeking to develop a practice or further their knowledge in functional medicine.

At times, email newsletters promoted online docuseries featuring the functional medicine practitioner. These docuseries were oriented around particular topics—for example, reversing autoimmunity, improving gut health, stem cell therapy, and increasing longevity. The different series, delivered in daily episodes and generally lasting a week or so, were created by filmmakers who either suffered from the particular disease being investigated or who have a family member who suffered from it. After personally experiencing the effectiveness of functional medicine for reversing chronic disease and promoting health, these filmmakers used their skills to conduct in-depth interviews with functional medicine practitioners, and sometimes recovered patients, on the topic.

The filmmakers then lace together video excerpts from interviews to document the curative power of functional medicine approaches with respect to the disease or issue at hand. The films unfold like extended conversations among dozens of practitioners. In reality, each functional medicine practitioner was interviewed separately, in different locations, often separated by great physical distances. In order to obtain these interviews, filmmakers traveled across the country and even around the world. The only people with whom each practitioner conversed during filming were the filmmakers. Nonetheless, the responses of the practitioners are stitched together to give the illusion of a continuous conversation among everyone featured in the film. These docuseries are an indispensable discursive form in the functional medicine community precisely because they allow for a variety of voices to converge on the topic at hand.

As I became more interested in the perspectives of particular functional medicine practitioners, I began looking for them in increasingly public digital spaces. While the HealthMeans summits are free and readily accessible to anyone who signs up, the platform is not a well-known space of public engagement. The summits, eCourses, and online trainings in which I had been participating were mostly geared toward health professionals, and they provided me with valuable insight into how different functional medicine practitioners interact with one another. Through my virtual attendance, I was conducting participant observation among a closely (albeit digitally) knit community of functional medicine practitioners. But the question remained: How did these practitioners engage with potential patients in public digital spaces? To answer this question, I turned to YouTube and Facebook.

The YouTube videos I watched were often the video extension of functional medicine practitioners' audio podcasts. The videos sometimes took on even more of a public presence, as was the case with Dr. William Li's 2010 TED Talk, "Can We Eat to Starve Cancer?" and the TEDMED series. Meanwhile, I joined a few Facebook groups created by particular functional medicine practitioners and health educators as a platform for directly engaging patients, followers, and the public. These multiple strategies provided me with a clear picture of how functional medicine practitioners engaged with each other and their patients online.

However, I was still curious about how functional medicine unfolds offline. To understand how functional medicine discourse circulates in print, I read books by the functional medicine practitioners I was already following. For the most part, my ethnographic research does not include the studies published in scientific journals by the same doctors and researchers. I made the decision to focus on books intended for a wide audience, many of which are *New York Times* bestsellers, because, as an ethnographer, I am interested in public discourse and the social life of ideas. I wanted to understand how functional medicine is portrayed and explained to the public—a project that extends beyond the ways the etiology of particular diseases is described

## TABLE 1. DATA SOURCES

| Data source type | Number incorporated into this ethnographic research project |
|---|---|
| Hours of coursework in nutrigenetics and nutrigenomics | 60 |
| Functional medicine interlocutors' newsletters | 29 |
| Continuing medical education credits | 27 |
| Books intended for a wide audience | 19 |
| Webinars, eCourses, and master classes | 18 |
| Online summits and conferences | 16 |
| Company newsletters | 16 |
| YouTube channels | 11 |
| Facebook groups (totaling 241,100+ online group members in December 2020) | 9 |
| Docuseries | 6 |
| Podcasts | 6 |
| Blogs | 4 |
| Magazine and newspaper subscriptions | 3 |
| Online health education platforms | 2 |

among academics in the ivory tower. This choice reflects my descriptive and analytical aims for this book, and my hope that its non-prescriptive framework will encourage readers to critically reflect on their own understandings of health and disease and to consider how they might position themselves more agentively regarding their well-being.

Finally, I felt the need to directly observe how functional medicine practitioners interact with one another as colleagues. When conducting standard ethnography, the anthropologist describes the behaviors and experiences of those observed. Thus, I conducted in-person participant observation while completing continuing medical education credits from the American Medical Association. This in-person participant observation provided me with the opportunity to connect with numerous functional medicine practitioners in a face-to-face setting.

While I considered many more sources of ethnographic data—especially with regard to webinars, eCourses, master classes, summits, and docuseries—I stopped when I felt my data had reached saturation; that is, I

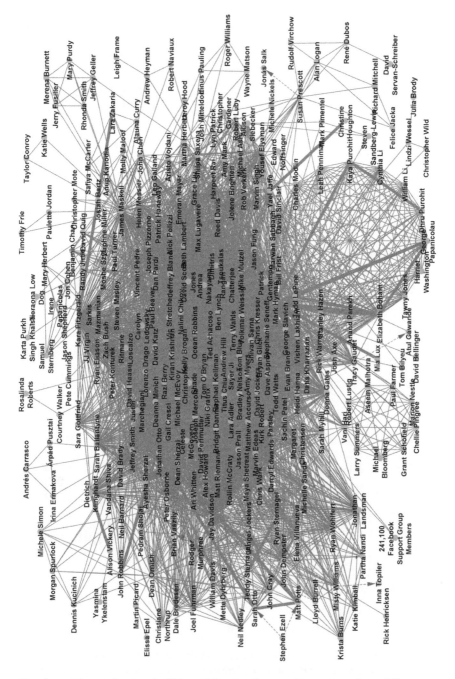

*People-centric social network. This social network map demonstrates how different interlocutors are connected to one another. Bold lines represent "real-life" connections (e.g., individuals who are coworkers, siblings, or spouses). Dashed lines indicate when an individual referenced another individual. Credit: Jason Vega. Full-color image hosted at https://tinyurl.com/Nested-Ecologies-Images.*

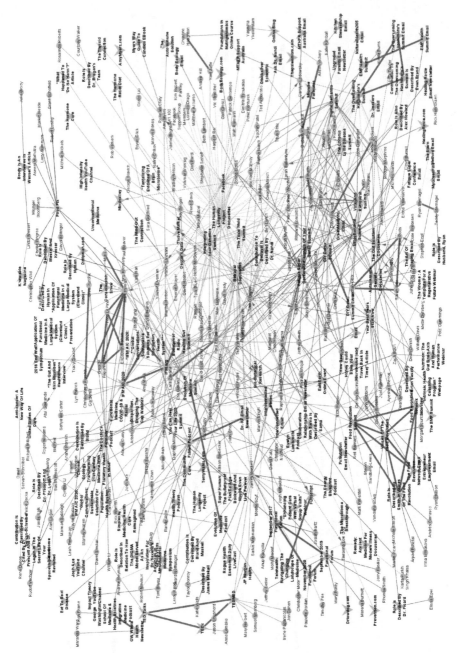

Source-centric social network. This social network indicates how individuals are connected to one another through their participation in different sources (e.g., podcasts, webinars, summits). Bold lines represent "real-life" connections (e.g., individuals who are coworkers, siblings, or spouses). Dashed lines are indicative of "promotional relationships" (individuals or platforms that promoted the products or services of companies or of other individuals). Credit: Jason Vega. Full-color image hosted at https://tinyurl.com /Nested-Ecologies-Images.

concluded my research when each additional online event no longer exposed me to new faces or ideas. Over the course of my ethnographic fieldwork, I recognized that the individuals I was observing form a cohesive community whose discourse revolves around common themes. I had become digitally familiar with almost all the functional medicine practitioners who have a significant online presence, and I had listened to virtually every aspect of their discourse.

Functional medicine, as a discursive field, includes individuals from numerous professions. I have included interlocutors with diverse backgrounds in this study in an effort to accurately represent functional medicine's heterogeneity. Thus, some of these interlocutors have been trained in alternative medicine and a few have not studied past the bachelor's level. Some readers may discount these alternative forms of expertise. However, more than 60 percent of functional medicine practitioners included in this study possess the type of advanced training that even the most skeptical readers will likely appreciate: out of 241 practitioners, 32 percent possess a medical doctorate (MD) and 27 percent have obtained a doctorate in science (PhD) or pharmacy (PharmD). (For detailed information on each interlocutor and their academic training, please see the appendix.)

I have decided to include the true names of individuals whenever my data collection occurred in a large group setting (i.e., professional conferences) or via a publicly available source (e.g., online summits, docuseries, podcasts, blogs, YouTube channels). In contrast, I have provided pseudonyms for individuals included in this ethnography whenever interactions referenced took place in private settings (e.g., my personal health care providers).

## DIGITAL AUTOETHNOGRAPHY

This book challenges readers' existing notions regarding ethnographic research and anthropological writing. Some of my research occurred while I was in lockdown due to the COVID-19 pandemic, potentially leading the reader to assume that circumstances motivated my endeavor into digital ethnography (Miller 2020) and necessitated an added layer of reflexivity regarding the constitution of sociality during social isolation (Navaro 2020). This is somewhat true. However, it is more accurate to say that pre-existing discursive forms and social assemblages, not the era of COVID, caused me to rethink my research methods, my role as an anthropologist, the type of data that is relevant to my project (Ramos-Zayas 2020), and how my interlocutors are configuring social relations (Strathern 2020).

## TABLE 2. RESEARCH SUBJECTS

| Profession/Role | Number of individuals included in this ethnographic research project* |
|---|---|
| Medical doctors (MD) | 77 |
| Health and science doctorates (PhD) | 63 |
| Entrepreneurs, health advocates, and consultants | 39 |
| Patients | 28 |
| Nutrition experts (PhD, CCN, CN, FACN, DACBN, MS) | 26 |
| Health coaches and educators | 18 |
| Chiropractors (DC) | 15 |
| Naturopathic doctors (ND) | 13 |
| Filmmakers and show hosts | 10 |
| Health science journalists, editors, and authors | 9 |
| Administrators of functional and integrative medicine clinics and organizations | 6 |
| Osteopaths (DO) | 6 |
| Nurses (RN, CNS) | 6 |
| Acupuncturists | 6 |
| Politicians | 5 |
| Oriental medicine practitioners (DOM, MSOM/MSAOM) | 4 |
| Dieticians (RD, RDN) | 3 |
| Pharmacists (PharmD and Registered Pharmicists) | 3 |
| Food activists | 2 |
| Ayurvedic doctor (AD) | 1 |
| Institute for Functional Medicine Certified Practitioner (IFMCP) | 1 |
| Other allied health professionals | 6 |

*Here, I am only including individuals whom I quote or refer to directly in my research. I am not including the hundreds of thousands of other individuals who participated in online summits and conferences, appeared on YouTube channels and podcasts, belonged to Facebook groups, were featured in docuseries, attended continuing medical education, or delivered presentations on online health education platforms but are not directly referred to in my work.

In the case of functional medicine, conducting digital ethnography was vital to my project since the majority of functional medicine discourse has been taking place online since well before the COVID-19 pandemic. Furthermore, while some functional medicine patients may travel great distances for an initial intake or once annually to meet with providers, functional medicine practitioners often transition patients to videoconference consultations to alleviate some of the expense, the demands on time, and the physical burden associated with travel. Nonetheless, functional medicine practitioners aim to accomplish "person centeredness" by setting aside time—up to three hours for the initial intake and thirty to ninety minutes thereafter—to listen to patients' stories and explore their concerns.[2] Similarly, in the absence of proximity, functional medicine patients use online support groups to create a sense of community, thus redefining what it means to be held by a social collective by engaging in a digitized biosociality (Rabinow 1996).

## WRITING IN THREE REGISTERS

The following chapters are filled with the voices and opinions of approximately 140 functional medicine interlocutors, my experiences as someone seeking recovery from chronic disease, and my critical perspective as a medical anthropologist. To that end, I write in three different registers (see Mol 2003).

The first register is what I refer to as "meta-ethnography." In coining this term, I am extending the format of epidemiological meta-analysis to ethnographic research. In epidemiology, a meta-analysis is a study that assesses all existing studies on a particular topic in order to produce an average outcome or consensus from their findings. When conducting research for this book, I quickly realized that the various online sources I was examining—podcasts, summits, YouTube channels, and docuseries—were actually composed of interview after interview with members of the functional medicine community. Perhaps the most salient examples of this are functional medicine docuseries. For example, during the opening scene of the docuseries *Autoimmune Secrets*, Dr. Tom O'Bryan, a physician and host of the series, tells the viewer, "You are going to learn from eighty-five of the world's foremost experts, including scientific researchers, who are considered the fathers and grandfathers in the field of autoimmunity." Even more important, Dr. O'Bryan says, "You are going to hear from people who have turned their autoimmune conditions around and have found optimal health." Referring to Jonathan Otto, a filmmaker who has created several prominent docuseries in the functional medicine space, Dr. O'Bryan notes that "Jonathan and I, with our film crew, have teamed up and have traveled all across the country and all around the world—through England, Germany, Portugal, Spain, and Brazil—to gather the stories." In this docuseries, viewers accompany Dr. O'Bryan and Otto on their journey to discover the true cause of autoimmune disease and its true solution. As I watched these docuseries, it struck me that I was watching *ethnography* unfold before my eyes. This led me to also consider interviewers on podcasts, YouTube channels, and online summits—usually functional medicine practitioners interviewing their colleagues—as ethnographers.[3] By positioning these online venues as the sources of my ethnographic data, I conducted a meta-analysis of ethnography—that is, an ethnography of ethnography.

By writing in the register of meta-ethnography and textually simulating the functional medicine docuseries, I contribute to my overarching approach of simultaneously *demonstrating* and *describing* the effect of particular modes of communicating information in the functional medicine realm.[4] Given this book's textual form, I cannot replicate the audiovisual nature of the docuseries, but I aim to preserve elements of the docuseries' discursive structure. I similarly weave together the voices of numerous functional medicine practitioners, thus creating a textualized simulation of the ethnographic docuseries.

Second, I write in the register of anthropological theory, thus connecting emerging arguments within functional medicine to long-standing perspectives in medical anthropology. While docuseries and other online sources are meant to educate their audiences about functional medicine and convince them of the merits of functional medicine—usually with regard to a particular category of disease—I reorient the data culled from these ethnographic sources in order to analyze functional medicine as a series of paradigm shifts. According to Kuhn (1962), a paradigm is the totality of concepts, techniques, and values shared by a scientific community. In this vein, I illustrate how functional medicine practitioners critique the basic principles of conventional medicine, position themselves as "scientific revolutionaries,"[5] and advocate for the mainstreaming of lifestyle medicine. At the same time, I examine how social inequalities determine who is able to access health-sustaining resources, such as a clean environment and nutritious food, and critique how functional medicine practitioners have invested more time and energy validating their approaches—to each other, the scientific community, and the world—than acknowledging how privilege facilitates access to these resources.

Finally, I describe my method as a digital autoethnography because my recovery story is embedded in this book. Illness autoethnography uses the ethnographer's own experience as a source of ethnographic data (Murphy 1987; Nowakowski and Sumerau 2019; Ettore 2005; Richards 2016). My story is braided together with the stories of other functional medicine patients and practitioners because, frankly, including my own healing journey is the only honest way to write this book. At the same time, this book is not a memoir. I do not provide every detail of my ill health and recovery, and the glimpses I provide into my personal experience are not necessarily in consecutive order.

This tripartite methodological approach gives new meaning to "multisited ethnography." I create a cartography of functional medicine in the United States, thus identifying different "windows" through which recent paradigm shifts in medicine can be examined (see Marcus 1995; Menéndez 1996; Rapp 2000; Wilson 2004). To accomplish this task, I weave together my stories and those of others as they unfold across multiple physical and digital spaces. As a whole, this "braided tale" (Lester 2019) tells a much more important story about unequal access to health. It emphasizes that recovery is possible, but that in our society, healing is facilitated by privilege.

## USING AUTOETHNOGRAPHY TO DESTIGMATIZE DISEASE

Between certain chapters, you will find "interludes" that provide glimpses into my healing journey. These interludes preface the following chapters, add autoethnographic texture, and demonstrate what is at stake for patients of functional medicine. When writing in this autoethnographic register, I provide "thick descriptions" (see Geertz 1973) of how I experienced illness and recovery. By including my own story, I am acknowledging that the observed and the observer are inextricably intertwined. Furthermore, I expand the potential purposes for conducting ethnography to include personal healing and recovery.

Given the great lengths I went through to conceal my health struggle, it may seem counterintuitive that I am using my own experience as the thread that ties all the chapters together. I hid my illness from others because I was afraid they would see me as less capable, and they would judge me and the judgment would be something from which I could not recover, long after my illnesses had subsided. I had internalized the stigma against illness, so much so that my fear kept me from being transparent with those around me. Thus, while I initially planned to examine the processes leading to unequal health outcomes solely through the experiences of others, I have since reflected on the mysterious workings of stigma and have decided to use my own experience as a resource when arguing for a destigmatization of illness and disease.

A vast literature in anthropology problematizes practices of "othering" (Brons 2015). Those who are not "Self" are "Other." That is, people who fall outside of the familiar social category of "us"—people who don't belong and are referred to with the distancing pronoun "them"—are social Others. Thus, the term "othering" describes the discriminatory behaviors that are directed at individuals labeled as outsiders and outcasts.

Throughout history, horrendous acts of violence and abuse have been unleashed on people who were considered as not belonging to the dominant social group. Examples include the Holocaust, concentration camps, segregation, and apartheid, to name a few. Medical anthropologists turn the lens of othering on to illness and disease. Often, people with disease are treated with discrimination. By weaving my personal story into the pages of this book, I hope to diminish the potential for othering. I am not writing about people struggling with some mysterious disease in a faraway place. I am writing about the chronic diseases that affect 51.8 percent of Americans who struggle with a chronic disease and the 27.2 percent who have multiple chronic conditions (Boersma, Black, and Ward 2020). I am writing about myself. If my readers judge someone in this text, let it be me—but better yet, let my readers receive my message of why illness and disease should not be stigmatized.

Turning again to my own story, I will use infectious diseases as an example since they tend to be among the most stigmatized conditions. Different diagnoses are overlain with particular social narratives (Leach and Scoones 2013; Lonardi 2007), and, as a result, different diagnoses elicit reactions ranging from empathy to disgust. I am choosing to focus on the most highly stigmatized diagnoses I have—viruses—so that we can think critically about the nature of stigma. In so doing, I am simultaneously demonstrating how an anthropological approach transforms how we think about everyday situations.

While it is all too easy to fall into dichotomous thinking—labeling people, behaviors, beliefs, practices as good or bad, right or wrong, familiar or strange—an anthropological approach challenges us to critically analyze our own assumptions. That is, anthropologists are trained to identify and examine the narratives that are socially inscribed onto situations, hold them at a distance, and ask why and how certain moral judgments are made. By carefully examining that which seems all too obvious, anthropologists often uncover mechanisms that allow our preconceived notions to erase and naturalize intersecting types of social inequality (e.g., race, class, gender). By not recognizing these mechanisms, individuals can inadvertently participate in the reproduction of social inequality. However, by examining the harmful effects of particular social narratives, individuals can proactively contribute to creating a more equitable future.

In the "Prelude," I *admitted* to being a carrier of herpes simplex 1, the human papillomavirus, and Epstein-Barr. Here, I am using the word "admitted" because I am acknowledging that these viruses may be regarded by some as a cause for shame. By sharing my own story, I hope to dispel stigma ascribed to certain health conditions.

These three viruses all belong to the herpes family of viruses, along with other viruses such as chicken pox and shingles (the reactivation of chicken pox). They are all extremely common—meaning each virus is carried by the majority of Americans at some point in their lives, even though most carriers are asymptomatic. In fact, 50 to 80 percent of individuals become infected with oral herpes over the course of their lives (Johns Hopkins Medicine, n.d.), 80 percent of sexually active people are infected with papillomavirus at some point (Cleveland Clinic. n.d.), and 90 percent of young adults are *already* infected with Epstein-Barr (Duke University Medical Center 2010). While these herpes-family viruses are ubiquitous, most people only come to know they have them when they begin to have symptoms, which tends to occur when people have compromised immune systems.

And despite all these facts, we tend to assign different meanings to different viruses. The oral herpes virus is the butt of disparaging jokes, while genital herpes (HSV-2) is even more deeply mired in stigma. The human papillomavirus is regarded with disgust if it results in genital warts, but is mostly disregarded if it manifests as plantar warts. Chicken pox is not stigmatized at all—until recently when vaccines for chicken pox were introduced. Contracting chicken pox and being painted with the "pink medicine" was considered a rite of passage for most school-age children. Many people are unaware of Epstein-Barr, but, like chicken pox, it is often a pediatric virus and it affects 50 percent of children by age five (Sureshbabu 2021). Shingles usually affects the elderly and is considered very painful; thus, this diagnosis often elicits empathy. Why are herpes-family viruses assigned meaning based on the age group they affect and the body part on which they manifest?

Different health conditions and diseases are overlain with particular narratives about the people they afflict. For example, at the time of this writing, the coronavirus pandemic has produced racialized narratives that cast Chinese individuals as suspected vectors of disease. University Health Services at the University of California, Berkeley went so far as to say, in an infographic posted on Instagram, that xenophobia is a "common" and "normal" reaction to coronavirus. The infographic, which was quickly removed in response to a backlash from students, defined xenophobia as "fears about interacting with those who might be from Asia and guilt about these feelings." On March 18, 2020, the Asian Pacific Policy and Planning Council launched Stop AAPI Hate, an online reporting forum. Within one week, the forum received more than six hundred and fifty direct reports of discrimination against Asian Americans (Kandil 2020). In early 2021, anti-Asian violence included numerous fatal attacks on Asian elders and women.

Racialization and xenophobia are just one type of narrative that can emerge around a virus. I argue that, from a more general standpoint, stigmatization structures the social life of infectious viruses, while masking a lot of the biological etiology of these viruses (Ablon 1981; Hopper 1981; Singer 2009b). In the process, stigmatization also desocializes our understanding of the social inequalities and historical influences that shape not only who contracts infectious disease, but also who is more likely to suffer from its worst effects (see Farmer 2001). Resisting these narratives, a large body of work in medical anthropology centers around overlapping vulnerabilities that structure the transmission of infectious disease and play a determining role in outcomes (see Farmer 2006; Martinez 2018).

While I have never had the symptoms that people associate with these viruses—for example, oral lesions in the case of HSV-1—I discovered their presence in my body through lab testing. My immune system is compromised due to a genetic predisposition, which was only made worse by a series of assaults over the course of my life. At my worst, I had Epstein-Barr titers up to thirty-one times the cutoff for a positive result.

At the age of twenty-one, when I received my first herpes diagnosis (HSV-1), I bought in to this stigma. For a long time, I considered it "unfair" that I—someone trained in the health sciences, committed to monogamy, and determined to use every precaution—would be infected with a "sexually transmitted disease." The strain I had was primarily transmitted via saliva, not sexual contact, but I nonetheless felt deep personal shame. Like an invisible predator, the virus knocked me off my feet for years. At the time, I was unaware of how viruses interact with my genome—the complete set of genes that are unique to me—and I thought I had caught a particularly potent strain of the virus. Knowing how debilitating HSV-1 had been for me, I was unwilling to risk infecting anyone else. These misconceptions left me feeling isolated for years. It was not until I came to terms with the fact that everyone, including my mother and grandmother, has a herpes virus and that I contracted papillomavirus from my husband while we were both in a monogamous relationship that I began to let go of my self-stigmatization. Eventually I learned that viruses don't discriminate—only people do.

In addition to herpes-family viruses, I also have typhus, a virus carried by lice, ticks, fleas, mites, and rodents. I discovered this when I was at my sickest and the local night clinic physician tested me for any possible culprit for my strange symptoms. The lab result identified antibodies for the virus, but was equivocal in determining whether the virus was latent or reactivated. I probably would have never discovered these antibodies had I not gone to that particular night clinic.

The clinic was one of my only options for middle-of-the-night internal medicine, and low-income patients are its primary demographic. Furthermore, as a clinic in the US-Mexico borderlands, many of its patients are of Mexican origin, and some are from rural contexts. When the doctor, a white man, entered the consultation room, he addressed me in Spanish, "Amiga, ¿cómo sientes? Vamos a ver como te podemos ayudar." ("Friend, how are you? Let's see how we can help you.") He assumed that I am primarily a Spanish speaker—an easy assumption to make given the local demographic and my phenotype—and I did not correct his assumption by telling him that Spanish is actually my third language after Toishanese and English. We carried out the rest of the visit in Spanish. I am strangely grateful for having been profiled in this way because his assumptions about me led to a diagnosis—a virus that I was likely infected with while conducting research in rural Mexico for my first book.

Again, a large body of medical anthropology literature points to how race- and class-based inequalities determine who will be infected and who will be spared (see, for example, Farmer 2001; McElroy 2015). In a stealthy sleight of hand, those who experience racial discrimination and for whom local governments have failed to provide basic infrastructures are often blamed for their plight (Briggs and Briggs 2003).

Lastly, autoethnography is a way for me to argue for the destigmatization of disease and to reveal my lived empathy for those who suffer with similar diagnoses and chronic illness in general. Acknowledging how the topics at hand are deeply personal to me helps to resist portraying those afflicted as Others.

## (HYPER-)SELF-REFLEXIVITY

Self-reflexivity in anthropology acknowledges the many ways the ethnographer is not, and can never be, a "fly on the wall." Ethnographic observations do not manifest from an omnipotent view from nowhere. Instead, an anthropologist's interpretation of the goings-on under observation is in every way refracted through and shaded by personal experience.[6] Anthropologists must use all their senses to obtain ethnographic data and to learn about frameworks that are unique to a particular culture or community. They then use theoretical perspectives and, importantly, their own experiences to assign meaning to the data. Furthermore, self-reflexive anthropologists reflect on their identities and life experiences in relation to others and consider how these factors shape their interactions and relationships with the people they study.

This type of embeddedness allows anthropologists—especially those concerned with the philosophy of science—to keep the following questions at the forefront of their minds: Who are the authors of scientific "discovery"? Do they face conflicts of interests? Who profits from scientific findings? Who is harmed? Does the way science is conducted sustain social inequality or obscure environmental justice?

I am inspired by Bruno Latour (1987), among other scholars specializing in science, technology, and society who explore how scientific work unfolds in practice. I furthermore argue for a critical epidemiology that uses mixed methods and interdisciplinary teamwork to incorporate the unique skills of anthropologists. These include throwing into question existing perceptions of disease, challenging existing structures that frame "askable questions" and "publishable results," seeking to identify scapegoats and victims, and, ultimately, uncovering the differential valuation of human life (see Farmer 2001).

For this research, I used many of the techniques I describe on my journey toward wellness, and I am better because of it. As a health scientist, I identify with the functional medicine practitioners, many of whom experienced chronic disease themselves and who learned a new medical paradigm in order to find the answers that conventional medicine could not provide and heal themselves. The emergent discursive themes and functional medicine techniques I feature in this book often echo medical anthropological theory and methods, thus reflecting my own opinions as a participant observer. This book, then, is both an ethnography and an autoethnography, meaning I used participant observation as a technique to gain access to the stories of others while also incorporating my own.

It is important for me to acknowledge how my "ethnography at home" mimics the ways in which privileged patients exercise their economic and cultural capital by accessing the internet, attending webinars, reading newsletters, and purchasing vitamins. I use hyper-self-reflexivity (see Spivak 1988a, 1988b; Spivak, Chakravorty, and Harasym 1990; Kapoor 2004) to critique overarching structures that frame social inequality and attempt to minimize my role in reproducing these structures. Hyper-self-reflexivity is thus integral to both my ethnographic method and my ethical commitments to society. In order to enact hyper-self-reflexivity in this book, I must continually reveal my own privilege vis-à-vis the topics at hand. I would not be as well as I am today if it were not for the economic capital that my family and I were able to invest in my healing. To begin with, I would likely have had less access to educational opportunities had I not grown up middle class. Second, my being born one generation removed from the actual experience of immigration gave me the luxury of increased choice when it came to selecting my career. My mother immigrated to the United States. She worked as a field hand on California farms as a child and as a secretary and tutor through college. Members of her generation were pushed to choose professions that would guarantee financial stability. She encouraged me to choose the career that would make me the happiest, and thus I became a medical anthropologist.

Furthermore, I am able to write this book today because of the vast out-of-pocket expenses we paid at every turn of my healing journey. During 2019, the year the majority of my healing occurred, my out-of-pocket health expenses totaled $22,898.[7] This figure includes a few medications, lots of supplements, occasional doctor visits, nutrition counseling, and extensive lab testing. This figure excludes research-related costs, like registration for continuing medical education and fees for online courses. Although I am genetically vulnerable to environmental toxins, I have also excluded from this amount indirect, health-related expenses such as organic food at the supermarket and "clean" cosmetics. Furthermore, I have excluded expensive modifications we made to our house, including exchanging old carpet for tile and installing a whole-house water filtration system. Thus, the true costs of holistic health are actually much greater than what this enormous figure suggests.

By recognizing that I *purchased* my recovery—an option that is out of reach for most people—I am calling out and critiquing my own privilege. Privilege is a form of ignorance (see Rogerson 2020, 167). The privileged elite can afford to live unaware of how the majority struggle economically and how certain resources and types of care are inaccessible to many. Since

I possess a certain degree of privilege, I must use hyper-self-reflexivity as a method, thus allowing me to shed some of my ignorance and critically analyze how my life-altering experience of disease reversal is, sadly, not available to most people. Health inequalities and unequal access to health resources are instantiated and reproduced at the intersection of "race" and class. I am thus attentive to how intersecting race- and class-based inequalities structure who is able to recover from chronic disease and how these inequalities are, at times, inadvertently reinscribed by well-intentioned functional medicine practitioners seeking to reverse chronic disease.

Sharing my own story is a way to enact (hyper-)self-reflexivity and to honestly and transparently reveal my positionality vis-à-vis the topics at hand. My story brings to life some of the larger issues at stake in this book: the process of "science in action" (Latour 1987), the limitations of our current medical paradigm, and alternatives for the future. In this book, I question what counts as medical science and explore scientific frontiers in health care. In so doing, I examine the limits of conventional medicine as a significant locus of authority in our society. What would happen if medicine embraced a spirit of humility and was already ready to be wrong (Fuentes 2012)? Concepts from functional medicine problematize the randomized controlled trial as the most valuable method of inquiry and the gold standard for knowledge production. They suggest that not everything real—for example, stress—can be measured and quantified. They ask about the limitations of current technologies and open up a space for other systems of perception, including those offered by emerging technologies. The goal is not to discard conventional medicine, but to introduce a complementary model that fills in the gaps where conventional medicine falls short.

## WHAT IS TO COME

In the next two chapters, I analyze the ways functional medicine represents a much-needed complement to conventional medicine. Functional medicine practitioners do not disregard the value of conventional medical interventions, especially for treating acute conditions. Rather, they propose functional medicine as the appropriate alternative to conventional medicine when it comes to reversing chronic disease. In chapter 1, these practitioners describe functional medicine as a series of paradigm shifts and position themselves as scientific revolutionaries who are going against conventional wisdom in order to lead the way toward the future of medicine. These paradigm shifts require significant changes in medical education and health

care delivery. Then, in chapter 2, I explore what functional medicine practitioners call "systems biology." From this perspective, the body is viewed
as an interconnected system, and chronic disease can only be reversed
by addressing its root causes. The body is equated to a walking, talking
ecological universe. I offer the concept of nested ecologies as a heuristic
for describing how systems biology extends beyond the body to the surrounding environment, thus linking internal and external ecologies. When
describing external ecologies, I emphasize how contexts of social inequality
frame health and disease.

The following chapters turn to how functional medicine serves as a fresh
lens for understanding human biology. Chapter 3 explores informational
biology in the era of "Big Data" and how functional medicine interlocutors have reconceptualized disease based on emerging epigenetic science. I
argue that, given the rise of genomic profiling companies such as 23andMe,
individuals' access to informational biology is premised on their relative
privilege-disadvantage as bioconsumers. I thus position epigenetics as a
molecular biological framework for assessing structural inequality. I use the
analogy of "structural myopia" to critique how well-intentioned efforts at
effecting epigenetic change through lifestyle medicine inadvertently ignore
issues of inequality. I use the concept of nested ecologies to emphasize how
physical and social environmental factors shape health and to avoid blaming victims. In this vein, I expand the concept of sociogenomics to include
the epigenetic effect of social inequality. Chapter 4 builds upon chapter 3 by
exploring how microbes—tiny microorganisms including bacteria, archaea,
fungi, protozoa, and viruses—act upon human genes to produce epigenetic effects. Turning to functional medicine discourse on the microbiome, I
problematize binary assumptions regarding human vs. non-human, Self vs.
Other, social vs. biological, mind vs. body, and good vs. evil. Ultimately, this
chapter presents humans as walking, talking ecosystems consisting of trillions of microbes. Chapter 5 delves deeper into the microbiome by examining functional medicine critiques of conventional approaches to nutrition
and hygiene. The chapter presents a quadripartite "social microbiome," thus
describing how microbes are social life forms, how each person's microbiome is determined by their social circle, how socially ingrained habits affect
the microbiome, and how the microbiome is a lens for analyzing social
inequality. I explore the Anthropocene and how environmental degradation unleashes its detrimental effects along intersectional structures of vulnerability, and I thus argue for greater environmental stewardship (Swistun
and Auyero 2009; Petryna 2003). The exposome (the sum total of toxic
exposures individuals face from the time of their conception until death)

is shaped by social inequality, thus resulting in health disparities based on class, race, and gender.

In the concluding chapter, I delve deeper into how the food system is described by functional medicine interlocutors in order to further illuminate the Anthropocene and how human health is nested in political ecology. In so doing, I leverage nested ecologies to critique current food policies and propose changes for the future. Our current food system produces significant exposome variability, thus illuminating the intimate relationship between poor diets and poverty. I argue, along with a subset of functional medicine interlocutors, that the existing food system renders low-income minorities and minority children especially vulnerable to poor health outcomes. At the same time, I signal how functional medicine interlocutors have often promoted "consumption-based activism," a neoliberal strategy that inadvertently reproduces inequality. In so doing, I point to the state's responsibility for ensuring access to healthy food.

*~ Interlude ~*

# THE BIRTH OF AN
# ANTHROPOLOGIST

When I was four years old, a family friend came to visit my Chinese maternal grandma, Popo. The visitor squatted and asked me, "What do you want to be when you grow up?" I confidently responded, "A dermatologist!" not having the faintest idea what being a dermatologist entailed. I knew a dermatologist is a type of doctor, and in the Chinese immigrant community in which I was reared, children are constantly reminded they have two options in life: become a doctor or an attorney. Three family members—my mother and two uncles—are attorneys. I think being an attorney requires an assertive personality—something I do not possess—and I imagined it as a career filled with daily conflict. Instead, I wanted to heal people! Also, my favorite aunt is a dermatologist, and I wanted to emulate her.

For the next fifteen years, I was certain I was on the path to a career in medicine. In high school, I completed a concentration in science, technology, engineering, and medicine (STEM). I was fascinated by the human body and earned top marks in anatomy and physiology. When I was seventeen, I was accepted to the Brown University Program in Liberal Medical Education (PLME), an eight-year medical continuum. The program selected approximately fifty high school students each year from around the world. After being offered admission to Brown's undergraduate program, PLME students are additionally granted admission to its medical school. While PLME students are required to complete undergraduate courses in chemistry, physics, biology, and calculus, they are otherwise encouraged to pursue a liberal education and even select a nonscience major. The program does not require students to take the MCAT. Undergraduate PLME students are given hospital privileges for medical observerships and are also invited to enroll in elective courses at the medical school beginning in the first year.

I loved being a PLME student and was so enthusiastic about the program that I was elected class representative year after year. Starting my very first month as a PLME student, I began taking advantage of the opportunities to shadow physicians in different specialties and hone in on the specialty that most interested me. I was innately drawn to children and human reproduction, so I spent my first year in PLME shadowing in the departments of OB/GYN, pediatrics, reproductive endocrinology, and neonatology, among others. After my freshman year, I headed home to California for summer break. Eager to continue my shadowing in OB/GYN, I reached out to my own gynecologist and shadowed her for a brief time. Hoping to explore a new field, I sent letters to pediatric surgeons and was fortunate to receive a positive response from a local pediatric surgeon, a Chinese man who, as a child, had been given the options of becoming a doctor or an engineer, and he chose doctor. He created a student intern position for me that allowed me to shadow all surgical specialties at both the UC Davis Medical Center and Sutter Medical Center in Sacramento. I will forever be indebted to him for his generosity.

As it turned out, I was most inspired by pediatric surgery. I had noticed that in certain specialties and fields—for example, cardiac surgery, oncology, and internal medicine—patients didn't really get better. Even if the cardiac surgery is executed perfectly, in many cases this invasive intervention merely buys the patients a little time. Similarly, the side effects of chemotherapy are often torturous, and the results can be grim. Finally, I was struck by the response of an internal medicine physician who rejoiced when she discovered a bacterial infection she could treat with antibiotics. Why was a "positive" result on a urine test something that warranted celebration? I realized then that the vast majority of her day was not about "curing" patients, but rather about managing chronic illnesses using pharmaceuticals. In all these areas of medicine, patients usually didn't get better—most times, they gradually got worse. It was a grim perspective.

Newborn babies born with congenital birth defects could undergo significant operations and have a chance to grow into healthy children and adults. I observed the surgery of a baby born with an omphalocele, a defect of the abdominal wall that causes an infant's internal organs to stick out through the belly button. The surgeon tucked the infant's organs back into the abdominal cavity, securing them in their proper place, and closed the abdominal wall with carefully placed stitches to maximize aesthetics. A few weeks later, a baby who underwent the same surgery as an infant came in for a follow-up appointment—all smiles, gurgling with pleasure and wiggling with excitement. Small children often do get better. Given my childhood dream of healing people, I needed my chosen specialty to be one where patients get better. As I discovered, the options were few.

Fortunately, or unfortunately, depending on one's perspective, the more I observed of conventional medicine in action, the more I became disenchanted. Looking back, those hundreds of hours observing doctors practice medicine were my first ethnographic project. What can I say? I was always meant to be a medical anthropologist; I was already one from the start.

During my extensive observations of pediatric surgery, I seized every opportunity to engage the surgeons in conversation about themselves. They shared some harsh truths with me about their lifestyles. The conversations that affected me the most were with two female pediatric surgeons with regard to their family lives. The first of these impactful conversations took place in Providence at one of the university hospitals. The surgeon, who guest lectured in my fetal medicine elective course, never married and has no children. She confided that, given her profession, she didn't have time to have a family. The second conversation was with a surgeon in my hometown. She explained her husband was, for all practical purposes, a single father as she was often absent from family dinners and their children's extracurricular events. When she walked through the door, her children did not greet her with excitement because they knew, at any moment, her pager might go off and she would run right back through the door to the hospital. She told me, "You have to make the choice between being there for your own children or saving the lives of other people's children." I've always been maternal—this trait is nailed to the core of who I am—so her words haunted me.

After summer break, I returned to Brown for my sophomore year and enrolled in Culture and Health, my first medical anthropology course. During that introductory course in medical anthropology, I was exposed to books like Anne Fadiman's *The Spirit Catches You and You Fall Down* (1997)—books I affectionately refer to as the gateway drugs to medical anthropology. As I began thinking about the social factors shaping disease, I questioned my chosen profession even more. If many diseases result from deeply entrenched social inequalities, and conventional medicine fails to consider these extrabiological causes, was a degree in medicine worth pursuing? During that semester, my future in medicine faded away as a medical anthropologist was born. Thirteen years later, when I faced my own health issues, my training as a medical anthropologist would be my salvation.

In the years after leaving PLME, I joked that I would have been a terrible physician. After hearing the patient's concerns, I would have put down the prescription pad and asked questions like, "How is your sleep? Are you getting enough rest? What do you do for exercise? What strategies do you use to de-stress? Do you have good social support? Is there conflict in any of your relationships? What is your diet like? What type of nutrients are you consuming every day?" In my hypothetical situation, the patient responds and I carefully listen to their response. Then I tell them, "You don't need a doctor. What you need is better quality sleep, more exercise, a routine that helps you manage stress, the resolution of tensions in your close relationships, and a more nutrient-rich diet." I explain how to do each of these things, taking up far too much time for each patient, and send them off, usually with no more than lifestyle instructions in hand. I often ended my joke saying, "I would have been fired because I wouldn't have made the hospital any money!" Years later, when I was conducting research for this book, I discovered that the hypothetical situation I was describing was the reality of functional medicine. My joking fantasy closely resembles how functional medicine doctors treat their patients.

# CHAPTER 1

# PARADIGM SHIFTS

Medical anthropologists have studied "alternative medicine" for decades, thus signaling the varieties of medical experience (Lock 1984), problematizing "the hegemony of orchestrated pluralism" (Lock 1990), and positioning alternative medical practice as a source of empowerment and pleasure (Farquhar 1994). Functional medicine is a curiously different type of alternative because it is an *outgrowth* of mainstream medicine. At the same time, it defies old vs. new, traditional vs. modern, and non-scientific vs. scientific binaries. Practitioners of functional medicine consider their approach to be *even higher* science than that of mainstream medicine. Tom Blue, strategic advisor at the Institute for Functional Medicine, suggests that the integration of functional medicine into the health care system will lead to "the accelerated application of much more modern science in the day-to-day of medicine." At the same time, functional medicine practitioners root their practice of medicine in ancestral wisdom. My growing familiarity with functional medicine, its basic principles, the variety of tools it uses, and its practitioners reaffirmed my lifelong faith in traditional Chinese medicine and herbalism, while also sharpening my biomedical acumen and elevating my understanding of environmental and temporal context with regard to the body. How do these seemingly contradictory elements come together in functional medicine?

I must provide some historical context to explain how functional medicine formed into the discipline it is today. Functional medicine emerged in the early 1990s, after Dr. Jeffrey Bland and some of his contemporaries held a fateful meeting to define and consolidate their new approach in medicine. Dr. Bland is regarded by many functional medicine practitioners as the "father of functional medicine." He is founder and president of the Personalized Lifestyle Medicine Institute, co-founder of the Institute for Functional Medicine, and author of more than one hundred twenty peer-reviewed research papers on nutritional biochemistry and medicine.

It was Dr. Bland who proposed that this new paradigm in health care be called "functional medicine." At the time, different medical specialties (for example, radiology, cardiology, and endocrinology) were using the adjective "functional" to describe a commitment to finding and addressing underlying causes instead of merely treating or masking symptoms. Dr. Bland wanted to use the adjective to describe the new medical model that he and his colleagues were envisioning. However, the term "functional" also had a derogatory meaning at the time. He explains, "'Function' in medicine [was a type of] pejorative terminology that was related to psychosomatic illness or geriatric dysfunction." Nonetheless, Dr. Bland intentionally chose to redefine the term as something desirable, and the Institute for Functional Medicine was born in 1991. His approach represented a risk, but thus is the nature of "scientific revolution" (Kuhn 1962).

While functional medicine practitioners would prefer to be considered thought leaders rather than be exiled from the medical community, they run the risk of ridicule when they introduce ideas that counter the conventional paradigm. Dr. Bland describes the people who inspired him, lifelong mentors like Dr. Linus Pauling, as individuals who "were never comfortable with the status quo and . . . were willing to travel a sometimes difficult road of being an outlier." Thus, in positioning themselves as "scientific revolutionaries," functional medicine practitioners do not allow this risk to deter them.

According to Kuhn (1962), revolutionary science must always face resistance from "normal science" before a paradigm shift is achieved. Dr. Mark Hyman, medical director at the Cleveland Clinic Center for Functional Medicine, provides an example of the resistance Kuhn identified when he describes how, for decades, the medical community considered it nonsense that doctors' lack of hygiene could be to blame for childbed fever. When Ignaz Semmelweis suggested that doctors wash their hands before surgery and childbirth, Dr. Hyman says, "[h]e was basically exiled and ended up dying in disgrace with no money and excommunicated from the medical community." He continues, "It took fifty years for them to go, 'Yeah, maybe we should wash our hands.'" Given these types of historical examples, functional medicine practitioners understand that it is difficult to change paradigms.

For functional medicine "revolutionaries," however, the risk is worth the potential benefit. Pointing to leaky gut as an example of how this willingness to go against the status quo can, over time, produce benefits for medicine at large, Dr. Bland notes, "We invented the term 'leaky gut'. That was considered a heretical term when we first used it." Dr. Bland describes how, for the first fifteen years of using the term, he faced disapproval and was often overtly criticized. However, he says, "Over the years, this also became fairly well documented. Now these are acceptable terms in immunology and gastroenterology." Naturopathic doctor Kara Fitzgerald concurs. "We in [functional medicine] were vindicated time and time again as the microbiome, dysbiosis, intestinal permeability, and systems concepts became mainstream ideas in science." While Dr. Fitzgerald acknowledges that these mechanisms are largely not acted upon in mainstream medicine, she points to how they have become recognized concepts.

The drive to be "revolutionaries" among functional medicine thought leaders is tempered by the desire to properly vet new information. Responding to the question of when it is the right time to introduce new concepts, Dr. Bland indicates, "There's always an interest in bringing everything new in because you want to be at the front of the pack, but you have to be a little cautious not to bring too much that's new that hasn't been properly vetted [where] you don't know exactly what you're really dealing with so later you're having to say, 'I made a mistake. I didn't fully understand what was going on.'" In the same vein, Dr. David Servan-Schreiber, a neuroscientist who survived brain cancer twice before succumbing to the disease, suggested avoiding "treatment whose effectiveness has not been proven but that has proven risks" (2009, 103). Functional medicine practitioners aim to revolutionize how medicine is practiced, while also ensuring that changes are based on sound scientific evidence. Dr. Hyman asserts, "You have to rejigger your whole paradigm because all of a sudden the world was flat and now it's round and we have to think differently. . . . I'm hoping we're going to see something like the Berlin Wall come down or some cataclysmic shift in how we do things." Although functional medicine proponents face enormous resistance, they argue that the time is ripe for a paradigm shift in medicine.

## FUNCTIONAL MEDICINE CRITIQUES OF BINARY THINKING

In my classroom, I tell my students that anthropology teaches us that issues are often not as black and white as they may seem. If we take a step back and distance ourselves from our own perspective—that is, our own set of life experiences and our position in society (Haraway 1988)—we can come to understand many other ways of knowing, feeling, and being (see Bateson 2000). Instead of seeing in black and white, I tell my students to "see the world in color." In this same vein, Dr. Bland explains how functional medicine resists binary thinking: "The preconception[s] in medicine is [are] you're well until proven sick and disease is a binary function." Then, pointing to how integral nonbinary thinking is to the functional medicine model, Dr. Bland admits, "If I was to really ask what's the most important singular takeaway from the Institute for Functional Medicine curriculum . . . it's principally how to move our minds away from thinking of things as binary, as true/false, yes/no, multiple choice, [and] disease or no disease." According to this view, the total absence of health is death. Anyone who is alive experiences health and disease as unfolding on a spectrum and not as a binary.

Functional medicine practitioners apply this nonbinary thinking to the issue of how to vaccinate children against disease. While "anti-vaxxers" and pro-vaccination advocates engage in heated debates on the national stage, functional medicine practitioners advocate evaluating each vaccine on a case-by-case basis.[1] Dr. Bland addresses the question of whether the positive outcome of vaccines exceeds the relative risk on average for the world population. "From my perspective, anybody that argues unequivocally against vaccines hasn't looked at population statistics. Immunization against smallpox was a lifesaver for millions of people over the last fifty years." However, he then clarifies that the risk-to-benefit ratio depends on the individual being inoculated. Individuals experience a range of unique effects due to how different immune systems react when exposed to a foreign substance.

According to this model, problems occur while administering vaccines to a particular patient if convenience factors outweigh critical considerations. Dr. Bland points to shortcomings in how the existing vaccine schedule is universally applied to all newborns: "Now, what happens when you start adding multiple [vaccines together]? You want to immunize against everything. You want to do [that] on an infant, an unknown immune system, for efficiency reasons because you want to get [the vaccines done] before they get to school." Dr. Bland critiques how health providers assume this practice to be safe because each individual vaccine has been proven safe in clinical trials. In so doing, these providers do not consider how trials only confirmed the safety of individual vaccines when administered in isolation and over a longer period of time. Answering his question, he continues, "Your relative risk evaluation might be changed by the level of assumptions you're making without knowing exactly what the effects of multiple [vaccines] given rapidly to a young immune system would have on that individual." He likens this approach to "doing a study without really a lot of data" since the effects to the patient's long-term health are unknown.

Instead of asking whether or not parents should vaccinate their children,

Dr. Bland reframes this issue from a nonbinary functional medicine perspective. Pointing to diseases like measles and mumps that were deadly during his childhood, Dr. Bland notes, "There is no question in my mind that the right immunization, given at the right time, at the right dose, can be beneficial." However, in a critique of present-day vaccine schedules that prioritize efficiency over individual considerations, Dr. Bland states, "There's also no question in my mind, that you could take the same [vaccination] model and make it dangerous, in which the risk equation went toward risk and went away from benefit."

Functional medicine resistance to binary thinking also extends to the mind-body dualism referred to in medical anthropology as the "Cartesian split." The adjective "Cartesian" is a reference to philosopher René Descartes, who proposed in his *Discourse on Method*, originally published in 1637, "Cogito, ergo sum" (I think, therefore I am). His proposition gave way to ongoing debates about where to locate one's sense of being in the world—in the mind or in the body. This either/or framework—or "split"—has been discredited by medical anthropologists who emphasize that the mind *is* a part of the body.

While general acceptance of the Cartesian split has tended to shape how doctors understand and treat stress, mind/body separatism is currently being debunked within the realm of functional medicine. Dr. Andrew Heyman explains, "We could probably trace that back to even Decartes in the seventeenth century when we split the mind from the body. The priests and then later the psychologists would inhabit the domain of the mind." As a result of this history, contemporary talk therapy aims to help patients develop coping skills and emotional resiliency. As program director of Integrative and Metabolic Medicine at the George Washington University School of Medicine, Dr. Heyman aims to direct greater focus to "the physiological components of the stress response and how they interplay with our ability to be emotionally resilient under times of stress." In so doing, he points to how much more work needs to be done, including by functional medicine practitioners: "Even though we provide some attention to the topic, I think that until we better understand the interrelationships of the physiologic components of the stress response, we tend to miss some important features of how to protect our patients from ongoing stress."

I argue that a total re-envisioning of health problems and a recharacterization of mind and body as thoroughly enmeshed is needed. For example, in *Gut Feminism*, Elizabeth Wilson elaborates on how the nervous system extends from the "central nervous system" to the "peripheral nervous system." These adjectives—"central" vs. "peripheral"—are themselves a false binary since what distinguishes the two is more arbitrary than concrete. Wilson uses the example of abdominal migraine. Since the gut is encased in the enteric nervous system, stomach pain, nausea, vomiting, or lack of appetite can be accurately described as abdominal migraine (Wilson 2015). This diagnostic category has gained acceptance by the medical community at large over the last few years. Wilson's example of abdominal migraine is useful since it demonstrates that asking whether a problem is "psychosomatic" (in the mind) or "real" (in the body) misses the point. Both mind and body are part and parcel of the whole person, and they are fundamentally inseparable in how we experience health and disease.

Just as the mind is in the body, the body is also in the mind. Health problems that are generally located in the head can be rooted elsewhere in the body. Psychiatrist and author Dr. Kelly Brogan describes the case of a patient who was admitted to the hospital for catatonic depression. "She was largely non-responsive, hallucinating, delusional. She was treated with antipsychotics and antidepressants to no avail. It wasn't until she was transferred to another hospital that they bothered to check a blood B12 level." The patient's acute symptoms were reversed when she received an injection of vitamin B12 in the form of cyanocobalamin. Dr. Brogan also cites the case of a thirty-seven-year-old woman, published in the *New England Journal of Medicine*, who was treated with medication for delusional psychosis. The treatment was to no avail until she was diagnosed with celiac disease. Describing the case, Dr. Brogan explains, "When they put her on a gluten-free diet, all her systems reversed." These cases document that problems in the body can produce symptoms in the head.

Despite the oneness of mind and body, decades of medical anthropology, psychological anthropology, and medical humanities research have demonstrated how, in the absence of clear biological etiology, patients may be stigmatized for "psychosomatic" issues (see Kleinman and Becker 1998; Kirmayer and Gómez-Carrillo 2019). In a similar vein, internist and author Dr. Cynthia Li describes how she concealed her autoimmune symptoms because she was afraid of "getting stigmatized as a difficult patient." She explains, "I knew from the other side what doctors did with patients like me."

Reflecting on his training in medicine, Dr. Hyman admits, "We were subliminally trained to have a dismissive attitude to many categories of patients." From the perspective of mainstream medicine, diagnoses like irritable bowel syndrome, chronic fatigue, and fibromyalgia were indicative of "trouble patients" who physically manifested psychological issues "in their head." Dr. Hyman continues, "In medicine we have a very perjorative way that we talk about these patients. We use a fancy medical word. We say it's 'supratentorial,' which means that it is in your brain, it's in your head. It's very nasty and not true." He notes, "[Regarding] the implication that the patient is crazy . . . [one of] two things [is] true. Either the patient is crazy, or the doctor is missing something. I am going to bet the doctor is missing something." He argues that the root cause of disease can often be identified using thorough, advanced laboratory testing.

## FUNCTIONAL MEDICINE CRITIQUES OF PHARMACEUTICALIZATION AND MEDICALIZATION

Functional medicine doctors, themselves trained in conventional medicine, identify important limitations in the way they were taught to practice medicine. As the keynote speaker at the 2019 Advances in Mitochondrial Medicine Symposium, Dr. Robert Naviaux, professor of medicine at University of California San Diego, pointed to one simple, yet significant limitation in medical education: medical textbooks describe biological states instead of processes—or, at best, pathways instead of networks. According to Dr. Naviaux, "life is dynamic and always in motion," thus physicians cannot rely on textbook knowledge. He indicated, "Our textbooks give us things in photographs, not in videos of the way natural history changes over the course of a person's lifetime."

The problem with viewing disease as a biological state instead of a systems-level process is that it leads mainstream medicine doctors to assuage symptoms with pharmaceuticals instead of identifying the root cause and reversing the disease. Dr. Nalini Chilkov, a doctor of Oriental medicine, uses the analogy of a tree to clarify this point: "We might see little yellow leaves at the tip of a branch and go, 'That's a disease.' Then we go and we get some green paint and we paint it over and go, 'We fixed it.'" She emphasizes how creating health requires addressing the root causes of disease. In the absence of addressing the causes—fixing the water, the soil, and the conditions that determine the tree's health—the tree will simply produce more yellow leaves, necessitating more green paint. In contrast, by fixing the root causes of disease, "we get beautiful flourishing green leaves at the tip of the branch." Extending Dr. Chilkov's point, Dr. Susan Prescott argues that while "risk factors" may be determined to be the "cause" of disease (e.g., poor diet and chronic stress), social, cultural, and economic factors are "causes of the causes." I could not agree more.

Dr. Joel Fuhrman, family physician and nutritional specialist, argues that doctors' role as prescribers ultimately allows patients' underlying disease processes to continue advancing, and many of his colleagues are reevaluating their careers as a result. Speaking to Dr. Fuhrman's assertion, Dr. Pete Cummings, a forensic pathologist, describes how he constantly witnessed preventable causes of death. The experience led to a mid-career crisis that Dr. Cummings self-diagnosed as "Profound Life Frustration (PLF)" due to his inability to help others. Dr. David Scott Jones, president emeritus, Institute for Functional Medicine, similarly admits, "Medical school was not what I expected it to be." According to Dr. Jones, medical school curriculum is "about a certain heuristic [in which] you evaluated a patient, not as a whole person [but] as a system of [independent] organs, and you ask questions to try to single down on which organ is having the most trouble." In this heuristic, doctors make a diagnosis and then look up what drugs can be used in the treatment of that diagnosis. Clinician and author Chris Kresser laments, "The saddest thing to me is that the default approach to these conditions is just prescribing medication." This method does not identify the root cause of disease, nor does it reverse the disease process.

This prescription-based model led Dr. Jones to become deeply unsatisfied with his profession. He reveals how two years into practice he realized how unhappy he was prescribing pharmaceuticals for all his patients, only for them to then suffer from side effects. Dr. Jones recounts, "I looked at the list of who was coming the next day, and I didn't even know who to call to say, 'I'm only going to do mischief in your life.'" Looking back, he confesses that he didn't know enough at the time to truly help patients with their health problems. His confession underscores how, for many patients, pharmaceuticalized medicine can have serious iatrogenic effects.

Iatrogenesis, a topic of great interest among medical anthropologists (see, for example, Inhorn 1993), refers to patients suffering the unintended side effects and consequences of therapies meant to benefit them. It is, in essence, worsening health caused by the doctor and the medicines or interventions provided by the doctor. "For chronic conditions, acute care medicine, which is basically the scalpel or the prescription pad, are probably some of the more toxic things that you can have," says Dr. Todd LePine. "A lot of what I see in my patients here is *iatrogenic imperfecta.*" Dr. LePine, an internist, turned to functional medicine after becoming frustrated with pharmaceuticalized medicine and the ways in which medications cause health problems such as mineral and vitamin deficiency. In his current practice, he works to minimize the iatrogenic effects of pharmaceuticals: "The less drugs you use in medicine, the better off the patient is."

The majority of these interlocutors are trained in conventional medicine, but their critiques are not aimed at their colleagues, but rather at how medical education primarily teaches doctors to turn to pharmaceuticals to treat disease. As Dr. Hyman explains, "It's hard because that is what we know how to do." Furthermore, doctors are bound by bureaucratic and juridical structures that limit and determine how they are able to treat patients. Dr. Heyman indicates that, when prescribing medications, he gets to "click the boxes" because he is following standard of care.

Similarly, functional medicine proponents with a research background critique the process of determining the safety of pharmaceuticals. In terms similar to how Dr. Bland critiqued vaccine trials, Dr. Datis Kharrazian emphasizes, "They never look at polypharmacy, or how these medications all interact with each other." Furthermore, clinical trials do not consider how drugs affect different genotypes, that is, the different genetic constitutions of individual organisms. Dr. Kharrazian, a clinical research scientist and professor, explains that pharmaco-genotype interactions can produce a completely different response from one person to the next. Thus, real-life polypharmacy results in diverse impacts to individuals' receptor site responses, brains, and microbiomes in ways that are still unknown. Despite the fact that clinical trials do not document the effects of drugs under real-life conditions, these trials are legitimized as evidence-based research.

This critique of clinical trials raises the question of whether pharmaceuticalized medicine is the most appropriate model for society. Dr. David Katz, the president of True Health Initiative, poses the following hypothetical situation:

> Imagine if the news were to break tomorrow, on whatever glowing screen you happen to like best these days, "There is a new drug available, approved by the FDA . . . it's available in bountiful supply, it is stunningly free of side effects, it is shockingly inexpensive, safe enough for children and octogenarians alike, and, taken once daily for the rest of your life, will reduce your risk of ever getting any major chronic disease by 80 percent." Who do you call first? A doc for a prescription or your broker to buy stock? Frankly, both would be excellent decisions.

Switching back to reality, Dr. Katz states that not only is there no such pill, but also, in his professional opinion, "there never will be any such pill."

At the Advances in Mitochondrial Medicine Symposium, Dr. Heyman similarly characterized the problem of disease management to his colleagues via a series of rhetorical questions: "Through conventional methods, do you ever reverse chronic fatigue? Do you ever reverse fibromyalgia?

Do you ever reverse chronic migraines?" Then, answering his own questions, he exclaimed, "No! You do lifestyle management, and you give them a couple meds, and you tell them to exercise, and you tell them to come back in a few weeks. [Then] you tell them the same thing . . . for the next thirty years of their life." Speaking on his podcast, Dr. Hyman agrees that chronic disorders like fibromyalgia are not something patients recover from unless they seek help within the functional medicine paradigm.

These examples allude to how functional medicine doctors turn to functional medicine after feeling frustrated with the "limited toolkit" they were offered in medical school. According to Dr. Cynthia Li, "I knew that the tools that I had in my doctor's bag were really limited. I already knew that, but that's kind of the best I could do." In his symposium address, Dr. Heyman noted, "Once you walk through that clinical door and you start trying out all this stuff, you can never go back! You can never go back to just the prescription pad! How limiting would that feel? If I forced all of you . . . to only use the prescription pad again for a month, you'd probably quit." In fact, many functional medicine providers assert that the prescription pad is the least necessary tool in their repertoire.

Within the functional medicine model, it is usually not appropriate to prescribe a drug to a patient indefinitely. Initially, this approach may seem jarring to patients since, as Dr. Hyman puts it, "That's what [patients have] been taught. 'You have to live with this. You have to manage your disease.'" To this, he responds, "I don't want to manage it, I want to get rid of it!" Entrepreneur and health economist James Maskell echoes Dr. Hyman: "The goal is full resolution of symptoms and to be able to live a healthy lifestyle without long-term dependence on medication." Stated differently, the goals of functional medicine are to address root causes and promote healing. The goal is *not* disease management. This critical approach to pharmaceuticals does not mean, from the perspective of functional medicine, that medications should never be prescribed. Instead, they should be carefully assessed for risks vs. benefits and then used cautiously when deemed necessary. When medications are introduced into treatment protocols, they tend to be used sparingly and temporarily.

Some functional medicine proponents frame the reduction of pharmaceuticalization as an economic imperative. Maskell explains that pharmaceuticalization drives up health care spending, especially in chronic, autoimmune diseases. According to the American Autoimmune Related Diseases Association (AARDA) and National Coalition of Autoimmune Patient Groups (NCAPG) 2011 report, the annual costs of autoimmune diseases are likely well over $100 billion. The report reads, "While $100 billion is a staggering figure, it is likely a vast understatement of the true costs of autoimmune disease as the annual costs of only seven of the 100+ known autoimmune diseases, Crohn's disease, ulcerative colitis, systemic lupus erythematosus (SLE), multiple sclerosis (MS), rheumatoid arthritis (RA), psoriasis, and scleroderma, are estimated through epidemiological studies to total from $51.8 to $70.6 billion annually" (American Autoimmune Related Diseases Association, 2011). According to Maskell, reducing the use of prescription medication would be beneficial for patients' health, would increase doctors' job satisfaction, and would reduce health care spending.

However, other functional medicine proponents critique a hyper-capitalist financial structure that incentivizes overmedicalization and what Atul Gawande refers to as "superloading" (Gawande 2009). Dr. William Davis, a cardiologist, suggests that healing has been subverted in the name of both personal and system-level profit.

> A lot of my friends are employees of hospital systems and they tell me . . . "I'm an employee . . . and the more revenue you generate for the hospital system, the larger your end-of-quarter bonus." So, generate as many MRIs, neurology consultations, electrophysiologic studies, heart catheterizations, surgeries, transplants, etc. as you can and your bonus will be much bigger. It won't be ten thousand, it will be fifty thousand or seventy thousand at the end of the quarter.

According to Dr. Davis, this financial structure encourages doctors to churn *people* for revenue. He continues, "People [are] being used for profit . . . and it's just plain wrong."

Comparative health spending statistics demonstrate that exorbitant health expenses in the United States have not produced better health. According to Dr. Davis, Americans have dismal health outcomes while paying more for health care than every other developed country. Dr. Emeran Mayer, director of the G. Oppenheimer Center for Neurobiology of Stress and Resilience, indicates that the United States has seen more than a twenty-fold increase in per capita health care expense since 1970. According to the World Health Organization's 2000 report, the US health care system was the most expensive out of the 191 member nations included in the study; however, it ranked seventy-second in the overall level of health (see Mayer 2016, 7–8). At present, health care consumes almost one-fifth of the US gross domestic product (see Roehr 2013).[2]

Despite an explosive increase in health care spending, chronic diseases are increasing at pandemic proportions (see Terzic and Waldman 2011). Dr.

Mayer writes, "We have made little progress in treating chronic pain conditions, brain-gut disorders such as irritable bowel syndrome (IBS), or mental illnesses such as clinical depression, anxiety, or neurodegenerative disorders. Are we failing because our models for understanding the human body are outdated?" (Mayer 2016, 8). Reacting to these statistics and similar to medical anthropologists, functional medicine practitioners resist medicalizing natural life stages caused by the aging process and normal human emotions.

Some functional medicine practitioners are actively working to reconfigure notions of aging in both the clinic and the laboratory. The work of Dr. Marwan Sabbagh, a neurologist at the Barrow Neurological Institute, emphasizes that Alzheimer's can be prevented and reversed, thus dispelling the notion that cognitive decline should be accepted as a normal part of aging. Dr. Peter Osborne dismisses the misconception that disease is a natural part of the aging process. "We try to create diseases out of natural things in life." Dr. Osborne, a clinical nutritionist, characterizes his patient population as "brave" because they choose not to believe conventional doctors who suggest that ill health is a normal part of aging. Thus, resisting conventional medicine "myths" not only requires boldness on the part of functional medicine practitioners, it also requires patients to resist biomedical authority in marked ways.

Dr. Osborne then describes how the natural process of menopause is treated as a disease. While he coins the term "diseasify" to describe the problematic pattern he observes, medical anthropologists have been critically analyzing the same phenomena—under the name "medicalization"—for decades (see Browner 1999; Lock 2001). He explains, "When a woman goes through menopause, we try to create a disease out of that and say that that somehow now needs to be medicated." Dr. Osborne identifies the medical industry's financial interests as the underlying reason why menopause is treated as a disease. "It's a perfect idea if you want to make money." Dr. Osborne thus extends medical anthropologist Margaret Lock's 1993 argument in *Encounters with Aging: Mythologies of Menopause in Japan and North America*. Using ethnography, statistics, historical data, medical publications, and popular culture materials, Lock challenges North American assumptions about menopause and demonstrates how the experiences, meanings, and endocrinological changes associated with menopause are largely culturally determined. In Japan, menopause is seen as a normal part of the aging process, not a disease-like state.

Dr. Osborne then turns to the medicalization of affective states—for example, depression. "There is nothing wrong with being sad and going through a period of depression. That's part of life experience." He describes how individuals may experience depression in response to difficult situations—for example, when grieving the loss of a loved one. In his view, depression can be an important emotion that individuals need to experience in order to make sense of what they have experienced. Dr. Osborne notes how doctors are trained to treat depression as a disease, instead of acknowledging deep sadness as a human state. His opinion is clear: Treating every anomaly as if it were disease is a "horrible" and "dehumanizing" approach.

Dr. Osborne is again speaking to topics that have a rich history in anthropology. For example, Arthur Kleinman's 2004 essay, "Culture and Depression" illustrates how cultural meanings and practices shape how depression is confronted, discussed, and managed. Many cultures classify the symptoms of depression in a different way from mainstream Western medicine. Since the meanings of pain are specific to different cultures, so are depressive experiences in those cultures (Kleinman 1982). Kleinman uses the somatization of depression in China as an example for how different these experiences can be. It is not that Chinese people do not experience deep sadness. Instead, they manifest their pain through chronic pain syndromes—a tendency Kleinman refers to as a "biologically patterned illness experience" (Kleinman 1982). Taken together, Dr. Osborne's assertions about and Kleinman's extensive research into depression suggest that deep sadness, however it manifests, is part and parcel of being human.

Functional medicine practitioners' resistance to medicalization also extends to geneticization, the tendency to attribute disease purely to genetic inheritance. Dr. Servan-Schreiber noted, "We all live with myths that undermine our capacity to fight cancer. For example, many of us are convinced that cancer is primarily linked to our genetic makeup, rather than our lifestyle. When we look at the research, however, we can see that the contrary is true." Instead of attributing the cause of many chronic diseases to the patient's genetic fate, functional medicine practitioners attempt to create health by intervening upon the interaction between genes and the environment.[3]

## FUNCTIONAL MEDICINE FOCUSES ON CREATING HEALTH

While at first glance, the two goals of treating disease and creating health may seem like the same thing, functional medicine practitioners explain how, in actuality, this represents a major paradigm shift. Fatigue specialist Ari Whitten asserts, "The entire medical system—every layer of it—from the actual care that you are receiving, to the insurance, to the actual research that is being conducted by very well-intended, altruistic, great, very smart people who are . . . trying to help people is fundamentally focused on disease and illness." Whitten continues, "That seems like a reasonable, somewhat logical approach to health until you realize that health isn't actually built by popping pills to interrupt abnormal biochemical pathways. Health is built by focusing on what are the things that actually create optimal cellular function, and metabolic function, and hormonal function." In a similar vein, Dr. Chilkov emphasizes that by focusing on treating symptoms instead of creating health, "we've misplaced where the focus should be." In making these comments, Whitten and Dr. Chilkov highlight the shortcomings of the existing paradigm.

Viewing patients through the lens of creating health rather than that of treating disease produces entirely different answers. Neurology researcher Dr. Martin Picard describes how this focus on disease leads to a pharmaceutical-oriented, palliative treatment: "You study disease and then that leads to wanting to fix disease, and then that leads to developing very targeted, specialized molecules—drugs—and then that leads to the way that we practice medicine, which is palliative." In essence, the lens one is looking through— the paradigm that structures one's thought process—determines the actions that one will take.

Functional medicine doctors who were trained in conventional medicine describe how their medical school education did not address how to create health. As physician, scientist, and author Dr. William Li notes, "We need to have the humility to recognize that we know quite a bit about disease and we have some good medicines to treat them. But when it comes to health, we need to keep our eye on the ball. We need to focus on what we are learning." What Dr. Li is proposing sounds simple, but in fact, it requires doctors to see through the lens of health and become familiar with a new paradigm.

This topic is the focus of a joking exchange between Dr. Hyman and his guest, Dr. Sabbagh on *The Doctor's Farmacy* podcast.

SABBAGH: You and I are both physicians. Part of our day job is taking care of people with disease. So here we are saying, "Let's step back from that. Instead of treating disease, let's [create] health."
HYMAN: Did you take the course in medical school called Creating Health 101?
SABBAGH: I did not! I did not take that course!
HYMAN: I didn't either! We didn't learn that!

Dr. Kirk Robert Parsley similarly describes how health care providers are taught *disease care*. Reflecting on his own experience in medical school, he explains, "I learned how to recognize disease, name it, and then I can follow an algorithm to treat it." His personal reflection is strikingly similar to Dr. Jones's disappointment with contemporary biomedicine. However, expanding on Dr. Heyman's comment about checking the boxes and following the standard of care, Dr. Parsley explains, "If I go outside of the algorithm, I lose my medical license because this is the only way you do it, because a bunch of gray-haired old men in a boardroom decided that this is the only way it's to be done."

Dr. Parsley analogizes health insurance to car insurance to further emphasize his point about how health care is, in fact, disease care. He points to how auto insurance does not pay for maintenance, such as tire rotations and oil changes, since it is reserved for catastrophic costs. Dr. Parsley asserts, "That's what health care is, and what we call health care in the [conventional] sense. That's what the medical community is good at. All of the maintenance stuff is really on you. . . . There is no other option." Dr. Parsley's analogy sums up the consequences of "disease care" in the absence of "health optimization medicine."

Disease care aims to increase longevity—that is, keeping people alive for longer, even if this entails a steady decline in function during old age. Dr. Mayer writes, "Our disease care system . . . has focused almost exclusively on treating the symptoms of chronic disease" (Mayer 2016, 266). This inattention to health is so deeply ingrained that, as Kresser points out, "[i]f you look in the index of a medical textbook that a medical student would see in their program and you look for 'health' in the index of that textbook, you're not going to find anything. There is no definition of health in most medical textbooks. The primary focus is disease. That's true in any branch of medicine." While he readily acknowledges that it is important to address disease when it occurs, he emphasizes prevention as the true measure of medical success.

Functional medicine practitioners argue that the health care system is not set up to prioritize prevention. Virology researcher Dr. Paul Turner comments, "What fascinates me about medicine is, of course, you turn a lot of attention to it when things aren't going well. That almost by definition causes us to sit back and rest on our laurels when things are going well." According to Dr. Picard, that "resting on our laurels" is not due to indolence, but rather because "we don't know what to do when there is no disease, so we need to wait for disease to happen." When disease does occur, doctors are taught to use pharmaceuticals to suppress symptoms.

In contrast, health optimization increases "healthspan," which is defined by functional medicine interlocutors as the amount of time an individual can live with optimum *quality of life*. According to Dr. Mayer, "Optimal health has been a popular topic in the lay media, but it's not a goal that physicians are trained to help their patients achieve" (Mayer 2016, 266). Doctors' frustration with their disease care, combined with their desire to optimize health, has prompted some (including the interlocutors in this book) to advocate for functional medicine. Dr. Hyman explains, "I'm interested in thriving, not just surviving. Functional medicine is really about how to create a thriving human."

Over the course of my research, I noted how interlocutors sometimes expressed hope that in the future, functional medicine will become the primary mode of health care. For example, Kresser imagines a future where, under this new medical paradigm, "instead of just putting Band-Aids on symptoms by using drugs or surgery . . . we actually orient toward identifying and addressing the underlying cause of the problem." In this same vein, Dr. William Li asserts, "The science of health is really the future of medicine." Blue reiterates these hopes, saying, "I really think that we're at a tipping point where . . . we'll find that we aren't looking at two types of medicine; this is just medicine."

At other times, however, interlocutors have positioned functional medicine as an outgrowth of mainstream medicine and a complementary approach to existing treatment protocols. These individuals have pointed to how "disease care" and "health optimization medicine" can be complementarily combined for the benefit of certain patients and have advocated for the team-based approach. Speaking about cancer treatment, Dr. Chilkov says, "You need a disease expert who understands what tools can go after the tumor, and you need a health expert to say, 'How do we actually orchestrate this so that we have the best outcome possible, not just cell kill?'"

Similarly, Maskell emphasizes how disease care and health creation are separate projects. "One of the things that I am becoming more and more clear on is that by leaving health creation in the hands of people who were never trained for it and also don't really understand it . . . we are ultimately capping the potential of health creation by saying that it has to go through the same channels as disease care." At the same time, Maskell clarifies that he is not dismissing the value of treating disease. "We have to honor disease care in its rightful place as necessary and awesome. And we have the best part of it here in America." Like Dr. Chilkov, Maskell argues that both conventional and functional medicine are necessary: disease care and health creation should be pursued by health care teams, with each provider focusing on what they do best.

When advocating for team-based care in the future, these interlocutors acknowledge that paradigmatic differences between disease care and health optimization medicine approaches will persist due to disparate goals. For example, functional doctors and their mainstream counterparts may order some of the same tests. The range that is reported as "normal" on conventional lab results is the range within which mainstream medicine practitioners consider their patients to not be ill. In contrast, Dr. Ted Achacoso, a health optimization specialist, indicates that functional medicine practitioners "do not use illness-medicine ranges." Instead, they "are actually looking at balancing the subtle toxicities and borderline deficiencies that are not necessarily disease." In the functional medicine approach, doctors often aim for a more restricted range of values because their goal is to optimize their patients' health by correcting metabolic imbalances and preventing disease.

Thus, some functional medicine proponents argue that functional medicine can flourish within existing biomedical spaces because it augments, but does not replace, what existing medical treatments accomplish. Describing increased acceptance of the functional model, Blue explains, "We now have legions of success stories and practices all around the country and now the world that are applying it." Blue offered the Cleveland Clinic's Center for Functional Medicine (CCCFM) as one such "success story."[4] Dr. Fitzgerald likewise highlights the Cleveland Clinic, citing the *Journal of the American Medical Association* issue describing its positive health outcomes (Beidelschies et al. 2019). Although CCCFM is ambivalently emplaced in a mainstream clinic—evidenced by how the center struggles to be reimbursed for the "value" it provides to the system—Dr. Fitzgerald points to how, in comparison to a decade ago, functional medicine has made "extraordinary strides . . . in mainstream medicine."

More and more doctors are seeking out additional training in functional medicine. Despite functional medicine's current ambivalent emplacement in mainstream medicine, it is not viewed by these doctors as incommensurable with their training. Rather, they view functional medicine techniques as "added value" to their existing repertoire. Dr. Fitzgerald's Clinic Immersion program, which trains doctors in the functional model, has drawn increased interest from the greater medical community. In an email newsletter, she writes that "more and more docs are craving the possibility of [functional medicine.]" Doctors who enroll in her Clinic Immersion program value how functional medicine diversifies their tool kit, thus allowing them to denormalize illness and create the conditions for patients to experience resilient health.

## DENORMALIZING ILLNESS

From the functional medicine perspective, many patients do not seek optimal health because they normalize their illnesses. Dr. Osborne asserts that many people are sick without knowing it because their norm is some degree of illness. "I can't tell you how many times my clients will tell me something like, 'My norm is that I've always had diarrhea. I've had diarrhea since I was a kid. I've had stomachaches and pains ever since I was a kid. I've had headaches for as long as I can remember. That's just who I am.'" People accept illness as part of their identity as long as they are functional; however, their illness limits their capacity for joy, vibrancy, and health.

Thus, the problem does not begin with how disease is treated, but rather with how it is (not) identified. Dr. Osborne contrasts "health as resiliency" with what he calls "functional illness." From his perspective, health resiliency does not mean perfect health, but rather one's ability to adapt to the changing environment without getting sick. According to Dr. Osborne, most people are not resilient because they live in a state of functional illness. "They can get up, go to work, put on their clothes, make breakfast, whatever it is they have to do for the day. But they don't feel well—their health is not really all that optimized or they don't have resiliency." From Dr. Osborne's perspective, a great number of people are "functionally ill" without even knowing it. Revealing to patients how they ignore their illnesses and allow their poor health to define their norm potentiates the possibility of health optimization.

So what would happen if the focus of health care was expanded beyond only treating disease to include health creation? What foundational steps would have to occur to initiate this change and what would be the potential outcome? For Dr. Martha Herbert, professor of neurology at Harvard Medical School, the first step is to convince the public and the public health and medical systems that healing is the goal. Dr. Herbert notes that successful recovery stories are often dismissed as anecdotal. "People will have their kid recover, and then they will tell the story. But no one is taking measurements in real time while the process is going on." Dr. Herbert indicates that integrative practitioners know that individuals can recover from "lifelong conditions" such as autism, but the public is not aware because of a lack of published scientific evidence.[5]

To remedy this situation, Dr. Herbert is tracking recovery as it happens. "We are . . . going to be tracking the laboratory measures and the changes in the course of [recovery] so that we can write a scientific paper or a number of scientific papers. We are going to do brain scans and gene expression and microbiome studies." Through tracking multiple laboratory measures over time, Dr. Herbert hopes to document the systems biology of getting better and how this is seated within the context of the family.[6] From this perspective, changes made at the household level (for example, diet) will not only lead to improvement for the autistic child, but will also likely produce health benefits for everyone in the household.

The ultimate aim of her research is to create actionable knowledge for patients, providers, and public health professionals. To this end, Dr. Herbert proposes a multi-pronged approach. By working with an electronic health record, her team has established a mechanism for disseminating their findings. She underscores the participatory nature of functional medicine:[7] "We will open it up to the public so the public can participate in learning how to get better." Dr. Herbert further indicates, "We want to conduct an educational campaign and a scientific campaign to make recovery the goal that we all reach for, and [to] transform the medical and public health systems."

As many functional medicine proponents indicate, changes to medical education are needed. Harking back to Kresser's lament regarding the absence of "health" in the indexes of medical textbooks, Dr. Naviaux argues that doctors cannot seek what they cannot name—that is, the problem can be traced back to a missing vocabulary. "[We] have trouble maintaining focus on a process or a problem unless it has a name. So this is a fundamental gap in our medical vocabulary—there was not a name for healing!" Dr. Naviaux aims to fill this gap by offering the term "salugens," which he defines as "the molecules, the natural products, the metabolites, the herbs that naturally promote healing." The word "salugens" is rooted in the Latin word for health (*salutem*, or *salud* in Spanish) and offers a counterpart to pathogens, where none currently exists.

The vocabulary that one uses potentiates scientific inquiry. Providing salugens with a name is valuable because it does something: it allows practitioners to see possibilities and imagine therapeutic strategies that they otherwise would not be able to conceive. Dr. Naviaux continues, "It adds a new job, and that's the job of not just finding the pathogens, but the salugens." In essence, by coining the term "salugens," Dr. Naviaux created a way for practitioners to focus on actually promoting health instead of just alleviating symptoms. The term "salugens" allows practitioners to see health not as a black box, but as something that has regulatable steps (see Latour 1999).

Words shape thoughts, which in turn shape actions and the fabric of our reality (see Lévi-Strauss 1963). Entrepreneur Vishen Lakhiani refers to anthropological and historical studies to explain this point. Describing the Himba, a tribe in Africa that has multiple words for the color green but no word for the color blue, he says, "When you show them blue and green squares, they're unable to pick out the blue square because they cannot see blue. This raises the question: can we see something if we don't have a word for it?" He extends his example to other cultures and other parts of the world. "If you look at ancient Chinese texts, if you look at ancient Greek texts such as *The Iliad*, there is no such word for the color blue. Even Homer described the ocean back then as the 'wine dark sea' but there was no mention of the color blue." In turning to these examples, Lakhiani is incorporating observations from anthropology regarding how language structures our perspective of the world around us. Specifically, medical anthropologists have studied how the use of metaphors silences and shames patients (Sontag 1978), how narratives can reify culture (Taylor 2003), how drug users' relationship to language can reconfigure their relationship to drugs (Summerson Carr 2011), and how words can shape ideas about health, immunity, patient-provider relationships, and the relationship between psyche and soma (Martin 1994; Good et al. 1990).

In a similar vein, functional medicine proponents underscore the importance of naming salugens. At the same time, they argue that while introducing new vocabulary potentiates novel inquiries and therapeutic approaches, it is not enough to guarantee a shift in the medical paradigm. As more and more salugens emerge, doctors will have to pay careful attention to avoid lapsing into medicine's current reductionistic model wherein each symptom is isolated and treated using a nonsystems biology, one-to-one approach.[8] As entrepreneur and health consultant Dr. Matthew Accurso explains, "If I believe the body is the sum of parts—for instance, your heart is not working, I need to address your heart; your kidney is not working, I need to address your kidney—then I'm going to be very mechanistic in my approach. I'm going to give you a pill, a potion, or lotion, a supplement." He goes on to explain why supplements—even when they are considered salugens—can lose their health-promoting potential if they are not prescribed as part of a systems biology approach. "We know that there are supplements out there that are wonderful. There are exercise regimens that are wonderful out there. There are so many things we can apply to the body that are wonderful. But the fact is that if I'm addressing the body mechanistically, then it's a glorified drug." A whole-person approach is needed.

Thus, in functional medicine, salugens are being promoted as an integrated part of a systems biology approach. Dr. Bland points out that when salugens—what he refers to as "wellness promotors"—are incorporated into medical education and medical therapeutics, they would also have an economic effect that shapes the business of medicine (see Good and Good 1981). He explains, "It's going to have an enormous effect on an emerging new industry, which is going to be a wellness-based industry that's based on these parameters." In the future, Dr. Bland envisions a wellness-based industry scaled for the masses. While he argues that industry will allow salugens to become a regular part of health care provisioning by encouraging investments in health creation instead of disease care, I am wary of how a "wellness-based industry" may inadvertently reinscribe neoliberal logics, thus determining who can afford to be well. How might industry-based opportunities for wellness exacerbate "race," class, and gender inequalities?

While Dr. Bland envisions the development of a wellness-based industry in the future, other functional medicine interlocutors signal major obstacles. Geneticist Dr. Moshe Szyf notes how existing financial incentives favor the research and development of pharmaceuticals while presenting obstacles for research into salugens. Dr. Szyf explains, "It's very hard to get a patent on a natural product. And it's very hard to protect it. If you want to invest a billion dollars in research, you want to get some sort of reward, a return on investment. . . . So, there's a bigger incentive for a drug company to develop a new poison than to reinvestigate some safe compounds. Because there's no return on such an investment." In his view, the existing structure financially incentivizes the hyper-pharmaceuticalization of medicine (see Bell and Figert 2012) and discourages a paradigm shift toward health creation.

I argue that in the context of neoliberalism, even if financial incentives were to favor research into health creation, substituting salugens for pharmaceuticals would primarily benefit the privileged. Currently, the most privileged can afford the best treatments, thus facilitating their ability to buy their way out of sickness. The most privileged could also afford the most effective salugens in a wellness-based industry, thus allowing them to buy their way into optimal health.[9] Thus, I ask, can functional medicine proponents reframe wellness so that it is more accessible and not an exclusive resource for the most privileged? Leaders within the functional medicine space identify changing health insurance as the place to start. However, they fail to challenge neoliberal structures by simultaneously suggesting that changes in health insurance may create a domino effect that provokes change in adjacent industries.

Harking back to Dr. Jones's comments about how his colleagues "super-load" patients to create greater revenue for the hospital and larger bonuses for themselves, Maskell notes that conventional medicine doctors are paid by health insurance for every "disease care" intervention they provide. Meanwhile, the services provided by functional medicine doctors for health creation are not paid for by health insurance. Maskell argues that changing how health insurance operates can make doctors accountable for creating health instead of allowing medicalization to drive up health costs. Dr. Molly Maloof, physician and lecturer at Stanford University, agrees: "I do think we need to build a system on top of it that is about . . . investing in your health rather than putting money into an insurance policy that you don't get to see until you actually break." Dr. Hyman similarly asserts that reimbursements shape how doctors practice medicine. "If we are now accountable for the health of our population, not just doing more stuff . . . that's a very different incentive, which is going to change practice. I think, where money goes, practice follows." He adds, "If we get paid to do things, like angioplasties and surgeries, we will continue to do them. But if we get paid for doing lifestyle things, then we will start doing that." In this view, the difference between doctors earning more money for doing "more stuff" vs. earning more money for doing "the right stuff" is at stake.

Here, I point to a potential slippage: What if doctors become incentivized to do more of the right stuff? At first blush, this may seem like a nonsensical question. How could doing more of the right stuff possibly be a bad thing? By pointing to this slippage, I am signaling how the journey to wellness is unending. Health can never be optimal—rather, it is constantly in the process of optimization. Even those who have already recovered from chronic disease may wonder if there is more they should be doing to prevent potential relapses in the future. This harks back to Lakoff's (2012) notion of "preparedness," albeit in a different context. As a person seeking wellness, how can you prepare for an unknown future? How do patients and their providers prevent all potential illnesses that have not occurred and may never occur? What are the criteria for sufficient prevention?

Health can always be further optimized and more prevention can always be done, so doing more of the right stuff may inadvertently create a meritocracy in which individuals with the best insurance and the greatest access (read: the most privilege) engage in an ongoing quest for optimal health and prevention. This would be beneficial to them and, as functional medicine proponents argue, would likely cost less than pharmaceutical treatment and surgical intervention. However, I argue that the most privileged do not suffer the most from chronic disease. Rather, the most disadvantaged populations bear the greatest disease burden. Unfortunately, disadvantaged populations would continue to be the most vulnerable in insurance models that prioritize wellness.

If changes to health insurance do take place, they will likely occur through the gradual introduction and solidification of health creation as a legitimate pursuit. Thus, functional medicine proponents are advocating for changes to medical education—especially changes that rely on emerging evidence to lessen the "translational gap."

## FUNCTIONAL MEDICINE AIMS TO CLOSE THE TRANSLATIONAL GAP

In medicine, advances in science are often not reflected in clinical practice for seventeen years—the time it takes for emerging findings from medical research to make their way into medical school curriculums and for a new generation of doctors to complete their training and begin putting those findings into practice (see Morris, Wooding, and Grant 2011). Reacting to this gap, Blue says, "It's insane. Where else in our entire economy would you find the breakthrough thing taking seventeen years to make it into your household, your new smartphone, your computer, or whatever? The pace of the application of innovation in medicine is tragic." The time lag between when research findings emerge and when they are reflected in clinical protocols is referred to as the "translational gap."

Functional medicine practitioners do not attribute the translational gap to doctors' indolence. Given the enormous number of new scientific papers published each year—approximately 2.5 million according to research from the University of Ottawa (Boon 2017)—doctors are forced to read primarily within their specialty. Nonetheless, as Dr. Hyman asserts on *The Human Longevity Project*: "There are enormous amounts of information that we're not able to assimilate and use." Thus, doctors must develop effective methods for determining which studies to read. Dr. Fitzgerald describes how she browses her inbox for articles that directly shape clinical practice, writing, "I am most likely to open and read (i.e., actually click on) those heavy on the science, especially featuring new research."

Since pharmaceuticals are not functional medicine practitioners' primary resource for treating disease, the papers of most interest to them focus on topics such as systems biology,[10] lifestyle interventions, environmental toxins, epigenetics, the microbiome, diet, food, and nutrition. While the number of papers that interest functional medicine practitioners are a small subset of the total being published, these papers also address a wider array of topics than would generally be of interest to most specialists. Furthermore, the mode of discourse that functional medicine practitioners use to communicate emerging scientific discoveries extends far beyond papers published in scientific journals.

As I have mentioned, the ideas rapidly circulating and evolving in the functional medicine community take on a vibrant social life in digital spaces—through, for example, webinars, master classes, podcasts, YouTube episodes, online summits, email newsletters, and listservs—that are often open to the public. In the case of Facebook groups, sometimes hosted by a functional medicine practitioner, the intentional aim is to bring patients into the digital-social discourse. When functional medicine researchers do publish their findings, they often prioritize books written for public audiences over scientific papers that may be read by only a few colleagues in their area of expertise. Dr. David Sinclair, professor at Harvard Medical School, indicates, "I've been so busy, I haven't written a lot of these ideas down in scientific publications. I've been working on the book. So it could be that the world will be able to read about all this science before scientists do." This emphasis on publishing for the public signals how functional medicine has reconfigured the role of bioconsumers.[11]

Functional medicine practitioners also make it a priority to close the translational gap by introducing new therapeutic techniques into their clinical practices in real time. According to Blue, "[w]hat functional medicine is accomplishing is an acceleration of the application of modern science in the day-to-day practice of medicine rather than a divergence." As soon as there is enough literature to support clinical efficacy, functional medicine practitioners implement changes in their practice.

By pointing to the role of medical education, Blue is careful not to demonize doctors who have only received conventional training and place their functional counterparts on a pedestal. "It's not so much a failing of conventional doctors and the superstars that are functional medicine doctors. It is that there are a growing number of doctors who are deciding, sometimes at their own expense . . . to go out into the world after their education [and] invest more money and more learning." Only through this additional time and financial investment do functional medicine providers understand how to reverse chronic diseases by addressing underlying causes.

Dr. Volkmar Weissig, professor of pharmaceutical sciences at Midwestern University, offers his personal experience of seeking out further education in order to understand the root causes of disease. Dr. Weissig learned about mitochondrial DNA diseases by attending lectures offered by specialists and basic scientists at the United Mitochondrial Disease Foundation meetings. He notes, "I myself teach in a college of pharmacy, and we educate future doctors of pharmacy. . . . Mitochondrial diseases are not yet in the curriculum." In the absence of change to medical and pharmacy school curriculums, doctors become personally responsible for seeking out advanced knowledge.

Many of the bodily systems that functional medicine attempts to optimize and restore are not currently taught to health professionals. While Dr. Weissig notes that mitochondrial diseases do not figure into pharmacy school curriculums, Dr. Achacoso confirms that "metabolomics, epigenetics, bioenergetics dealing with mitochondria, the gut immune system being the gut microbiota, [and] exposomics" are not presently taught in medical schools. In order to incorporate these new scientific discoveries into their clinical practices, functional medicine practitioners must train themselves to use technologies that they were not familiarized with in medical school.

While this self-led training allows functional medicine practitioners to expand their toolkit and use advanced diagnostics, it also presents significant shortcomings and concerns. Dr. Heyman explains, "This is the promise and peril of integrative medicine, which by definition is that we integrate diet, and exercise, and stress management, sometimes meds, and botanicals, and supplements, and acupuncture needles . . . ." He pokes fun at how functional medicine practitioners ignore the protocols they were taught in medical school when they learn of something new that produces better results "and pixie dust, and we even sacrifice some virgins occasionally . . . if we can find them!" Dr. Heyman's remarks use humor to hyperbolize how functional medicine practitioners attempt to close the translational gap in medical research.

As Dr. Heyman indicates, functional medicine practitioners' dismissal of discrete treatment paths (i.e., protocols) introduces both disadvantages and advantages. On the one hand, he admits that while "there is evidence for each thing that I do, I'm not always certain which were the steps that were the most responsible for improvement. And it might be different in different patients. So, you do feel like it's a little bit of a kitchen sink approach." While Dr. Heyman maintains that there is an order and a rationale to his work, Dr. Robert Luby, director of Medical Education Initiatives at the Institute for

Functional Medicine, fears that, in the absence of medical school education on salugens and systems biology, "[i]ndividuals without medical/training licensure (or with limited training) will practice as mavericks and/or outside the scope of their licensure, especially as diagnostic and therapeutic intervention 'products' become more available to the public." Both doctors advocate for the incorporation of functional medicine into medical education.

On the other hand, functional medicine personalizes treatment to each individual patient in a processual manner. While Dr. Heyman admits that this approach may seem "weird" or "voodoo" from an outsider's perspective, he asserts that it is based on the provider's practical willingness to "do whatever it takes" to help the patient improve, including "suspending their own disbelief" when trying new technologies. Dr. Heyman's words hark back to anthropologist Claude Lévi Strauss's foundational 1963 work, "The Sorcerer and His Magic," in which Quesalid, a novice Kwakiutl shaman, begins as a doubter. However, as Quesalid starts believing in shamanism, his belief potentiates his healing power as a shaman.

The theme of delayed self-belief resonates with many functional medicine practitioners. On *The Doctor's Farmacy*, Dr. Hyman recounts his transition into functional medicine and how he began instructing patients to do things that were "outside the box" of what he had learned in medical school—for example, dietary changes. When patients returned for a six-week follow-up and reported improvement, Dr. Hyman describes his thought process as, "You are? Really? ... What? That worked? ... Okay, fine." He explains, "It really took me years and years to expect that people would get better because I thought, 'I don't know what I'm doing. It seems to make sense, and it's not going to hurt them.' And people just recovered. It was just amazing to me!"

Dr. Hyman's retelling of his experience casts a spotlight on the enormous potential benefits when functional medicine practitioners exercise a readiness to experiment with new techniques. Dr. Fitzgerald describes this as "an open-mindedness and a willingness to jump in and try something out." This open-mindedness extends to what counts as legitimate scientific knowledge. While functional medicine doctors continue to value evidence-based medicine—that is, protocols designed after large trials—they also value evidence-informed clinical care. In the absence of large trials, functional medicine physicians are guided by the results they see in clinic.[12] By resisting preconceptions, accepting that what they know may be wrong, and validating clinical observations as "evidence," functional medicine practitioners are again adopting an anthropological perspective.

## "ALWAYS READY TO BE WRONG": RESISTING PRECONCEPTIONS AS AN ANTHROPOLOGICAL APPROACH TO PATIENT CARE

Like anthropologists, the originators of functional medicine set out to identify preconceived notions in medicine and to critically analyze their usefulness. When teaching introduction to sociocultural anthropology, I tell my students I am always ready to be wrong (Fuentes 2012), and I invite them to offer perspectives that may contradict my own. As an anthropologist, I acknowledge that my perspective is situated within my own life experience (Haraway 1988). It is only one limited perspective of the world, and it can always be expanded through my interactions with others.

My perspective can change at any moment based on what I observe in the world around me and what my students teach me. Like anthropology, functional medicine incorporates the same willingness to discard or critique what one has learned and replace it or improve upon it based on what is being observed. Dr. Bland maintains, "Preconceptions often spear how we see [and] how we interpret observations." He adds, "Don't accept the norm as a standard of identity for the future. . . . You've got to continually push forward in understanding and not get too comfortable with what you already know because it probably, in retrospect, will turn out to be fairly naïve." This anthropological perspective is what drew me to functional medicine as a patient.

At the same time, when incorporating new techniques into their treatment protocols and seeking to close the translational gap, functional medicine practitioners must embrace an ongoing readiness to be wrong. For Dr. Heyman, this readiness is folded together with a healthy dose of humorous self-deprecation. The speed of scientific discovery means, at any given moment, the protocols being used in functional medicine clinics are, in his words, "old school." At the 2019 Advances in Mitochondrial Medicine Symposium, he provided the following dialogue for a comical, imaginary interaction between a functional medicine doctor and a chronic fatigue syndrome patient:

Functional medicine doctor: "Oh, if you have a fatiguing illness, I know what to do because I'm functional! I'm functional! You are going to take your CoQ10, ribose, carnitine, and alpha-lipoic acid. I'll see you in eight weeks. I know you are going to feel great!"
Patient at follow-up appointment: "Dr. Heyman, I'm as tired as I

ever was, I'm a little poorer because you sold me these stupid supplements, and I don't even know what mitochondria are, but I'm sure they are not working for me!"

He wrapped up his archetypal account by acknowledging, "That was where we were. That was all we knew." Dr. Bland and Dr. Heyman's assertions also indicate that current functional medicine approaches are inadequate when seen through the lens of the future. Both emphasize that the commitment to constant learning is not just about increasing the layers of knowledge about different molecules, but also about readiness to acknowledge that existing understandings of the body and its functioning are "incredibly limited." In the same vein, Dr. LePine admits, "The more I learn, the more I realize how little I know." Through this admission, he makes a public commitment to continue learning through emerging research.

This commitment is integral to the practice of functional medicine since, according to Dr. Bland, functional medicine practitioners must work to reframe concepts in novel ways and prove their points by "convinc[ing] other people from evidence." At the 2019 symposium, Dr. Heyman began this work by walking his colleagues—medical professionals who, by attending the symposium, were earning continuing medical education credit—through a new, "cutting edge" model for treating chronic disease. Scanning the room, Dr. Heyman reassured his audience, "If this is new to you, it should be! It is new to everyone. This is the new sort of language and science and medicine that is beginning to converge in very interesting ways."

Dr. Heyman probed the audience with questions that required a sharp memory of what they had learned in medical school, only to then explain how recent research showed that understanding to be outdated and false. Learning this new model for treating chronic disease meant that symposium attendees had to be reschooled. While implementing the model he was presenting required learning about emerging research, Dr. Heyman insisted that the endeavor is "very exciting because as we push ourselves in the scientific side, we are getting closer and closer on the clinical side." According to Dr. Heyman, implementation of actionable insights from emerging science directly improves clinicians' ability to resolve chronic disease among their patients.

At the same time, actionable insights are often gleaned from the patient's self-report. Thus, the functional medicine approach begins with asking a question. While doctors are trained to identify *what* the problem is, anthropology and functional medicine ask *why* things occur. Dr. Brogan illustrates this distinction:

The way that I was trained was fundamentally never to ask the question "Why?" In the existing medical model, doctors exclusively seek to match a diagnosis with an intervention; thus, the patient's life history is irrelevant for providing treatment. We never have been taught to ask, "Why is the person depressed? Is this a psycho-spiritual issue? Is this a nutrient deficiency? Is this some sort of endocrine imbalance? Is this some sort of medication adverse effect?"

While Dr. Brogan characterizes the question of "why" as a "distraction" in mainstream medicine, this question lies at the heart of functional medicine.

## LISTENING AND OBSERVING: ADOPTING ANTHROPOLOGICAL METHODS

Dr. Naviaux describes how functional medicine researchers conduct bench science in anthropological terms. In the lab, these researchers are using new technologies to "listen to" and observe the communication among human cells. Dr. Naviaux explains, "It's just like when an anthropologist goes to the Amazon and wants to learn the language of the Yanomami Indians. You have to begin writing down what you hear, and then you write the words that come together, and then you start beginning to understand the syntax of the language." Dr. Naviaux's research team is applying this anthropological approach to cell-to-cell communication. "We are literally using mass spectrometry to . . . document the words that cells are using to communicate with each other and we are beginning to build that up in patterns and pictures." Teams like Dr. Naviaux's are uncovering novel biological structures and mechanisms at a dizzying pace, necessitating a new lexicon to describe what they are observing and learning.

During patient consults, functional medicine practitioners also use a method resembling that of anthropologists. They aim to listen and observe because only by understanding the complete context can they begin to untangle a web of symptoms and get to the underlying systemic cause. Describing the effects of this approach to medicine, Maskell says, "[Doctors] fall back in love with medicine. They love sitting with patients for a long period of time. They love helping people get to the root cause of their issues." In a similar way, anthropologists conduct in-depth interviews and use participant observation as primary research methods. Deep engagement with a community context allows anthropologists to identify and analyze broader issues of social inequality.

In functional medicine, the patient's story is a valuable diagnostic resource (perhaps even more valuable than a medical textbook or lab result). Dr. LePine describes how he spends the first hour-and-a-half consult with a new patient primarily listening to the patient's story. During those initial ninety minutes, Dr. LePine asks open-ended questions and allows the patient to tell every facet of their illness narrative (Kleinman 1988). This (anthropological) method of obtaining a detailed history differs markedly from how Dr. LePine was trained in medical school. In the existing medical model, physicians are trained to obtain an "exclusive history" about the one symptom in question. This exclusive history places the symptom, instead of the patient, at the center of the story. In contrast, a detailed history shifts the focus from the symptom to the patient and, furthermore, recasts the patient as a whole person.

In addition to paradigmatic and methodological differences between mainstream and functional medicine, the ability to obtain a detailed vs. an exclusive history is based on the amount of time the physician has with each patient. Kresser highlights the constraints of mainstream medical consultations. "The average time that a primary care doctor spends with a patient is now eight to ten minutes." According to Kresser, short consultation times restrain doctors' abilities to ask meaningful questions about symptoms, much less discuss diet, behavior, or lifestyle changes that may lead to improvement. Harking back to the problematic pharmaceuticalization of medicine, Kresser concludes that "[t]here's just enough time maybe to figure out what drug or medication could be used to address those symptoms and write that prescription and hurry the patient out the door before the next one comes in."

In contrast, in the realm of functional medicine, patients' illness narratives provide clue after clue regarding underlying causes and thus potential therapeutic approaches. Dr. LePine describes the questions that go through his mind when he is listening to the patient's history: "Where were they when they got sick? Where are they now?" To this, Dr. Hyman responds, "They will tell you what's wrong, and when, and what." Dr. LePine concurs, explaining that he resists the temptation to interrupt patients to ask for further details on a particular topic. He clarifies that allowing patients to talk more is ultimately very productive since "[w]hen you really do that, and let the patients tell their story in their own way, in their own terms . . . you really find out all of the little details and you can . . . play detective and piece . . . the puzzle together." From the perspective of functional medicine, listening to the patient is fundamental to providing proper care.

Functional medicine practitioners describe conducting discursive analysis, paying careful attention to the order in which the patient's illness narrative unfolds. Dr. Chilkov explains, "When I have a new patient, I try to ask an open-ended question, like, 'What brought you here? How can I be of service to you?' Then I just sit back and listen because a lot of times, as the patient tells me what's of concern to them, whatever they say first is I know what is the most troubling to them." Many functional medicine doctors agree that the very first concern the patient expresses is what requires the most attention.

While the anthropologist gathers ethnographic data by conducting in-depth interviews and engaging in participant observation, functional medicine physicians gather data through what Dr. Hyman describes as "very detailed histories [and] very advanced diagnostic testing." Laboratory results allow the physician to "observe" the patient beyond the scope of clinical interactions. While the patient's illness narrative provides detailed social and environmental context, laboratory results offer detailed insight into the patient's internal biology.[13]

In anthropology, informants' accounts of their experiences and life history are as important as what the anthropologist observes. Likewise, since the functional medicine paradigm places high value on both qualitative data *and* quantitative data, the patient's unique illness narrative provides as many diagnostic clues as lab markers on advanced diagnostic tests.[14] The patient's report of symptoms, or lack thereof, may even take precedence over laboratory results. For example, if a laboratory test suggests dysbiosis (an imbalance of intestinal flora), but the patient does not report having any gastrointestinal symptoms, there is no need to immediately intervene. Doing so could provoke symptoms where previously there were none. In the end, laboratory tests can help provide clues as to what may be going wrong, but the patient's lived experience in their own body predominates.[15] Positioning the patient's self-report as equally as valuable as or more valuable than laboratory results—similar to basing clinical interventions on observed outcomes and not just clinical trials—represents a significant shift away from what has previously counted as evidence.

At the same time, prioritizing the patient's lived experience signals a substantial reconfiguration of doctor-patient interactions. Many functional medicine practitioners have themselves struggled with chronic disease or have cared for a loved one who has. Within the functional medicine realm, providers often make claims to cultural capital—resulting in greater social capital—on the basis of these experiences. Furthermore, functional medicine practitioners describe feeling betrayed by their own training and diagnose a need for embodied empathy among doctors (see Sletvold 2014).

Dr. Cynthia Li, a former autoimmune sufferer, refers to an essay, "Arrogance," by Franz J. Ingelfinger, published in 1980 in the *New England Journal of Medicine*.[16] In the essay, Ingelfinger posed the question, "What would medicine look like if one of the prerequisites for entering medical school was having had a serious illness?"[17] Dr. Li asks, "Would there be more empathy? Would there be more belief? How do we start with that as a doctor—just believing all patients?" The ability to listen to someone's story, to empathize with them, and to suspend one's own preconceived notions in order to fully engage with that person's reality are foundational skills in both functional medicine and anthropology.

While functional medicine practitioners advocate for validating patients' concerns, I argue that they must simultaneously consider how power imbalances between the doctor and patient structure what is perceived and heard. This issue has been analyzed by medical and linguistic anthropologists (see Matthiessen 2013; Hasty et al. 2012); however, it is absent from functional medicine discourse.[18] Multiple social factors—for example, the patient's gender and language proficiency (Lebrun 2012)—can ameliorate or exacerbate power imbalances between patients and providers. Thus, these power imbalances are intersectional in nature (Crenshaw 2014).

When specifically examining the patient's income, education, or occupation, differences in verbal and nonverbal behavior have been termed "the social gradient in doctor-patient communication" (Verlinde et al. 2012). In essence, when the patient is higher on the social gradient than the doctor (for example, a white male patient and a Hispanic female doctor), a larger portion of the consultation time is devoted to the patient's concerns. When the doctor is higher on the social gradient than the patient (for example, Hispanic female patient and a white male doctor), the patient is more likely to be interrupted by the doctor and speak fewer words overall. Doctor-patient communication is one area in which functional medicine can benefit from engaging anthropological perspectives on social inequality.

## THE FUNCTIONAL MEDICINE MATRIX: THE NEED FOR ENGAGEMENT WITH ANTHROPOLOGICAL THEORY

As with doctor-patient communication, the functional medicine matrix (and functional medicine discourse in general) largely neglects the issue of social inequality. In making this critique, I argue that while functional medicine resembles anthropology in many ways, it can be strengthened by greater engagement with anthropological theory. While certain functional medicine practitioners and proponents analogize their work to that of linguistic anthropology or cite cultural anthropologist Margaret Mead and medical anthropologist Paul Farmer, as a whole, functional medicine is often unaware of anthropological theory, even when functional medicine proposals closely resemble those presented in published anthropology literature. For example, by proposing a spectrum of wellness and disease, Bland, Jones, and Leo Galland, among other colleagues, suggest that patients can move in the direction of wellness through integrative approaches. In so doing, they unwittingly echo medical anthropologist Eduardo Menéndez's (1994) theorization of the health/disease/medical care process.[19]

Menéndez's argument that health is humans' primordial state is further echoed by functional medicine proponents. In both views, only when health is disturbed will an individual progress along the continuum toward disease, which in turn prompts the individual to seek patient care. At the same time, Menéndez highlights the many attempts of individuals and their families to address the health problem within the domestic sphere before seeking the assistance of a medical professional.[20] Menéndez focuses on the home remedies, dietary measures, herbalism, and traditional medicine techniques that individuals turn to before seeking help in a clinical context. These healing strategies, and a focus on "patient-activated care," also figure into the functional medicine paradigm.

In the late 1990s, Dr. Bland and his colleagues introduced a new model for patient care with the hope of disrupting medical practice. This new model rested on the functional medicine matrix, a template for understanding the root causes of a patient's illnesses. When compared to conventional medicine, the matrix considerably expands the scope of functional medicine's therapeutic considerations. However, I argue that if the functional medicine matrix were to systematically incorporate the insights of medical anthropology, it would be more attentive to issues of privilege and disadvantage, thus imbuing the model with more disruptive potential.

The functional medicine matrix asks practitioners to consider a series of interrelated biological systems in each patient: defense and repair, energy, biotransformation and elimination, transport, communication, structural integrity, and assimilation. The "rough cut" of this model was originally drawn out by Dr. Bland and Dr. David Scott Jones on the back of a napkin. Inspired by the extremely popular films starring Keanu Reeves, *The Matrix* (1999), *The Matrix Reloaded* (2003), and *The Matrix Revolutions* (2003), Jones coined the term "functional medicine matrix" to describe the model.

Dr. Bland and Dr. Jones collaborated with Dr. Galland, an internal medicine physician and integrative medicine leader, on the matrix. Dr. Galland introduced the "patient-centered concept" and advocated for attentive listening to the patient's illness narrative (Kleinman 1988). Emphasizing the importance of the patient's story, the matrix requires practitioners to identify disease antecedents, triggering events, mediators, and perpetuators. Practitioners ask what happened before the onset of illness, what triggered the illness, what other elements are involved in how the illness manifests, and what factors contribute to its perpetuation.

The functional medicine matrix also serves as a template for identifying lifestyle factors that can be "modified: to produce better health. So-called 'Modifiable Personal Lifestyle Factors'" include sleep and relaxation, exercise and movement, nutrition, stress, and relationships. When using the matrix, functional medicine practitioners ask how each of these lifestyle factors can be modified in individual patients to help create and maintain optimal health. Dr. Bland characterizes this emphasis on lifestyle—and the recognition that there is no genetic on-off switch for disease and wellness[21]—as "a revolutionary new concept that we're still learning about." Focus on lifestyle is central to functional medicine and has inspired the naming of both the Personalized Lifestyle Medicine Institute (PLMI) and the Lifestyle Matrix Resource Center. Modifiable lifestyle factors also inform group-delivered functional medicine—regarded by Maskell as the future of functional medicine.[22] Maskell asserts that the health creation moving forward will involve groups of people empowering themselves through health by exercising together, eating well, and sleeping well.

My training in medical anthropology and epidemiology prompts me to critique the institutionalization of lifestyle within functional medicine. I signal that it is not lifestyle, but social, political, and economic factors that determine health outcomes by first structuring how people live their lives.[23] These political, economic, and social causes of illness and disease are referred to within public health and epidemiology as "social determinants of health." Thus, from the perspectives of medical anthropology and social epidemiology, the degree to which lifestyle is modifiable largely depends on the individual's relative privilege-disadvantage.[24]

In using this hyphenated term, as opposed to a binary presentation of privilege or disadvantage, I am using Kimberlé Crenshaw's concept of intersectionality to argue that vulnerability and privilege unfold on opposite ends of a spectrum (Crenshaw 2014; Atewologun and Sealy 2014). Crenshaw, a lawyer, philosopher, and critical race and gender theorist, posits that different axes of inequality are not additive. For example, a Black man may experience "race-based" discrimination and a white woman may experience gender-based discrimination. However, a Black woman's experience is not equivalent to that of the Black man's "race-based" discrimination plus that of the white woman's gender-based discrimination. Instead, Black women experience "race-based" discrimination, gender-based discrimination, *and* discrimination that is unique to them as *Black women*. Using intersectionality as a lens, I suggest that most people are not *wholly* privileged or *wholly* disadvantaged, but experience varying degrees of privilege and disadvantage based on intersecting social factors (e.g., "race," class, gender).

Since the vast majority of functional medicine patients tend to enjoy a relative amount of privilege, most functional medicine providers tend not to be faced with the lived realities of those for whom lifestyle is not modifiable through choice. As a result, functional medicine practitioners often neglect how social, political, and economic factors shape "lifestyle choices." In pointing out how the matrix fails to consider the determining effects of social inequality on lifestyle, I do not mean to discredit the idea that health and disease result from a mixture of biological and social factors. This idea is central to both functional medicine and medical anthropology. Furthermore, the functional medicine matrix operates as a powerful diagnostic tool in the clinical practices of functional medicine practitioners, given their fairly narrow patient population.

However, as someone who was originally educated in the biomedical modality, I am aware of how rarely structural factors are considered when treating disease. Earlier in this chapter, I recounted how I acritically and irreflexively joked about my hypothetical future as a failed physician due to my emphasis on sleep quality, diet, exercise, stress management, and interpersonal relationships over prescription medication. I recognize that, by including nonbiological factors into their clinical considerations, functional medicine practitioners are expanding upon the existing medical paradigm in important ways. At the same time, the functional medicine matrix is missing an invaluable layer: structural inequality (Farmer et al. 2006). Indeed, adding this layer to the functional medicine paradigm would potentiate it as a means for social change.

# ∾ *Interlude* ∾

# STUCK IN A WEB
# OF CHRONIC DISEASE

*In 2019, faced with an onslaught of diagnoses, I knew I needed holistic care. I had discovered the field of functional medicine and tried to find a functional doctor, but for months I encountered obstacle after obstacle. The care I needed was not covered by my insurance policy.[1] Functional medicine doctors charged hundreds or even thousands of dollars per visit—and that was if you were lucky enough to get an appointment! The functional doctors in highest demand were booking appointments up to two years out. I could not pay the steep prices many functional doctors were charging, and I could not wait two years for my first appointment.[2] Determined not to let these obstacles impede my recovery, I set out to learn everything I could about reversing my chronic diseases.*

*The more I learned, the more it became evident I was acting as my own functional medicine doctor. I began ordering lab tests for myself through a direct-to-consumer website. During our "Return to Wellness" workshop, Rikin and I analyzed the results and made therapeutic decisions from our dining room table. Rikin is trained in law and business and acknowledges his strengths are not in health and medicine. I am a teacher, so for me, the very act of explaining to someone else everything I had learned regarding my personal health issues and their underlying causes was extremely helpful. Rikin is sharp and he learns faster than anyone I know, and he asked me many questions that pushed me to dig deeper and recheck my thinking. Once in a while, I would run into something that was a matter of opinion—a supplement that would be beneficial for me in some ways but would pose a risk for me in other ways. In these cases, I would consult "Dr. Vega." I actually referred to myself as "Dr. Vega" in these instances—even though I am not a medical doctor—to validate my embodied knowledge and remind myself that I am the ultimate authority about my health.*[3]

After nine months, I had dug most of the way out of my health crisis. I was no longer struggling with chronic fatigue, migraine headaches, irritable bowel syndrome, or histamine intolerance/mast cell activation disorder. I had energy, and, overall, I felt better. But I still lacked resilience. As long as I followed a self-prescribed routine, I was fine. However, when I was unable to follow this routine—for example, when traveling—my body reminded me that I was not totally well. What I most wanted was greater resiliency, a pared-down health regimen I could sustain long term, and more freedom.

I was already doing everything I should be doing, based on the information I had available to me, so in order to fine-tune my treatment, I needed to expand into nutrigenomics and metabolomics—the study of how nutrition acts upon the genome and the study of how small molecules interact within the body's biological system, respectively. I felt like I had been running across a football field, jumping over hurdles and swerving past obstacles, and I was closing in on the ten-yard line. In order to get to the "end zone" of my healing journey, I needed the assistance of teammates. I needed to establish a relationship with a(nother) functional medicine practitioner for the first time.

This marked a turning point for me as a bioconsumer since I had to exercise my socioeconomic privilege in new (and expensive) ways. I identified one doctor I could afford, who had available appointments and is very well regarded in the functional medicine community. I also located a functional nutrition team that was willing to work with the doctor I selected. The doctor and nutritionists were located in different states and were all more than two thousand miles away from where I live in Texas. This did not pose a problem, since we were able to communicate as a team via video conferencing, telephone, and email.[4]

In the lead-up to my initial visit with a functional medicine team, the clinic receptionist emailed me a series of personal medical history intake forms and the clinic's office policies. As I opened each PDF attachment, I was surprised to find that one in particular, the Adult Medical Questionnaire, was twenty pages long. In addition to lab results, a timeline of medical complaints, and requested information regarding diet and supplements, my email response included ninety-four pages of attachments. The final section of the Adult Medical Questionnaire instructed: "Go back as far as you can remember—or even earlier if you have that information—and document any medical issues or major life events

*that have impacted your health—both favorably or negatively." The form
included spaces for descriptions of the patient's medical issues and life
events during the prenatal period, birth, early childhood, middle school,
teens, young adulthood, and adulthood.*

Instead of my recounting how I interacted with my functional medicine
providers after the fact and relying on my recall, I have chosen to share
excerpts from this intake form, thus providing an accurate view into how I
explained my medical history to my functional medicine practitioners for
our initial visit. By sharing excerpts from this patient questionnaire, I am
giving readers access to some of my ethnographic data in its raw form.

At first blush, this long narrative may seem superfluous or self-indulgent.
The level of detail I have included may be jarring for readers. However, I
wager that sharing these details publicly is even more unsettling to me than
it is to my readers! Having kept my health challenges private prior to writing this book—especially in professional circles and on social media, with
the exception of closed Facebook groups—I have found that sharing my
personal story now sometimes leaves me feeling disoriented and vulnerable.

Nonetheless, I have decided to share excerpts from my own intake form
because, as mentioned, my aim is to both describe and demonstrate the
issues at hand. Excerpts from the intake form demonstrate what is considered important and valuable information from a functional medicine
perspective. Through sharing these excerpts, I am demonstrating how foundational concepts in functional medicine inform patient care.

Functional medicine practitioners' reliance on patient narratives like mine
emphasizes how, from a functional medicine perspective, different symptoms and diagnoses can all be traced to a few underlying root causes. The
patient's illness narrative acts as a valuable diagnostic tool within functional medicine because each detail the patient provides is a clue about the
underlying causes of overall dysfunction. Every health issue a patient has is
interconnected. This focus on interconnectedness is encapsulated by what
functional medicine practitioners refer to as "systems biology." To clarify
how systems biology unfolds for individual patients, I will unpack the clues
in my own illness narrative. In so doing, I am applying anthropological
analysis to myself as a patient, as I would any other patient. Excerpts from
my response appear below:[5]

> *Before I was born, my mother was diagnosed with an "irritable
> uterus"—beginning in the fourth month of pregnancy, if she engaged
> in any physical activity she would have contractions. On one occasion,*

*she was having contractions that could not be controlled, even with increasing doses of various medications, so her doctors prepared her for transfer the following morning to a hospital with a NICU, giving her medications to develop my lungs as they anticipated I would be born very premature. According to my mother's telling of this story, she asked God to stop her contractions and . . . her prayers were answered. After being released from the hospital, she was placed on strict bed rest for the last five months of her pregnancy and was able to bring me to full term. According to her, if it were not for God's intervention, I would not be here today. I am grateful to be alive (!), but worry about all of the drugs I received in utero.*

My mother received betamimetics to stall her active labor. This included terbutaline, the most well known in this class of drugs. Short-term adverse effects of these drugs may include tachycardia and hyperglycemia, among others, for both the mother and the fetus. Less recognized are their potential long-term adverse effects. Two years before my birth, researchers in gastroenterology found that "[t]erbutaline decreased the sigmoid motility index both in healthy subjects and in patients with the IBS" (Lyrenäs 1985). At the time of my pending premature birth, the potential long-term consequences may have easily been outweighed by the urgent need to stop the labor progress. At the same time, it is likely that the obstetrician was unaware of gastroenterology research emerging out of Scandinavia. Either way, my decades-long struggle with IBS and constipation may be linked to this moment.

*During delivery, my mom had a retained placenta. She hemorrhaged and coded blue and was, fortunately, resuscitated. This was during the eighties when HIV/AIDS was [still not well understood],[6] so even though she had lost so much blood, she refused a transfusion and was discharged home against medical advice, but returned to the hospital two days later to receive a blood transfusion and stayed two weeks. . . . Meanwhile, I was home with my father and grandmother, and lactation was interrupted. When my mom returned home, she tried to breastfeed me but her milk would gush out, drowning me. She persisted until several weeks after she returned to work, at which time her milk dried up and she switched over to formula, but I "projectile vomited" every time she tried to feed me.*

*Eventually, and after my treatments at Kaiser failed to stop my projectile vomiting, she took me to my Chinese grandmother in Sacramento.*

*According to my grandmother Popo, I was not plump like a baby should be. Instead, my butt was just saggy skin, like a raisin, and my eyes were rolling around aimlessly in my skeletal head. (There might be a bit of exaggeration here, but I am just recounting what Popo told me.) She took me to a Chinese traditional healer—her uncle—and he wrote a prescription of dried duck kidney broth for me. I drank formula made with this broth in lieu of water for the rest of my infancy. When I transitioned to "solid baby food," I ate Popo's Chinese rice congee—not Gerber's or any of the stuff they sell in the supermarkets.*

Functional medicine practitioners ask whether the patient was born vaginally or via cesarean and whether the patient was breastfed or formula-fed. These details provide important insight into the beginnings of that individual's gut microbiome. Since I was born via vaginal birth, I was exposed to my mother's vaginal microbiome that provided me with the specific bacteria needed to digest mother's milk. Mother's milk contains microRNA that provides indispensable information for the baby's development, as well as bacteria that form the building blocks of the baby's microbiome. However, I did not breastfeed for any meaningful amount of time, thus making me more vulnerable to gut issues later in life.

*When I was six, I began having terrible cystic acne. My aunt, a Harvard-educated and Stanford-trained dermatologist (voted "Best Doc" in Sacramento Magazine multiple times!) put me on oral tetracycline as well as topical antibiotics. I can't remember how long I took the tetracycline—but [it was multiple years]. I used the topical antibiotics for nearly two decades.*

From the perspective of functional medicine, my childhood acne is a curious detail. Given what we know today, rBST-treated dairy products, steroid-injected beef, and BPA-laden food can expose children to unnatural levels of hormones and xenoestrogens. Furthermore, my genomic profile reveals that, due to my being homozygous for slow COMT, I am less efficient than "normal metabolizers" at ridding my body of harmful estrogen metabolites. Thus, both "natural" estrogens[7] and environmental xenoestrogens accumulate in my body. I was exposed to both, as were other children in my social circle. A teammate on my swim team began growing pubic hair and menstruating shortly after I began having acne. The concerning effects of conventional food on childhood health buttress advocacy among functional medicine practitioners for transforming our food systems.[8]

At the time, however, six years of age was considered too young for hormonal acne. In comparison, concluding my acne was bacterial in origin seemed more obvious. By offering me oral and topical antibiotic medications, my brilliant aunt was following the standard of care. She was also showing me compassion and love, since I was often ridiculed about my acne on the school playground. Unfortunately, regardless of whether my acne was bacterial or hormonal in origin, my long-term use of oral and topical antibiotics wreaked havoc on my microbiome, thus increasing my vulnerability to gastrointestinal issues even further.

> When I was about eight, I started to have migraine headaches and severe constipation. Almost on a daily basis, in the afternoons after school, I was sensitive to light and sound, so I would lock myself in my bedroom with the curtains drawn. Sometimes I would bang my head against the wall because the blunt force would distract me from the sharp migraine pain. I took ibuprofen every day, an adult dose (four tablets), sometimes more. My Popo would be banging and yelling on the other side of the door because she was concerned about me and didn't understand what a childhood migraine is. My constipation was equally severe.
>
> I remember there was a period in middle school . . . where I ate nothing but ramen for two weeks. It became like a "challenge" for myself— how long could I go just eating ramen? My mom worked really long hours, and when we moved to the new school district, we moved away from Popo—so I was often on my own [for meal preparation].
>
> When I was fourteen, I was diagnosed with IBS. In addition to constipation, I had stabbing pains in my abdomen. I switched to a diet that was very fat-restrictive and very focused on fiber-rich carbohydrates (like whole wheat bagels), Jamba Juice fruit smoothies (boosted with fiber), and salads.

Functional medicine focuses on the bidirectional relationship between the gastrointestinal system and the central nervous system.[9] Research has shown that individuals with a long history of migraine are more likely to be diagnosed with irritable bowel syndrome (see Arzani et al. 2020). Both diagnoses are due to a disrupted gut microbiome, which, in my case, can be traced to long-term use of antibiotics during childhood and very poor eating habits during early adolescence. I credit my mother with being the hardest-working and most loving single parent I have ever known. At the same time, I was left to my own devices while totally lacking education in nutrition during my early adolescence, representing another assault to my gut. In this way, my story is linked to broader initiatives in functional medicine to include nutrition in primary school education.[10]

Irritable bowel syndrome (IBS) is considered an "idiopathic condition." The Oxford dictionary defines "idiopathic" as "relating to or denoting any disease or condition which arises spontaneously or for which the cause is unknown." From the perspective of functional medicine, my IBS was far from idiopathic since it was the logical result of numerous assaults to my gut over a period of fourteen years. The gastroenterologist who diagnosed me suggested that a low-fat, high-fiber diet would help me with my IBS symptoms. Acting on this advice, I turned to a high-carb, wheat-heavy diet. From the perspective of functional medicine, this only worsened my future diagnoses of small intestinal bacterial overgrowth (SIBO), celiac disease, and leaky gut.

> *When I was thirteen, I had my first period. Five months passed before I had my second period. Then eleven months passed before I had my third period. Looking back, I know this was due to rapid weight loss and exercise-induced amenorrhea, on top of the normal process of menarche. . . . During freshman year of high school, I joined cross country and track and field and was immediately placed on varsity. I also joined the wrestling team and won the silver medal for California in my weight class. I ran faster and had an edge in the ring if I pushed my body to be "a lean, mean running machine," as my coach affectionately called me.*
>
> *At age fifteen, my OB/GYN recommended I take the birth control pill to "regulate my cycle." I took the pill for the next fifteen years—and, boy, do I regret it!*

Since 1960, adolescent girls have been placed on birth control pills for "menstrual regulation" (see Verma Liao 2012). When my gynecologist recommended the pill, she was also following the standard of care. However, due to my genetic uniqueness, my ingestion of synthetic estrogen on a daily basis in the form of birth control pills was definitely hazardous. As I have already mentioned, I am unable to clear harmful estrogen metabolites from my body due to slow COMT. Furthermore, birth control pills likely played a role in my worsening gut symptoms since they have been shown to increase leaky gut, contribute to gut dysbiosis (an imbalance in the gut microbiome), induce intestinal inflammation, and impair nutrient absorption (see Danner 2018).

*I went to college at Brown University. . . . I had transitioned from 5k races to sprint triathlons and half marathons, and spent up to six hours daily training for these events. I ran fifty miles each week; biked about fifty miles per ride (about once a week); and swam a 5k each time I went to the pool (about twice a week). It became increasingly difficult for me to train for my sports because I developed cholinergic urticaria and photosensitivity. This was either due to histamine intolerance or mast cell activation disorder—I've never been properly diagnosed—and lasted for the next thirteen years.*

By the time I reached college, imbalances in my hormones and microbiome were beginning to take a serious toll on my immune system. At the same time, my mast cells were overstimulated by excessive exercise, which, in turn, led to histamine flooding my system (see Kulinksi et al. 2019). Bathed in inflammatory chemicals, my immune system began reacting to multiple exposures in my environment, including everyday stimuli like heat and sunlight. Demonstrating how underlying causes can lead to multiple health problems, my total avoidance of the sun for years on end contributed to my subsequent vitamin D deficiency.

*When I started my PhD at Berkeley, I was ill most of the time. [My primary HSV-1 infection] put me in bed for a year. [Since I kept my infection a secret,] my professors began doubting my commitment to the program. To make matters worse, in that first year of studies at Berkeley, I was diagnosed with CIN-3 cervical dysplasia, despite having been vaccinated with Gardisil, receiving normal Pap smear results each year, and testing negative for HPV.*

*[After living in Mexico for several years while conducting ethnographic research], I moved back to California to write my dissertation—what is now my first published book. I was relatively "healthy" during these years, by which I mean I was a functional ill person. I adapted to my IBS and to my histamine issues and learned how to live "normally" for the most part.*

*[While writing my dissertation], I realized that it is very, very difficult to land a tenure-track job. The statistics were disheartening, and the numbers were really, really frightening for women of color. I decided to earn an MPH in epidemiology [in addition to my PhD in medical anthropology]—in case I didn't have any offers on the academic market and needed to switch to health care.*

*In March 2015, I was sandwiched in a four-car pileup on the freeway and my car was totaled. I sustained a neck injury and a concussion, while also discovering I had disc degeneration and arthritis in my neck. Starting three months after the car accident [and despite my concussion], I simultaneously enrolled in both the MPH and the PhD, taking 52 semester credits in a year. The dean had to waive the upper limit so I could take more credits than is allowed.*

*The concussion lasted six months, and looking back, I know it was because I was taking three semesters of biostats after ten years of not studying math, instead of taking the time I needed to heal. Also, while I was recovering from the concussion, my Popo, a primary figure in my life, passed away.*

*As it turned out, I was offered jobs on both the academic and health care job markets. I chose the lesser-paid option, in an underserved area, but I love what I do.*

Unfortunately, my already frazzled immune system endured numerous fresh assaults. The first was herpes simplex virus-1 (HSV-1). The hit to my immune system, combined with long-term oral contraceptives, arsenic-contaminated water in Mexico, multiple single nucleotide polymorphisms (variations in a single base pair in a DNA sequence; SNPs), and a three-generation family history of cervical cancer and dysplasia left me vulnerable to the spread of abnormal cells on the surface of my cervix (see Cancer Genome Atlas Research Network 2017).[11] Meanwhile, my immune system served triple duty, protecting me from diseases like typhus, which I was exposed to while conducting ethnographic research for my first book. My low-nutrient-density diet exacerbated the situation even further. As an ethnographer, I was committed to living a lifestyle that resembled those of my disadvantaged informants. Upon returning from ethnographic fieldwork, I subjected myself to an unhealthy amount of stress and ignored neurological trauma and psychological trauma. I struggled to recover from this web of attacks, and the slow speed of my recovery signaled an exhausted immune system reeling from continual assault. I was on the brink of disaster.

*I moved to Texas at age twenty-nine and bought a house. The place I moved to, McAllen, is scorching hot all year round. My aunt, the dermatologist who treated my acne as a child, recommended I take an over-the-counter antihistamine every day as a prophylactic measure to prevent my cholinergic urticaria. I followed her recommendation for the next two and a half years.*

*The same day I moved to McAllen, I met my husband Rikin, who moved to McAllen the same week. He is originally from Chicago and he also moved for a public service job. [He is] a federal public defender (which in McAllen means representing undocumented migrants). My husband and I fell in love very quickly—he is the reason why I believe in soul mates—and we married five months later.*

*In March 2018, I had an abnormal pap and I tested positive for HPV. Given my history with cervical issues, my OB/GYN decided to take a number of biopsies. She found abnormal tissue in some areas and not others.*

I was infected with human papillomavirus (HPV) by my husband. I am certain he was the source of my infection because I was tested for HPV during my annual pap smear mere days before meeting him and the result was negative. I am not acknowledging this fact in order to blame him. There is currently no way for a man to test for HPV. I am sharing these details about my HPV infection in order to dispel myths linking HPV to women's promiscuity. Also, my second experience with cervical dysplasia provides clues regarding the status of my immune system. Most people are infected with HPV at some point in their lives and are totally asymptomatic. For me, the experience was terribly different because my immune system was already in danger when I was exposed.

*The next month, my husband and I decided to store our embryos via IVF. We are both anxious-type personalities, although we've been making substantial improvements, especially in the last year. At the time, my husband told me he was not ready to be a father, and he might not be ready within the next five years. Having had an absent father myself, I believe both parents have to be ready—that chosen paternity for a man is just as important as chosen maternity is for a woman.*

*[During the IVF process,] I had ovarian hyperstimulation syndrome (OHSS). Fifty-seven follicles developed, from which the reproductive endocrinologist harvested twenty-three eggs. Of these, nineteen were successfully fertilized with Rikin's sperm, and fourteen developed to six-day blastocysts, grades AA and BB.*

*The experience was like a miniature pregnancy. Rikin was involved every step of the way—he got "misty" during an ultrasound, admiring out loud the "cute" follicles that were developing. I had to explain to him that those dark spots were sacks of liquid—not yet his future children. He gave me my injections each day. (I'm happy to inject others, but heck no [!], I'm not injecting myself!) I was bedridden for about a week after the procedure due to my OHSS. Rikin took excellent care of me, coming home each day on his [lunch] break to make my lunch and make sure I had water accessible by my bedside. The experience brought us closer and I was able to see his nurturing side like never before.*

*However, doing IVF came at a great physical (not to mention financial) cost. Although the IVF process was eighteen months ago, I have struggled to establish a regular menstrual cycle. I believe this to be due to multiple factors: never having allowed my body to establish a cycle at menarche; taking the pill for fifteen years; the influx of synthetic hormones during the IVF process leading to OHSS; a predisposition for estrogen dominance due to low COMT activity; and overdoing it with antioxidants, flavonoids, and polyphenols, which all inhibit COMT even further.*

Toward the end of my response, my patient's narrative provided details about the iatrogenic effects of conventional medicine. Given my lifelong history of hormone imbalance and my slow COMT, IVF was a very poor decision. I was injected with synthetic hormones that my body could not detoxify, and I suffered from OHSS—a painful and potentially dangerous side effect that causes the ovaries to swell and blood to leak through capillary walls into the abdominal cavity. IVF pushed my body beyond its natural capacity, leaving me temporarily crippled, bedridden, and in pain.

*Starting the month after we got married, I have been going through these cycles of extreme fatigue. Each episode lasts a couple months and the fatigue is so terrible that I can't get out of bed. During my first episode, a local doctor in McAllen discovered a borderline titer for typhus and treated me with two rounds of antibiotics. That didn't help, but the episode eventually ended on its own. In the months following IVF, I again started to feel chronically fatigued. This time, I just couldn't shake it.*

*We ended up driving to see an internist in San Antonio (an eight-hour roundtrip drive). This practitioner still works within the insurance model, so I was restricted to thirty minutes, if that, and told there is a strict policy of only three medical complaints at a time (which makes it impossible to give the practitioner a full history).*

*My first visit with this practitioner was in October 2018. She did a round of exploratory lab tests and by November she had diagnosed me with chronic fatigue, chronic Epstein-Barr (with titers 38 times the "positive" cutoff), hypothyroidism (low T3/free T3), vitamin D deficiency, an MTHFR SNP (heterozygous for C677T), and a burgeoning autoimmune*

*process [based on a positive lab result for antinuclear antibodies]. She
began treating me with liothyronine.*

    *That same month, on Halloween, I was in my second major car acci-
dent (my car was totaled for the second time). I sustained further injury
to my neck, which was already vulnerable from the first accident. I did
not receive any treatment. [Rikin massages my neck] once a week and
I do physical therapy exercises every night. That keeps most of the pain
at bay, but once in a while I engage in an activity that hurts my neck
(usually due to being in a posture my neck can't tolerate) and that causes
severe migraines.*

    *As the months passed, my . . . provider recommended I take lute-
olin; however, she did not suggest a dose. Long story short, I took too
much luteolin—a progesterone disruptor. This gave me terrible PMS
symptoms all cycle long, and at one point I was even a bit spastic. I
stopped taking luteolin and the provider gave me oral progesterone. That
canceled my period entirely—my body thought I was pregnant. Before
and after this experience, my cycles were averaging 63 days. During this
time, however, my cycle was 86 days. My period came as soon as I quit
the progesterone.*

    Given that my first episode of chronic fatigue occurred one month after
our wedding, my functional medicine doctor indicated to me that Rikin
may have been the source of my Epstein-Barr infection. We will never know
for sure, and, ultimately, it does not matter. Most people are infected with
Epstein-Barr, many before the age of five, and those who are infected earlier
in life are usually asymptomatic (Centers for Disease Control and Prevention n.d.). I am sharing my functional medicine doctor's supposition since
it demonstrates how, within the functional medicine paradigm, providers
attentively listen to the patient's illness narrative for clues that may reveal
the underlying causes of disease. Details embedded in the patient's illness
narrative include what was happening in the patient's life at the time of initial onset of disease symptoms. Regardless of how I became infected with
Epstein-Barr, my episodic experience of extreme fatigue furthermore indicates that my immune system was overtaxed and susceptible to external
stressors. Thus, after IVF mined my body for eggs, I again succumbed to the
effects of chronic Epstein-Barr.

    Unfortunately, my body continued to be on the receiving end of
attacks—some circumstantial and some iatrogenic. I sustained further neurological trauma during my second major car accident. Furthermore, my
hormonal imbalance was only aggravated by luteolin. While luteolin had

been prescribed to me for its antihistamine effects, it is a known progester-one disruptor, and my consuming it further disrupted my hormone balance. I've never used narcotics, but by following my doctor's recommendations, I became a "drug user"—the combination of medications and supplements I took left me feeling like I was living life on speed. When I called poison control, the agent explained the shocking chemical similarities between luteolin and methamphetamine. The prescribing physician tried to rectify this problem by prescribing progesterone, which made it impossible for me to menstruate.

> *In February 2019, my provider suggested I go to an allergist/immunol-ogist for my mast cell/histamine intolerance issues. When I visited the immunologist, I was tested for mastocytosis.[12] The result was negative. I was not given any further tests since the immunologist decided there is no practical difference between mast cell activation disorder and hista-mine intolerance. She would treat me the same way for both: three types of antihistamines (targeting H1 and H2 receptors, etc.) taken through five pills a day. I followed her orders for one week and then thought, "What am I doing? Heck no!" I quit all my antihistamines cold turkey.*
>
> *Around March 2019 I started to have some pretty severe anxiety—but the cause felt physiological to me. What I mean is, I wasn't emo-tionally or mentally anxious; however, I had all the physical symptoms of anxiety, including heart palpitations. [This turned out to be a side effect of my taking liothyronine, the thyroid medication the doctor in San Antonio prescribed.]*

At this point in my patient's narrative, I began resisting the conventional medicine approach. My prior experiences with luteolin and progesterone led me to be wary of the harmful iatrogenic effects of pharmaceuticals. I refused to take the antihistamines the immunologist prescribed because I did not want to become dependent on an increasing number of medica-tions. Meanwhile, I was "compliant" with my doctor's prescription of liothy-ronine for my low free T3, a thyroid hormone, but the medication caused a stress response in my body. All my muscles, including my heart, were con-tracting out of my control.

> *In June 2019, I started working with a functional practitioner. I asked him if it was okay to wean myself off liothyronine, and he agreed. This was my final prescription, so I am now prescription-free.*
> *I have discovered I am slightly fatigued if I don't take one serving of*

*D-ribose in the morning (5 g).[13] My San Antonio internist originally prescribed me 5 g three times a day for chronic fatigue, and I weaned myself down to one dose per day over time. I am still somewhat reliant on one dose a day to feel normal and energetic throughout the day.*

*In the interim, I have continued to take matters into my own hands regarding my pursuit of health. I ordered a number of direct-to-consumer lab tests to detect food sensitivities and use that information to guide a 5R protocol for myself. In general, I no longer experience GI discomfort. As I am writing this, I cannot recall the last time I had IBS-like symptoms—maybe one isolated occasion a couple of months ago . . . ?*

*Also, after discovering IgG reactions to BPA and mixed heavy metals, I took binders for several months to help remedy the problem. I've recently received test results from DNALife and have discovered that in addition to the MTHFR and COMT SNPs, I also have a GSTM-1 deletion!*

The patient's narrative I shared with my functional medicine providers concluded with additional clues. I have not been able to clear viruses and environmental toxins as quickly as the average person due to a GSTM-1 gene deletion and GSTP-1 SNP. The narrative also provides a clue about further damage to which I was not yet aware. My dependency on D-ribose, a type of sugar molecule that is a critical part of mitochondrial energy production, was the first sign that my mitochondria had been damaged by the numerous blows my body sustained during my first three decades of life.

*At this point in my return-to-health trajectory, I am hoping to minimize the number of supplements I take by maximizing nutrition. If I were to compare how I felt in November 2018 to August 2019, I would say the transformation was enormously positive. In August 2019, I felt normal on most days; however, I had a fairly low level of resilience. If I did everything correctly regarding rest, food, supplements, etc., I felt good overall. However, if any of these pieces were out of place, I would feel not so great in short order. . . . I am hopeful of establishing a lifelong pattern of health rooted in nutrition and overall wellness.*

My own story demonstrates how underlying causes like microbiome disruption, immune system vulnerability, and hormonal imbalance are knotted together in a way that results in multiple manifestations and progressively worsening health. It furthermore points to my role as a patient in defining the goals of the therapeutic relationship I was about to build with my new providers.

# CHAPTER 2

# SYSTEMS BIOLOGY

Systems biology—viewing every part of the person, and their environment, as thoroughly interconnected—distinguishes functional medicine from conventional medicine. Dr. Hyman comments, "It is actually amazing in [mainstream] medicine that our entire training teaches us the opposite— that there are all these organ systems. The GI system, and the liver, and the lungs, and the brain, and the heart, and the hormones." Dr. Susan Prescott and Dr. Alan Logan extend Dr. Hyman's comment, asserting, "The body has been dissected into separate pieces, more often considered separately than as part of a whole and commercialized beyond belief" (2017, 254).

In contrast, systems biology, to use the phrasing of Dr. Bland, is about "evaluating inter-organ communication" and "network physiology." Dr. Hyman simplified this concept to the most basic level when he sang to his podcast audience, "'The knee bone is connected to the thigh bone,' right?" While Dr. Hyman's musical description seems less than extraordinary, the concept of systems biology lies at the heart of functional medicine's paradigm-shifting approach to the human body.

Functional medicine practitioners offer the human microbiome as a compelling example of systems biology in action.[1] Dr. Bland explains, "Now we recognize that you can modulate, modify, or alter your gut bacteria—the so-called microbiome—by the way you eat, the way you live, the way you think, how you sleep, how you exercise, how you hydrate." He describes this as "fundamentally a paradigm shift in concepts" because, while conventional medicine relies on a mechanical model that views the body as the sum of discrete parts, emerging research on the human microbiome demonstrates that the body is one connected "super system."

Dr. Naviaux extends Dr. Bland's comment using the analogy of gears and cogs in a clockwork mechanism to describe how systems biology distinguishes the functional medicine model from existing understandings of the human body. In his analogy, metabolomics, transcriptomics, proteomics, circadian rhythm, and the adrenal-cortical-hypothalamic axis are all

separate gears, among others, working together to create health. Metabolomics describes the aggregate of all metabolic processes in the body.
Transcriptomics studies all the RNA molecules in a cell, thus allowing for
the identification of genes and pathways that respond to and counteract
environmental stressors. Proteomics is the large-scale study of all proteins
produced by the body. The circadian rhythm governs our sleep and wake
patterns—along with other mental, behavioral, and physical changes—
according to a twenty-four-hour cycle. The phrase "adrenal-cortical-
hypothalamic axis" signals the connections among the adrenal glands, the
hypothalamus, and the outer layer of the brain. By naming these multiple
processes together, Dr. Naviaux provides just a few examples of the many
"gears" and "cogs" that interact to produce the clockwork mechanism from
a systems biology perspective. In contrast, the existing medical approach
examines each gear in isolation. For each specialist, the gear upon which
they focus is the most important thing.

Dr. Naviaux attributes medicine's limited perspective to "reductionism,"
which he characterizes as "so strong in the West." At the same time, other
functional medicine providers argue that reductionism is more of a problem in medicine than in other professional disciplines. In engineering, for
example, different engine parts are not diagnosed separately, each assigned
to a different mechanic, without considering how the parts will work once
the engine is reassembled. As preposterous as that approach would be to an
engineer, this is precisely what is done through the organization of mainstream medicine into independent specialties. However, multiple functional medicine interlocutors argue that medicine is primed to embrace a
less reductionist approach to the body because of a historical shift in society
toward using computer informatics, matrixes, and Big Data to make sense
of information.

While some functional medicine proponents point to engineering
when arguing for a coordinated approach to the body, others advocate for
something even more radical—moving beyond the mechanistic approach
entirely. Dr. Mayer writes that we need to "move away from the dominant
yet outmoded ideas of the body as a complex machine with separate parts,
and toward the idea of a highly interconnected ecological system that creates stability and resilience against disturbances through its diversity" (see
Mayer 2016, 27). According to Dr. Mayer, this paradigm shift will reveal
new paths for treating and preventing common diseases and will require us
to demand more from our health care system.

Using the systems biology model, functional medicine practitioners approach the entire body as one biological system. To explain the

implications of this distinction, Kresser offers the example of a patient with brain fog, skin breakouts, gastrointestinal symptoms, insomnia, muscle aches, and fatigue. He explains that when that person visits their primary care doctor, they would likely be referred to a gastroenterologist, a dermatologist, and a psychologist. He then asks, "But what if the person is just gluten intolerant?" In the conventional medicine model, it is likely that this root cause will be missed since each symptom will be treated in isolation. Kresser continues, "The dermatologist will give some cream. The gastroenterologist will give some medication. The psychiatrist will give an antidepressant." As Dr. Hyman notes, "You go to specialists for every different part of you and nobody connects the dots." Because individual specialists are focused on different symptoms, they each offer a different treatment plan.

Even when the primary care provider attempts to treat the cluster of symptoms without referring the patient out to multiple specialists, the conventional medicine conceptualization of the body as discrete organ systems persists. Dr. Ben Lynch, naturopathic doctor and epigenetics expert, describes how primary care providers are trained: "If we had a liver problem, we would treat the liver. If we had a headache, we would treat the headache. We would forget the entire body is connected." In either scenario, no one is looking to determine what the common underlying cause might be of all the patient's symptoms, and therefore, the patient is unlikely to receive suggestions for a long-term cure.

Functional medicine practitioners contend that medicine's existing focus on organ systems was determined by limited available technologies in the past. According to Dr. Achacoso, "The technology that we had to diagnose things before was only relevant at the organ level. So we have the various different specialties in medicine: cardiology, and neurology, nephrology— because that's only the level that the technology actually could see at the time." From his perspective, scientific technologies have rapidly advanced, and the existing medical paradigm—including the organization of health care delivery into distinct specialties—has not adapted quickly enough to keep up with the rate of change. Where physicians were once only able to examine bodies at the organ level, emerging technologies allow them to examine cellular function.

This increasingly microscopic vantage point in turn allows functional medicine practitioners to see the whole picture. For example, mitochondria exist within every cell of the human body and how well they are functioning determines how well or energized a person feels. Chronic fatigue syndrome and other mitochondria-related disorders do not reside within one particular organ system and are impossible to understand without examining the body at the cellular level. Dr. Bland explains that, as the example of mitochondria demonstrates, a microbiological focus has allowed functional medicine to transition from "separatism and compartmentalization to more and more thinking of the body as a system."

Meanwhile, Dr. Hyman says, "I do wish [mainstream doctors] would understand that the paradigm that we learned [in medical school] is only part of the story . . . . There is another meta-layer of understanding how the body is organized." As a functional medicine doctor, Dr. Hyman relies on his medical training; however, he has also learned to ask, "What does the puzzle look like when you put it together?" When using this systems biology approach, "[i]t's just amazing the types of things that people can recover from." In the same vein, Dr. Lynch adds, "Your body is an amazing, beautiful system . . . . You have to use the whole picture and understand how everything is interconnected."

The systems biology approach disassembles (or, more accurately, reassembles) conventional diagnoses. Dr. Heyman explains that diseases that have been blamed on different organ systems (for example, the thyroid, adrenals, and, most recently, mast cells) are, in fact, rooted in disordered mitochondrial function. He jokes, "This is not a mast cell–based disorder. All of you mast cell junkies are mostly wrong. Sorry!" He then comically analogizes each particular organ system that had been singled out as a "has-been" in need of emotional support, saying, "So we now need to establish a support group for mast cells, and they may want to talk to the thyroid and the adrenals." Dr. Heyman's example points to how the lens through which the provider is viewing the patient determines the diagnoses: a focus on organ systems in the existing medical paradigm vs. systems biology in functional medicine.

Harking back to my description in chapter 1 of how our lexicon structures our reality, the medical paradigm furthermore determines the very nomenclature used in diagnoses. In conventional medicine, pharmaceuticals are used to suppress patients' symptoms. Given this approach, the nomenclature of conventional medicine logically applies descriptive labels to patients' symptoms. For example, "gastritis" is the combination of the prefix "gastr," meaning abdominal, and the suffix "itis," meaning inflammation. Since the conventional medicine system is not set up to ask how to resolve the root causes of the problem, its nomenclature does not need to explain the cause of abdominal inflammation. Simply naming the symptom is enough to commence pharmaceutical intervention.

Functional medicine practitioners, however, see little value in naming the symptom. As Dr. Hyman explains, "I always say, 'Just because you know the name of your disease doesn't mean you know what is wrong with you." In the same vein, Sachin Patel, founder of the Living Proof Institute and functional health coach, encourages others to, "[d]isconnect with the name of the disease or the dysfunction that's taking place because it's physiologically impossible to have a chronic disease isolated into one organ." The goal of functional medicine is to uncover and treat the underlying cause.

From the perspective of functional medicine, the nomenclature of mainstream medicine obscures and permits a certain degree of ignorance by cloaking unknown causes in legitimate-sounding terminology. "Idiopathic syndromes" are prime examples. As Dr. Hyman puts it, "We call something a syndrome in medicine when we don't actually understand anything." Dr. Bland agrees: "These names that we put on these conditions are really just manifestations of our lack of complete understanding of the personal disturbances that occur at the physiological level in the individual." To clarify this point, Dr. Hyman acts out a satirical conversation between a patient and a conventional physician:

> DOCTOR: Oh, you have irritable bowel syndrome.
> PATIENT: What does that mean?
> DOCTOR: It means your stomach hurts and you have diarrhea, or constipation, or bloating.

As a result of this lack of understanding, mainstream medicine aggregates individuals based on diagnosis (e.g., diabetes, heart disease, and arthritis). In mainstream medicine, Dr. Hyman says, "we just lump everybody with the same symptoms in the same categories, but that doesn't tell you anything about the cause." Dr. Bland further explains, "Each one of those individual people varies significantly in the way that they are actually presenting the disturbances in their own physiology that gives rise to those things that we call their disease." This grouping based on symptoms, in effect, erases important differences between varying underlying causes that produce the same effect.

Grouping patients based on symptoms makes sense, however, if the provider is operating from the existing one-to-one approach for symptom resolution. Dr. Lynch describes the existing medical approach in these terms: "One problem, one solution, everything's great, right?" As if responding to this question, Dr. Sabbagh explains, "You can't just say one thing, like 'It's taking a statin,' that cures everything else and you can just have bad behavior otherwise." Thus, while doctors are often taught in medical school to match different pharmaceuticals to isolated symptoms, functional medicine offers diverse strategies to begin unraveling the patients' network of symptoms.

Functional medicine's systems biology approach relies on its resistance to unidirectional notions of cause and effect. Nutritionist Andrea Nakayama rejects the illusion that there is one singular root to each patient's suffering. In an email newsletter, she writes, "Chronic conditions are multifactorial— many factors are involved in their expression." Dr. LePine concurs. "We talk about root cause, but it is actually root causes. There may be one major thing, but there are all these other things that play a supporting role." Expanding upon Dr. Bland's example of the microbiome, Dr. Lynch considers how diet, mindset, and environmental exposures may be contributing causes to most of his patients' health issues. Thus, the principle of multiple causality shapes functional medicine practitioners' diagnostic thought process. This means the functional medicine approach simultaneously examines all problems, searches for underlying causes, and attempts multiple solutions.

In so doing, functional medicine practitioners recognize that one cause can lead to many effects, any effect can be due to multiple potential causes, and the entire system can be alleviated by combining complementary therapeutic strategies.[2] Dr. Sabbagh indicates, "You have to exercise, you have to eat right, you have to sleep, you have to reduce your stress, you have to take the supplements, you have to do it all." His comments hark back to Dr. Heyman's remarks in chapter 1 about functional medicine being a "kitchen sink" approach. Like Dr. Heyman, Dr. Sabbagh clarifies that the integration of multiple therapeutic strategies is not only strategic, but also necessary for healing. At the same time, multiple therapeutic strategies produce universal benefits due to the interconnectedness of the body. Dr. Achacoso notes, "In a network, when you touch one thing, everything else moves." As Patel indicates, "The modality that you use for healing is going to heal every organ system in your body." From a systems biology perspective, it is impossible to develop a disease in isolation, and it is equally impossible to heal a disease in isolation.

Dr. LePine gives an example of how this systems biology approach unfolded in the case of a patient who has multiple sclerosis (an autoimmune disease) and infertility. After conducting a complete workup, Dr. LePine identified gluten sensitivity, toxicity due to mercury, and gut dysbiosis due to bacterial and yeast overgrowth. "So I worked on diet, worked on both prebiotics and probiotics, and cleaned up the gut. We got her completely off gluten. And, lo and behold, her multiple sclerosis went away." Harking back to the principle of multiple causation, he clarifies that not all cases of multiple sclerosis can be resolved by following the same steps since "there are many pathways to multiple sclerosis, just like there are many pathways to Alzheimer's . . . or any disease." However, as a result of Dr. LePine's treatment, this particular patient not only reversed her multiple sclerosis, she was also successful in becoming pregnant. Dr. LePine's example demonstrates that complementary treatment approaches are consonant with functional medicine practitioners' aims to examine the health of the entire person, within the context of their environment, over the scope of their life.

## LIVING HEALTHY

Functional medicine's systems biology model is specifically adapted for reversing chronic health problems, thus paving the way for denormalizing ongoing illness.[3] Blue describes his experience searching Google for the oxymoron "sick/healthy": "What you find is all kinds of books and apps and propaganda essentially designed to convince us . . . that we can be sick and healthy at the same time." As the former executive director and chief strategy officer of the American Academy of Private Physicians and the current strategic advisor of industry for the Institute of Functional Medicine, Blue is very aware of both how narratives regarding disease are scripted and the financial incentives that undergird these narratives. From his perspective, functional medicine practitioners will have to change the narrative by explaining that, contrary to what patients may be hearing and reading, they can expect more than "being sick well," "being well with chronic disease," and "living healthy with chronic disease." When patients seek the help of a functional medicine practitioner, the goal is to create wellness, not manage illness.

At the same time, existing medical techniques are highly successful at treating acute problems or injuries using pharmaceuticals and surgical techniques. Maskell emphasizes this point: "Putting the most trained physician with a prescription pad at the front of medicine is the best idea when you have acute disease." Echoing Maskell, Kresser states, "[Our existing medical system] does a fantastic job, by the way, of dealing with those acute problems." He goes on to provide a historical backdrop for the success of conventional medicine: "In 1900, the top three causes of death were all acute infectious diseases: typhoid, tuberculosis, and pneumonia. . . . [Our health care system] evolved in the context of acute problems and was really set up to deal with those." Unfortunately, due to a swift transition from acute to chronic disease as the predominating cause of death, the health care system is mismatched to the current needs of the population.

At present, seven of the top ten causes of death are chronic diseases.

Extending Kresser's remarks, Maskell explains that, even thirty years ago, taking the acute disease model of care and applying it to chronic disease seemed reasonable since people assumed that once the human genome was decoded, chronic disease could be solved with targeted pharmaceuticals.[4] Today, this notion seems absurd. Maskell indicates, "For chronic disease, the first person that you see should be a non-prescriber." Non-prescribers include health coaches, dieticians, and other health professionals who guide patients through evidence-based lifestyle changes such as diet, exercise, sleep hygiene, and stress management. From the perspective of functional medicine, chronic disease is largely caused by lifestyle, and thus requires lifestyle interventions.[5]

In essence, functional medicine proponents argue that acute disease and chronic disease are fundamentally different and thus require distinct approaches. Emphasizing the valuable role of functional medicine, Dr. Naviaux opines, "I believe that we need a fundamental paradigm shift in order to be more effective at caring for patients with chronic illness." This is not to disregard the value of acute care. As Kresser clarifies, "If I get hit by a bus, I definitely want to go to the hospital." However, in his view, acute care "fails miserably when it comes to these complex chronic problems." When the tools of mainstream medicine are applied to chronic disease, the mismatch leads to a situation where patients are either on expensive pharmaceuticals for the rest of their lives or undergo invasive surgical procedures or both.

Thus, functional medicine is beginning to gain traction in a time when many providers, patients, health economists, and politicians are asking how financial incentives shape health care, are interrogating both pharmaceuticalization and medicalization in terms of "value," and are examining the relationship between profit and patient outcomes. For functional medicine providers and proponents, the over-dependence on pharmaceutical "tools" is the result of how hospitals are administered, how insurance is reimbursed, and how research is funded, and it has resulted in our existing health care system's inability to effectively address the epidemic of chronic diseases in society. This epidemic comes with high economic and human costs in the form of health care spending and suffering. In this context, functional medicine practitioners suggest that their methods may add value to the system. While this might be true if functional medicine were to be fully integrated into health insurance, at present, patients generally pay a hefty out-of-pocket price for functional medicine services. This situation leads to de-pharmaceuticalization for the privileged.

The systems biology approach reconfigures existing notions of health, the human body, and disease etiology. However, it fails to tackle the questions of how social inequality affects the biological system and whom this paradigm shift is benefiting in practice. Instead, functional medicine proponents point to the inadequacies of pharmaceuticals, given the body's complexity. Dr. Heyman asked his Advances in Mitochondrial Medicine Symposium audience, "If we embrace this notion of this metabolic model where multiple parts are shifting simultaneously, why did we ever think dropping in one pharmaceutical into that mix would ever really matter?" He immediately answered his own question: "It can't, by definition." Almost as if in response to Dr. Heyman's question, Whitten remarks, "I would argue that the whole fundamental paradigm of seeking out some specific molecule or biochemical process that has gone awry and then developing a drug that is going to target this specific biochemical process and correct it is just myopic and so reductionistic and missing the big picture of how these systems are intertwined." In essence, the pharmaceutical approach ignores systems biology. Thus, functional medicine rejects pharmaceuticalization and instead aims to uncover how individuals' health is shaped by the environment.

## NESTED ECOLOGIES: EXTENDING SYSTEMS BIOLOGY TO THE ENVIRONMENT

Many functional medicine practitioners refer to every individual body as a unique ecosystem. Dr. Accurso uses the analogy of a pond to describe the human body. He states, "It's just one big pond. If I drop a little bit of heavy metals into that pond, it's going to pollute the whole pond. If I start to rip plants out of the pond, or take some native fish out of that pond, it's going to affect the entire pond." In his analogy, ripping out plants and removing native fish is akin to gallbladder surgery. According to functional medicine perspectives, there are no "unnecessary organs" in the human body. Organs are thoroughly and intimately interconnected as part of a system, and the body must be addressed as a whole.

This ecological thinking, applied to the human body, represents a paradigm shift in medicine. Separatism in the existing medical approach makes it difficult to identify connections among different symptoms and organ systems; it obscures from view connections between the body and the surrounding environment. According to Dr. Achacoso, in the existing paradigm, "people always fail to take a look at what's going on around them. They always take a look at what's going on inside them." Dr. Hyman links this oversight to silos and reductionism in medicine, which prevents doctors from asking questions like, "How do we produce energy and how does that affect climate? How do we grow our food and how does that connect to everything?" In essence, the very organization of the health care system obfuscates the effects of humans on the environment, and, conversely, of the environment on human health. In contrast, functional medicine practitioners draw concrete linkages between a person's internal and external ecologies.

However, ecological thinking does not, in and of itself, represent a change in social values or an awareness of privilege and disadvantage. Thus, I offer the concept of nested ecologies to describe how systems biology extends to the environment and to make space for issues of inequality. The concept of nested ecologies builds upon multiple concepts with a rich history in medical anthropology: namely, political ecologies of health, local biologies, situated biologies, exposed biologies, and syndemics. Hans Baer argues for a political ecology of health in medical anthropology. While political ecology studies how political, economic, and social factors effect change on the environment, Baer signals how political-economic factors—not just physical conditions—play a primary role in shaping the etiology of disease (see Baer 1996).

The term "local biologies" was originally coined by Margaret Lock in 1993 to indicate that while health at the community scale is biological, it is also shaped and determined by local culture and social factors (see also Lock and Kaufert 2001).[6] Abigail Neely (2015) combines the concepts of political ecologies of health and local biologies. In so doing, she mobilizes scales from the "internal ecologies" of individual bodies to the global, thus making way for a nested, place-based analysis that simultaneously understands health in the context of local understandings and global policies. Lock (2017) has argued that local biologies be recognized as a subcategory of situated biologies—how human biology is situated in time and space around the globe. The concept of situated biologies emphasizes how certain issues—for example, pervasive poverty, famine, oil extraction, radioactive waste, environmental toxins, dysfunctional governments, war, genocide, terrorism, and antibiotic resistance—affect the health of everyone, including through the intergenerational transmission of epigenetic effects. Coining the term "exposed biologies," Ayo Wahlberg (2016) specifically points to the role of industrially manufactured chemicals in a range of pathologies, including cancers, metabolic diseases, infertility, and sex development disorders. Together, these concepts serve as an invitation to engage with our contemporary challenges in our communities and worldwide.

Syndemics is a concept first developed by medical anthropologist Merrill

Singer in the mid-1990s (Singer 1994). The term "syndemic"—the merging of the words "synergistic" and "epidemic"—refers to how social, political, economic, and environmental drivers cause co-occurring diseases to synergistically interact in such a way as to produce an excess burden of disease. The concept of a syndemic extends beyond comorbidity due to its analysis of how overlapping diseases interact when nested in particular sociopolitical contexts.

Given this rich history, the concept of nested ecologies is neither a reinvention nor a corrective of the important conceptual work that came before it. Instead, I am offering nested ecologies as a heuristic tool for understanding how functional medicine uses systems biology to contextualize bodies within ecological environments. Thus, the term "nested ecologies" is shorthand for how functional medicine providers view complex environmental factors as forming part of, and playing a determining role in, the health of an individual's biological system.

Through nested ecologies, I am furthermore presenting a visual analogy since, like Matryoshka dolls, the internal ecosystem within the body is shaped by the external ecosystem that surrounds it. This multilayered analogy encapsulates situated and exposed biologies and the political ecology of health since my conceptualization of the external ecosystem includes political, economic, social, and physical factors.

Furthermore, nested ecologies simultaneously emphasize the role of physical ecology and critique functional medicine's neglect of political economy. That is, nested ecologies explore how social, economic, and political factors shape the health of the environment, which in turn shapes human health. In so doing, nested ecologies encourage biphasic analyses at the level of political ecology and political ecology of health. At the same time, I point to how functional medicine primarily focuses on systems-based etiology and thus pays insufficient attention to the social drivers of disease. While the systems biology model includes social, political, and economic factors, the explanations and examples offered by functional medicine practitioners demonstrate an overt emphasis on physical ecology and a de-emphasis on political economy. This inadvertent tendency belies many functional medicine practitioners' training in conventional medicine and the hegemony of how etiology is taught in medical schools. Thus, I offer nested ecologies as an invitation to functional medicine practitioners to refocus on how social, political, and economic factors figure into systems biology.

The concept of syndemics offers a similar invitation. When Singer chose *A Critical Systems Approach to Public and Community Health* as the subtitle for his 2009 introductory textbook on syndemics, he used rhetoric that is strikingly similar to that of functional medicine practitioners when describing systems biology. Some functional medicine practitioners are becoming aware of the close relationship between systems biology and syndemics as evidenced by the 2019 episode, "A Global Syndemic: Obesity, Undernutrition, and Climate Change" on the George Washington School of Medicine & Health Sciences Integrative Medicine podcast. This certainly is a step in the right direction; however, nested ecologies is a more appropriate concept for functional medicine since it possesses explanatory power for both health and disease.

From the perspective of nested ecologies, syndemics are the result of systems biology gone awry. The patient experiences a network of disease symptoms due to a network of root causes, including external factors such as the patient's political, economic, social, cultural, and physical context. Given that co-occurring disease is the first characteristic of all syndemics, this concept reflects how conventional medicine considers disease to be the starting point for all medical inquiries. In contrast, the concept of nested ecologies does not take overlapping disease as its point of departure. Healthy external ecologies encourage healthy internal ecologies. Meanwhile, inequitable external ecologies exact harm on individuals' health. Thus, nested ecologies incorporate functional medicine's view of health and disease unfolding along a spectrum (see Menéndez 1994). Nested ecologies acknowledge the "dark side" of systems biology (how noxious external factors can frame overlapping chronic disease) while also saving space for the possibility of health.

Functional medicine practitioners offer many examples of nested ecologies. For example, Dr. Bland characterizes autoimmunity not as an inappropriate reaction of the body to itself, but, instead, as an appropriate reaction of the body to an inappropriate, toxic environment. "I was looking at the literature and thinking about [autoimmunity] until I came to the belief that our body actually doesn't respond to itself; it is responding to something that is happening to our body that makes it a non-self." Expanding on these thoughts, he adds, "Then we say, which I find unbelievably suspicious, that the person is allergic to themselves." He clarifies, "They're not responding to themselves. They're responding to themselves that has been altered." From a functional medicine perspective, autoimmunity is "the model concern of our age," and it highlights the need for a paradigm shift in immunological principles.

Furthermore, the issue of autoimmunity points to the utility of a nested perspective that clarifies the effects of external ecologies on internal ecologies. Dr. Bland explains, "I think this construct of autoimmunity is . . . the intersection—it's the convergence—of all these principles of genes, life-styles, environment, diet, [and] the way that we manage children today." Pointing to how individuals are simultaneously exposed to an artificially sterile environment (due to societal obsession with antibacterial gels) on the one hand, and to an influx of toxic chemicals, processed foods, and geneti-cally modified plants on the other, he asserts that "[a]ll those things together create this increasing concept of autoimmunity."

While mainstream medical notions of disease etiology cannot explain sudden increases in the prevalence of autoimmunity, functional medicine proponents problematize existing definitions of autoimmunity by reconfig-uring this disease classification as a "construct" and a "concept." As Dr. Terry Wahls, clinical professor of medicine at the University of Iowa, suggests, "Over time we've been converting many more chronic diseases into possi-bly autoimmune, probably autoimmune, and then definitely autoimmune, and then treating it." In a 2005 report to Congress, the National Institutes of Health Autoimmune Diseases Coordinating Committee identified more than eighty autoimmune diseases (National Institutes of Health 2005). At the time of this writing in 2020, the Autoimmune Association lists 152 auto-immune diseases (Autoimmune Association n.d.). Given this upward trend, Dr. Wahls predicts, "Over the next twenty to thirty years, the vast majority of chronic diseases will have been reclassified as probably autoimmune in nature." Seen through the lens of nested ecologies, as larger portions of the population begin suffering the physiological consequences of an overly ster-ile *and* increasingly toxic environment, mainstream medicine will (errone-ously) reclassify more chronic illnesses as autoimmune diseases.

The nested ecologies lens is also useful for signaling how functional medicine proponents reconfigure notions of health and disease more broadly speaking. Kresser describes how, from an evolutionary perspective, humans primarily ate meat and fish, fruits and vegetables, nuts and seeds, and some starchy plants; were physically active throughout the day and lived in sync with the natural rhythms of light and dark; and formed close-knit tribal groups (see Gluckman and Hanson 2008). He encourages listeners to imagine what would happen if this evolutionary human was airdropped into New York where they are "eating pizza and drinking beer, sitting in an office for eight hours, [then] riding the subway home and sitting on the couch and bingeing on Netflix at night, and have the phone next to their bed [while it is] beeping and . . . emitting light that interferes with . . . circa-dian rhythms." Kresser concludes his hypothetical scenario by asserting that humans' internal ecology (our genes and our biology) is totally mismatched with our external ecology (the modern environment we have created).

Over the course of my ethnographic research, I noted how functional medicine practitioners leverage the issues of lifestyle and movement to critique what they see as increased individualism and loss of community. I can appreciate how this critique diagnoses fundamental problems with neoliberalism. Policies that favor deregulation and reduction of government spending dismantle the social safety net, leaving individuals to fend for themselves in the "free market." At the same time, people are losing their sense of belonging and security—the feeling of being held by a community.

However, what functional medicine interlocutors' critiques often fail to acknowledge is how functional medicine reiterates individualistic ways of being. The emphasis on (bio)individuality places the responsibility for healing on the individual and often sidesteps important issues of racialized and socioeconomic inequality. By positioning practitioners and bioentrepreneurs and patients as bioconsumers, functional medicine inadvertently perpetuates neoliberal notions of good citizenship, casts health as a bioconsumer item for purchase in private markets, and promotes individual responsibility at the expense of true social solidarity.[7]

Furthermore, I also signal how, when attributing the "pandemic" of chronic disease (see Terzic and Waldman 2011) to "industrialism" and an "American" way of life, functional medicine proponents inadvertently romanticize and exoticize impoverished Others, commodify non-Western knowledge, and describe non-Western cultures as frozen in an idyllic past. Functional medicine interlocutors suggest that non-Westerners are shielded from the evils of neoliberalism and capitalism, when, in fact, this respective philosophy and economic practice have formed a world system (Wallerstein 1976). Furthermore, these interlocutors attribute lack of access to technology and infrastructure to traditional cultural values rather than to penury and disadvantage. In reality, everyone alive today is living in the twenty-first century—although some have more resources than others. In proposing the concept of nested ecologies, I hope to flag and sidestep potential slippages into cultural essentialism by pointing to political, social, and economic inequality.

At the same time, I am offering a heuristic for how functional medicine practitioners examine an individual's toxic exposure when exploring the root causes of their disease. While a person's living environment may not figure into most mainstream medicine consultations, environments are an important feature of functional medicine consultations. Dr. Fitzgerald describes toxic exposures as "not just massive toxic dumps and these huge occupational exposures, but the perturbation of metabolic activity with what we could consider subclinical toxin exposures." She indicates that the amounts of toxins individuals are exposed to have increased exponentially with "the advance of using lots of plastics, and the eighty thousand chemicals, and [their] synergistic effects." Environmental toxins circulate through both internal and external layers of nested ecologies, thus providing a contextual backdrop for illness from a functional medicine perspective. Instead of viewing body and context as separate entities, the body exists in, with, and *through* the context in which it is situated. The body is an inward reflection of the environment that surrounds it.

This focus on environmental toxins requires functional medicine practitioners to situate individuals' health problems within a historical perspective. For example, Dr. Chilkov explains, "Baby boomers grew up in a time where lead was not regulated. As baby boomers start to have osteopenia and osteoporosis, the natural physiology of aging . . . , some of that stored lead is being liberated [from their bones] into the bloodstream." Toxic metals have an affinity for accumulating in fat, so when bone marrow is no longer the most viable option, these metals migrate to another place in the body that is primarily composed of fat. Functional medicine clinicians are noting that this other place is often the brain. Citing work done by Dr. Walter Crinnion and Dr. Joe Pizzorno, Dr. Chilkov concludes that "some of the rising levels of dementia are actually due, in baby boomers, to . . . endogenous lead exposure." In cases where functional medicine providers are unable to identify a clear source of environmental exposure, they turn to temporal clues within the patient's history and consider "the arc of time."

## SOCIAL INEQUALITY

I point to how some groups are more susceptible than others to an increasingly toxic environment. Simply put, social inequality shapes health outcomes and thus represents a crucial layer in nested ecologies. As Dr. Prescott puts it, "human health cannot be separated from the health of our physical, emotional, social, economic, and political environment." Furthermore, individuals make decisions about their health based on what they have access to. Therefore, "choice" is structured by intersecting axes of inequality (see Crenshaw 2014). Unequitable access leads to racialized and class-based differences in who suffers from chronic disease and who can *afford* to be well. I offer the food environment as one example.[8]

Functional medicine practitioners often echo Hippocrates in their claim that "all disease begins in the gut." From a functional medicine perspective, the gut is the part of the body with the most intimate and direct contact with the outside world since, through digestion, the food we eat literally becomes a part of our body. Food is not solely a source of energy—it also provides information to our bodies about the outside world. Adulterated food—food that has been sprayed with chemicals, processed, colored with food dyes, manipulated with genetic modification, and made to be addictive with artificial flavors—provides a particularly problematic set of information to the body. Certain foods—for example, gluten, dairy, sugar, and other refined carbohydrates—can cause the tight junctions in the gut lining to become "leaky," thus allowing for toxins to pass into the blood stream. When the immune system detects toxins in the blood, it begins producing antibodies to attack the invaders. According to functional medicine, if this process is left unchecked, it can trigger autoimmunity. Functional medicine practitioners thus adopt a "food is medicine" approach to healing disease and identify the problematic foodstuffs in the patient's diet that are leading to leaky gut. Functional medicine patients are then prescribed a diet that eliminates harmful foods, opting instead for foods that are healing, especially organic produce and lean meat.

By focusing so intensely on diet, functional medicine practitioners are not only advocating for eating patterns that they believe will reverse chronic disease, they are also underscoring how the existing food system is contaminated by environmental toxins. However, while functional medicine practitioners and patients emphasize the amazing results they have seen after changing their patients' diets, they tend to spend less time discussing the people for whom this approach is out of reach. That is, they fail to acknowledge the socioeconomic and racialized structures that undergird diet, culinary "preferences," and food access. Many people do not have access to organic produce in their neighborhoods or they may not be able to afford it. These same people are more likely to be exposed to other types of environmental toxins—a harsh reality that medical anthropologists identify as "syndemic vulnerability."

In making these assertions about functional medicine, I do not mean to discount the important work of functional medicine practitioners and advocates who are pushing for greater access to a safe environment and healthy food. I will discuss their ideas in further detail in the concluding chapters of this book. Instead, I argue that the concept of nested ecologies can strengthen the application of systems biology by holding space for critical analysis of how social inequality impedes the human right to health (Willen et al. 2017).

In the example I have developed, sustained emphasis on the social milieu not only asks how problematic food systems give rise to interconnected diseases, but also demands acknowledgment of who is inextricably embedded in those food systems and who can "choose" to opt out. Here, I am throwing "choice" into question since the ability to circumvent the conventional food system and "go organic" is buttressed by socioeconomic privilege. Unequitable food access is a form of social injustice, and many functional medicine practitioners and proponents can adopt an expanded role in fighting for a more equitable future.

Those living at the "bottom" of a society's social structure—whether in terms of, for example, socioeconomics, political voice, or status—are the most vulnerable in every aspect of health (Quesada, Hart, and Bourgois 2011; Marmot 2005). At the same time, individuals may experience divergent degrees of suffering even when exposed to similar political, economic, social, cultural, and physical factors. Due to their unique genomic susceptibilities, individuals are nested in their environments in distinct ways.

## CANARIES IN THE COAL MINE: A PRELUDE TO GENOMIC SUSCEPTIBILITY

From a functional medicine perspective, burgeoning diagnoses such as bipolar disorder, ADHD, and depression are occurring in response to harmful environmental stimuli.[9] Dr. Brogan indicates that, given our present environment, achieving population-wide health would require that individuals "show no signs that anything is wrong with our educational system, with our family units, with the total fracturing and disillusion of our community networks, with our food supply, [and] with exposure to chemical toxicants everywhere." Dr. Brogan's success in reversing these diseases through advanced testing and functional medicine therapies demonstrates that, often times, neurological pathologies and "mental illness" result from physiological processes caused by social and ecological environmental degradation. However, this finding does not explain why some individuals succumb to illness while others, faced with similar challenges, do not. Given the concept of nested ecologies, why are certain people more susceptible to disease?

In order to answer this question, many functional medicine practitioners refer to susceptible patients as "canaries in the coal mine." This phrase relates closely to individuals' genomic uniqueness. Dr. Bland notes, "We are asking the question . . . how resilient is the human genome to an unbelievably rapidly changing environment?" According to Dr. Bland, the ill health of "canaries" is an indicator that the human genome is not completely resilient since the "canaries are the first individuals with a genotype that is responsive to those changes." The recent eruption of certain diseases points to alarmed genes that, according to Dr. Bland, "are going into defensive battle against a hostile environment." This perspective, rooted in recent epigenetic research, transforms long-standing notions of genetic inheritance.

In the functional medicine approach to the human genome, it is incorrect to say that someone has inherited a gene for non-congenital disease. Offering the examples of rheumatoid arthritis or systemic lupus erythematosus, both autoimmune diseases, Dr. Bland explains that genes do not cause these diseases. Instead, it is the interface of genes with hazardous environmental inputs that results in these diseases. In a previous era, environmental triggers were absent and these same genes conferred selective advantage. Dr. Bland concludes, "The term 'disease' . . . makes a person unworthy or less than whole. But maybe they are actually super whole—it's just that the environment that they are in is not matched to their genetic uniqueness." His comments hark back to the destigmatization of disease, a theme of this book.

Given this epigenetic focus, rapid increases in chronic disease among American children are a topic of concern among many functional medicine practitioners. Children with autism spectrum disorder, attention deficit disorder, hyperactivity disorder, asthma, and food allergies are also often referred to as canaries in the coal mine. The recent rise in the incidence of these diseases cannot be attributed to genetics, but rather to an increasingly toxic environment. As Dr. Herbert explains, "These kids are showing us what we are all vulnerable to, but [not everyone is] as vulnerable as they are." Having studied toxicology during my epidemiology training at UC Berkeley, I understand that the smaller the person, the more that person is affected by exposure to environmental toxins. Thus, the sharp increase in children suffering from chronic disease is a red flag. It is a warning regarding our rapidly changing environment and a call to action for the whole of society.

Autism is one red flag that is frequently discussed in the functional medicine realm. From Beth Lambert's perspective, both genes and the brain are involved. At the same time, Lambert, executive director of Parents Ending America's Childhood Epidemic, frames autism as an environment-derived autoimmune condition, explaining, "It's a condition that's marked by increased inflammation, cellular toxicity, immune dysregulation, [and] gut dysbiosis—all these are medical things that are never really considered or taken into consideration when a child is treated for autism." Instead of arguing against existing medical techniques, Lambert argues that attention to nutritional deficits, cellular toxicity, microbiome imbalances, and immune dysregulation can increase the effectiveness of standard treatments. In so doing, she suggests that diverse treatments be combined in a systems-based approach.[10]

While the spread of chronic disease among America's youth warrants alarm, adults are not invulnerable. Turning to the example of cancer, Dr. Chilkov says, "When I'm asked the question, 'What do you think the three biggest contributors to the rising rates of cancer are today?' I say, 'Environment, environment, environment,' because it is the toxic environment in which we live that we are not biologically designed to cope with that is burdening our systems." For her, people who have cancer in the current environment are also canaries in the coal mine. While the toxic environment affects us all, those with health conditions like cancer and autism are more vulnerable due to the convergence of multiple factors, genetic and otherwise.

Seen through this lens, chronic disease represents a kind of opportunity. In presenting this idea, I do not mean to minimize the pain and suffering of those struggling with chronic disease. Instead, I am pointing to functional medicine perspectives such as that of Dr. Jay Davidson, a chiropractor, who suggests that even when it seems our chronically ill bodies are working against us, our bodies are, in fact, working for us by signaling dangers in our environment and lifestyle habits that need to be changed or eliminated. In this same vein, canaries in the coal mine alert the rest of society about environmental hazards that require urgent action. Dr. Brogan says, "I think of these people, my patients for example, as being highly sensitive beings. They are sensitive to toxicant exposures; they are sensitive to nutrient deficiencies. Meaningfully, they are sensitive to elements of our daily lives that are fundamentally wrong." By pointing to how the external environment shapes and determines individual health, the concept of nested ecologies is a plea for holistic ecosystems.

*Interlude*

# GENETIC FATE?

After having shipped my mouth swab specimen to Denmark a few weeks prior, I received an email from my doctor containing a PDF attachment of my DNA profile results. I held my breath as I opened the attachment. I felt anxious and excited at the same time. The last time I felt this way was probably when I received the decision letter regarding my application to the Program in Liberal Medical Education (PLME) at Brown University. I fingered the envelope from Brown, trying to assess its thickness and deduce whether it contained a "thick" acceptance package or a "thin" rejection letter. At the time, it seemed the words printed on the PLME decision letter would determine the course my life would take. This time, I felt like the words contained in the DNA profile would determine my health over the course of my life.

When I opened the results, I briefly glanced at the legend on the bottom of the cover page so I could interpret the results correctly. Then, I examined the "Priority Table," which indicated that methylation and oxidative stress were "moderate" priorities, while detoxification was a "high" priority. I continued scrolling and found the "Report Summary," which included dietary and nutrigenomic recommendations for supporting detoxification. The summary advised that I reduce exposure to environmental toxins, including cigarette smoke, smoked foods, air pollution, pesticides, heavy metals, and plastic.

On the next page was the "Summary Table" of all the specific single nucleotide polymorphisms (SNPs) tested by the laboratory. I scrolled through the table until I found a patch of SNPs that were accompanied by a cluster of twelve blue "impact circles." The circles followed a symmetrical pattern—1-3-2-2-3-1—that struck me as curiously aesthetic and worryingly ominous at the same time. The table indicated my "C" **and** "T" alleles for MTHFR-677 had "moderate impact" on my methylation. My CBS and COMT SNPs further hindered my ability to methylate. My detoxification was obstructed by CYP1A1-Msp1, CYP1A1-Ile462Val, and GSTP-1 SNPs—and a GSTM-1 deletion to boot! Like ornaments hanging on a Christmas tree, blue dots accompanied every SNP under the subheading "oxidative stress."

I scrolled down to the in-depth explanation of my methylation result. The PDF explained, "The process of DNA repair is called methylation." I already knew this, but I sassily thought, "Well, that would be important!" While the PDF did not explain all the functions of methylation, I knew it is also involved in, for example, epigenetic regulation of gene expression, central nervous system development (improper methylation can lead to neural tube defects in newborn babies), neurotransmitter biosynthesis and metabolism, histamine clearance, hormone biotransformation, cellular energy metabolism, and phospholipid synthesis.

The result indicated that, as a "T" allele carrier for MTHFR-677, I have "increased folate, vitamin B2, B6 [and] B12 requirements." I reflected on my out-of-range mean corpuscular volume (MCV) and mean corpuscular hemoglobin (MCH)—a condition called "macrocytic anemia" that can be caused by B12 deficiency. Due to my genetic predisposition for B vitamin malabsorption, could I be chronically B12-deficient even while consuming more than the daily recommended intake?

The result furthermore explained that an "A" allele for the COMT SNP is "associated with a three to fourfold reduction in the methylation activity of the COMT enzyme and is associated with increased risk for breast cancer." COMT is responsible for estrogen and neurotransmitter metabolism. I am a double "AA" allele carrier—a homozygote—what functional medicine practitioners call "slow, slow COMT." Knowing that the relative risk with two alleles is the square of the relative risk with only one allele (Rédei 2008), I began to calculate: If each "A" allele is associated with a three- to fourfold reduction in methylation activity and I have two copies of the "A" allele, that makes me . . . screwed.

I turned to my oxidative stress results, again holding my breath. Oxidative stress occurs when cells and tissues are unable to efficiently detoxify reactive oxygen species (ROS), leading to an accumulation of ROS in the body. According to the results, my "T" allele for eNOS-894 is "associated with atherosclerosis, essential hypertension, end-stage renal disease, and preeclampsia." My "CT" genotype for GPX1-Pro198Leu "has been linked to a disturbed anti-oxidative balance and has been associated with increased risk for chronic diseases, including certain cancers and coronary artery disease." Oxidative stress also plays a role in the development of dementia, diabetes, hypertension, stroke, and chronic fatigue syndrome.

These results explained a lot. I was struggling with high levels of oxidized LDL cholesterol. My Popo and Bok Bok (maternal great-grandmother) both lost a great deal to dementia. They were robbed of vital elements of personhood—memories, temporal continuity, and relationships with others—that are the sensations and ideations that solidify our existence. My grandfather had insulin-dependent diabetes. My mother is considered prediabetic and has been treated for hypertension. My Popo had a stroke, causing her right eyelid to droop. My mother and I have both experienced chronic fatigue, a weariness that puts "feeling tired" to shame.

I kept scrolling. My result for the BDNF gene was heterozygous for the rs6265 "T" allele. The BDNF gene is responsible for providing the instructions for making brain-derived neurotrophic factor, a protein that promotes the growth, survival, maturation, and maintenance of neurons in the brain and spinal cord. The results stated that my genotype is "consistent with reduced activity-dependent secretion of BDNF from neurons and impaired BDNF signaling." I scoffed out loud, "Hey! What are you trying to say?" As a scholar, I rely on my BDNF signaling to earn a living. I imagined that reduced BDNF secretion is to a scholar what having one hand might be like for a pianist. I acknowledged how this result could be the reason why my mother, grandmother, and great-grandmother have all experienced dementia.

My detoxification results indicated that certain SNPs—CYP1A1-Msp1 and CYP1A1-Ile462Val—also place me at risk for cancer. I asked myself, "Who has been diagnosed with cancer in my family?" My Popo is a cancer survivor. Her sister died of cancer. My mother and I have both struggled with cervical dysplasia.

Diving deeper into my detoxification results, I began reading about the glutathione S-transferase (GST) genes. These genes encode for glutathione S-transferase. Glutathione is referred to by functional medicine practitioners as "the master antioxidant." When glutathione conjugates to toxins, it escorts them out of the body. My results indicated that my "G" allele for GSTP-1 decreases the conjugation activity of the enzyme. I furthermore read that my GSTM-1 deletion results in absence of the enzyme, leading to reduced capacity for hepatic detoxification and "increased risk of various cancers, chemical sensitivity, coronary artery disease in smokers, atopic asthma, and deficits in lung function."

This was striking. I had been living with constant stinging in my esophagus and none of my conventional medicine providers were able to offer me an explanation that made sense. Contrary to their suppositions, I knew it was not heartburn or gastroesophageal reflux disease (GERD). The symptoms were not triggered by certain foods, nor did they ebb and flow with my meals. Could my GST genes be at the root?

According to my genetic profile, I was more susceptible to all kinds of respiratory issues and needed to be vigilant about airborne chemicals and carcinogens. Given the burning sensation was in my esophagus and not in my lungs, I didn't think I had atopic asthma, which is triggered by allergens such as pollens, pets, and dust mites. But, then I remembered that my best friend, also a PhD/MPH who struggles with chronic disease, had suggested I consider a closely related condition—eosinophilic esophagitis (EoE). I located a study on PubMed that equated EoE to "asthma of the esophagus" (see Virchow 2014). According to the study, both EoE and asthma are chronic immune-mediated conditions that are characterized by inflammatory changes in the mucosa and submucosa. Up to 80 percent of patients with EoE also have atopic asthma. Doctors often use an elimination diet and upper gastrointestinal endoscopy to make a diagnosis. I had already ruled out potential food triggers by doing an elimination diet on my own, and I did not need a doctor to stick a camera down my throat or assign me a disease label to confirm that my esophagus was inflamed. As a patient with embodied knowledge, I knew that the incessant burning in my airway was valid evidence of inflammation. The question was, what was I reacting to?

I had also described my symptoms to my mother, including the fact that they worsen in the winter months. She sent me articles about "cedar fever," an allergy to cedar pollen that can affect Texans from November through March. Connecting the dots, I decided to order a serum test for common respiratory allergens in the state of Texas to confirm her hypothesis. I thought, "If I couldn't access these diagnostic tools and if I didn't have so much support from the people who love me, I would never figure everything out!" At the same time, I recognized that my ability to order direct-to-consumer lab tests is a marker of my socioeconomic privilege.

I wondered if my GST genotype also made me more susceptible to viral and bacterial infection. Again, I turned to PubMed, thus narrowing my search to peer-reviewed, scholarly articles. The results unequivocally confirmed my suspicion. Morris et al. (2013) indicate that "[glutathione] works to modulate the behavior of . . . the cells of the immune system, augmenting the innate and adaptive immunity as well as conferring protection against microbial, viral, and parasitic infections" (3329). By encoding for glutathione S-transferase, GST genes are responsible for blocking the replication of, for example, the HSV-1 virus and the influenza virus (Smith and Dawson 2006; see also Palamara 1995). Furthermore, glutathione has been shown to block replication of HIV and has been identified as a "mechanism of indirect protection" against leukemia (Sanchez-Alcaraz et al. 2004).

These findings elucidated the underlying reason for some of my prior health struggles. My body had been ravaged by common viruses that most people never realize they have. While up to 80 percent (Johns Hopkins n.d.) of the US population has HSV-1 and most are asymptomatic, HSV-1 knocked the life out of me and left me mostly bedridden from 2009 to 2010. My GSTM-1 deletion and GSTP-1 SNP left me severely hindered when it came to blocking the replication of the virus. My GST genotype also left me vulnerable to chronic Epstein-Barr and post-viral inflammation (see Gao et al. 2017).[1] I needed to avoid becoming infected with viruses at all cost because I couldn't depend on my body to bounce back. My experiences with HSV-1 and EBV showed me that my body would fight to heal, but it could take years to turn the tide.

I was noticing a pattern, and I was starting to reach information overload. I began scrolling faster, and I barely noticed reiterations of my "increased risk for insulin resistance, diabetes . . . [and] hypertension." By the time I got to the "curious facts" that other genetic profiling companies advertise—for example, sensitivity to caffeine and bitter taste—I didn't care.

I had learned about this particular genetic profiling company while watching the "Interpreting Your Genetics Summit." A doctor of nutrigenomics spoke about the company's decision-making process regarding which SNPs to include. She indicated that including an excessive number of SNPs can cause inadvertent harm for a number of reasons. First, when bioconsumers turn to the internet to determine what they should do with an overwhelming amount of genetic data, they are quickly baffled by contradictory study findings.[2] Second, bioconsumers tend to consider individual SNPs in isolation when, in fact, SNPs must be considered in groups to assess their intersecting effects on a person's health. Third, bioconsumers may experience panic or despair if they are not counseled on the power of epigenetics to shape and reshape one's "genetic fate." For all these reasons, the company I chose only includes SNPs for which data are robust and conclusive. They group SNPs based on their intersecting contributions to different bodily processes. Each SNP result is accompanied by nutrition and lifestyle-based recommendations, thereby providing actionable information to the bioconsumer.

Despite the company's attempts to lead with "actionable knowledge"— the very reason I chose this particular genetic profiling service—my initial reaction was exactly what the speaker on "Interpreting Your Genetics" was hoping to prevent. Instead of jumping into action, I was dazed by the rhetoric of risk (Rapp 1988). Neither the tens of hours I spent listening to functional medicine practitioners discuss epigenetics nor the hundreds of pages I read on the topic could avert the sinking feeling in my gut. I was like a deer in the headlights.

I went outside to my backyard and began exercising in the sun—part of my everyday effort to raise my deficient vitamin D levels. But today was different. After reading what felt like an analysis of all the ways I might die, I felt the sunlight's warmth on my skin, reminding me that I was alive and (relatively) well. Compared to where I had been healthwise, I was the picture of vitality. I did push-ups, squats, and crunches, and the physical movement of my body helped to center me in my own strength. I had been analyzing my body from an intellectual distance as a specimen carrying multiple genetic "defects." Now I needed to reinhabit my body as the vessel for my very existence.

What had I learned, really? My genetic profile did not tell me what health problems I was going to develop or when. It merely stated that my SNPs are associated with an increased risk for a number of chronic diseases—cancers, dementia, diabetes, hypertension, atherosclerosis, stroke, chronic fatigue, respiratory illnesses, and chronic viral infections. Most of this I already knew from my family history. However, my profile did teach me more about the underlying mechanisms that lead to the health conditions affecting my family. As I mulled over this new knowledge, I decided to reframe my genetic information as empowering.[3] This moment marked a shift in my health journey. Instead of merely focusing my energy on treating the health conditions I already had—a project that was already producing promising results—I now needed to implement dietary and lifestyle changes to hopefully increase my "healthspan" and prevent a lot of pain and suffering.

Over time, knowing my DNA SNPs affected me in multiple ways. I looked back on my laboratory tests with new insight. Suddenly, my consistently low C-reactive protein (a marker of inflammation), despite then-rising antinuclear antibodies, made sense. I did not have any SNPs for the IL genes or TNF-alpha—genes associated with inflammation. It also made sense why I would have such high levels of antibodies to heavy metals and bisphenol A (BPA) in my blood. Since my detoxification pathways were severely compromised, toxic chemicals that are all too common in our contemporary environment had accumulated in my body with nowhere to go. As a result, I got sicker and sicker. I was the canary in the coal mine.

My genetic information also prompted me to think and act differently with regard to certain health conditions. With regard to my oxidized LDL cholesterol, understanding my genome helped me to step outside of public debates regarding the suitability of different types of fat. These debates are based upon the misassumption that particular foods are "good" or "bad" for everyone. I decided to take a different tack: I pursued a personalized diet based on nutrigenomic data. In my case, I needed to eat fewer saturated fats and more mono-unsaturated fats. Perhaps even more importantly, I needed to adopt lower-heat cooking methods and safeguard my cooking oils from oxidation by placing them in airtight containers, away from light and heat. I began steaming foods more often and applying oils as a dressing. The very next time I checked my cholesterol after making these changes, my oxidized LDL was well within the normal range.

My SNPs also explained why certain conventional approaches had not worked for me. As I dove into the literature, I realized that the birth control pills I took for fifteen years, combined with my slow COMT, could have contributed to my cervical dysplasia and my hypothyroidism. My provider prescribed liothyronine to help with the hypothyroidism, but this medication had severe side effects. For individuals with slow COMT, thyroid medications can cause feelings of anxiety, insomnia, irritability, elevated estrogen levels, and histamine issues. I experienced all these. In addition, my doctor at the time prescribed folic acid supplements, another synthetic substance that can slow down COMT even further.

My genetic profile not only clarified aspects of my past treatment, it also informed the therapeutic approaches I chose for myself moving forward. In particular, knowing my CYP450 profile—data regarding how my liver metabolizes different medications—guided my decision not to try low-dose naltrexone for my autoimmunity and saved me from potentially experiencing adverse effects.

At the same time, the results pointed to unimagined directions for potential intervention. I realized my years-long struggle with both histamine intolerance and oligomenorrhea were connected! Methylation, which is responsible for histamine clearance, is directly linked to catechol metabolism, which is responsible for estrogen clearance. The standout genes for these metabolic pathways are MTHFR and COMT, which encode methylenetetrahydrofolate reductase and catechol-O-methyltransferase enzymes, respectively. Furthermore, high estrogen stimulates the mast cells to release histamine, while high histamine stimulates the ovaries to release estrogen, causing a vicious cycle. With this new understanding, I

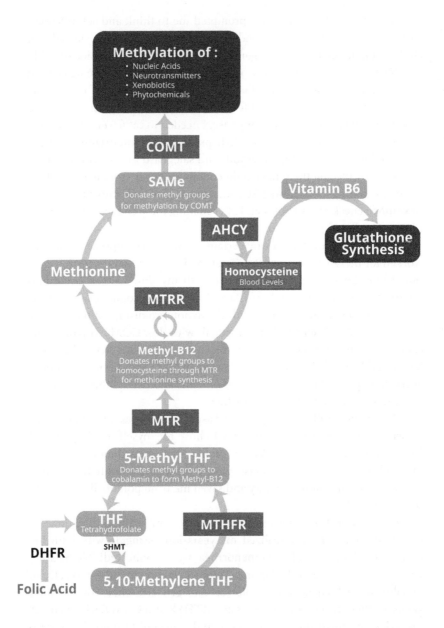

*Methylation pathways diagram. This diagram appears on the "Education" page of cellsciencesystems.com in Beth Ellen DiLuglio, "Why MTHFR Testing Is Not Enough," https://cellsciencesystems.com/education/news/why-mthfr-testing-alone-is-not-enough/. Full-color image hosted at https://tinyurl.com/Nested-Ecologies-Images.*

began experimenting with how certain foods affected my estrogen levels and how this, in turn, affected my histamine tolerance threshold in different ways throughout my cycle.

In October 2019, I changed my diet to include all the nutritional cofactors for healthy methylation and detoxification. At the time, my methylation was operating at a dismal 9 percent. Two months later, my methylation was operating at full tilt—100 percent! Also, over the course of 2019, my menstrual cycles fell from 86 days to 63 days to 42 days and finally to 39 days. While this was still outside of the "normal range" of 21 to 35 days (Cleveland Clinic n.d.), I was encouraged by the fact that I was only four days out of range—a far cry from where I had started.

Knowing my unique vulnerabilities—especially my GST genotype—also made me more cautious. When news of the COVID-19 pandemic broke, I immediately recognized the danger. COVID-19 emerged as the perfect predator: the coalescence of virus and respiratory illness. To evaluate my personal vulnerabilities to the pandemic threat, I sat down in March 2020 and reviewed information from my genetic, hormone, and neurotransmitter profiles; metabolic data; and serum biomarkers. At the same time, I recognized that the most valuable source of information was my embodied experience of decreased immune resilience to other, less deadly viruses. I had already suffered from chronic Epstein-Barr and chronic fatigue syndrome. I deduced that, if I were to become infected, my chances for succumbing to a "cytokine storm" were low to moderate. However, the potential for the infection to trigger long-term sequelae—for example, post-viral syndrome, autoimmunity, and respiratory diseases—was great.[4]

In June 2020, when articles began to emerge regarding the long-term consequences of COVID-19 infection, I felt like these articles were essentially road maps to what I might experience if infected. "Recovered" patients described ongoing abnormal heart rhythm, digestive problems, chest pain, shortness of breath, permanent lung damage, chills and sweats, chronic fatigue syndrome, headaches, dizziness, weakness, muscle pain—many of the symptoms I had struggled with in the past (Moffitt 2020; Steenhuysen 2020; Petri 2020). Although I was thirty-two years old and not at risk based on age alone, I knew being infected with COVID-19 could set me back years in my health journey—and that was the best-case scenario.

I started wearing a mask on March 8, 2020, while traveling to Cuba to present my research at a conference. I was the only person at the conference wearing a mask—it would be a month before residents living in my county were required by emergency ordinance to wear face masks. Part of me wondered if audience members thought I was overreacting, but I knew I could not afford to let my self-conscious feelings sway my proactive decisions to protect myself from the looming pandemic.

Back in McAllen, I put my training as an ethnographer into action. I attended functional medicine webinars to learn more about COVID-19 and to adapt my supplement protocol for greater immune resilience. One such webinar was aimed at providers. I was a provider with a patient caseload of one. Based on emerging research, I developed a protocol to use if I became infected with COVID. This involved purchasing supplements and a nebulizer and making sure I had everything on hand for immediate intervention. I knew exactly how I was vulnerable, so I took every precaution not to become infected.

Meanwhile, the world unraveled into chaos.

# CHAPTER 3

# (EPI)GENETICS AND ITS
# MULTIPLE IMPLICATIONS

For decades, medical anthropologists have analyzed the impact of genomics—the branch of molecular biology concerned with mapping genomes—on anthropology as a discipline and on society as a whole. Anthropological inquiry has often occurred through the lens of assisted reproductive technologies (ARTs). For example, Sarah Franklin (2013) queries how geneticization has led anthropologists to rethink consanguinity as the basis of kinship. In this vein, Joan Bestard (2004) examines the ovum—not blood—when pointing to changes in the Euro-American view of biogenetic substances as a symbol of enduring solidarity. Based on his ethnographic observations of egg donors and receivers in Barcelona, Bestard examines genetic links, gestational links, and descent links, ultimately noting how egg receivers appropriate biogenetic substances. For her part, Marilyn Strathern (2005; Edwards et al. 1999) explores the management of "kinship knowledge" and intellectual property rights in the context of claims over people.

The profound impact of genomics on society has prompted anthropologists to analyze what our discipline offers vis-à-vis how genomes are framed and understood. Gísli Pálsson (2008) argues for a relativized view of "genomic anthropology," indicating that genomic studies must engage with local notions of personhood and belonging. In response, Jonathan Marks (2013) suggests that anthropology is uniquely positioned to examine the ontology of genetic facts, which he frames as both natural and cultural. In the context of functional medicine, I signal how epigenetic facts are ascribed to "thoughts," "choice," and "behavior" in a way that obscures issues of structural inequality and privilege.

## INFORMATIONAL BIOLOGY

Functional medicine practitioners embrace genomic data, and informational biology in general, as clinical tools for designing personalized treatment protocols.[1] Dr. Bland optimistically asserts, "Genomics helps us move from diagnosis to prognosis, and, further, to transition from the disease industry to the wellness industry."[2] As someone who has used genomic information to transition from treating disease to creating long-term health, I identify with Dr. Bland's assertion. At the same time, as an anthropologist, I am hyper-aware of my own privilege. I therefore ask, who does the "genomics revolution" serve, and who does it marginalize?

To answer this question, I first turn to functional medicine practitioners' descriptions of informational biology in the era of Big Data, starting with Dr. Bland's description of why and how genomic science has progressed in recent years. He indicates that innovators and philanthropists such as Mark Zuckerberg, Priscilla Chan, and Bill and Melinda Gates are pushing the area of genomic research forward. Their strategy involves recruiting the brightest minds in biological and medical science. For example, the Gates Foundation wooed Dr. Leroy Hood away from his professorship at CalTech by offering him the directorship of the Institute for Systems Biology. Genomic research is being extracted from academic arenas and relocated to realms of technological innovation due to immense funding opportunities in Silicon Valley.

In order to elucidate and historicize the emergence of informational biology, Dr. Bland compares the genomic revolution to the computing technology revolution in the late 1970s and into the 1980s. During this period, novel types of software allowed people to do word processing, spreadsheets, and scheduling. Then, referring to Apple Inc., Dr. Bland notes that a "fugitive revolutionary company coming out of Cupertino, California, had a little bit of a different view of how to consumerize computing." According to Dr. Bland, Apple "empowered people" by reframing computers as personal instruments for information science, thus allowing people to have "access to their own information . . . and do things that were on their agenda." Over the course of a decade, "[c]omputer science then became personal computing, then became personal assistance, then became [an] extracorporeal brain." Today, 97 percent of Americans are computing on personal, super-powered smart devices (Pew Research Center 2021). This present-day reality was almost unimaginable in the late 1970s.

From the perspective of functional medicine experts like Dr. Bland, the genomics revolution will follow a similar path to the explosion of personal computing. "In the next years to come, and—I don't mean decades, I mean years—we are going to see [genomics] advance as rapidly in application and simplicity for the consumer as we saw with the complexity of microcomputing." When this does occur, Dr. Bland contends, "We are going to see a new understanding of the person." Informational biology is primed for mass consumption and holds the potential for transforming identities, individuals' relationships to self, and the face of medicine.

At the same time, mass marketing of informational biology is rendered possible by advances in data analysis. Dr. David Haase, founder and medical director of MaxWell Clinic, notes that "all of the interactions and interplays that happen in a single person . . . require computer analysis." Dr. Bland adds that at present, "We are starting to be able to do Big Data analysis of families of genes rather than one gene at a time." According to functional medicine, this transition from a single gene model to a genomic model is paving the way for lifestyle medicine interventions.

However, in order to achieve even greater actionability, the future of genetics may depend on artificial intelligence (AI). Dr. Helen Messier, a practioner with the Institute for Functional Medicine, argues, "AI has a greater capacity than the human brain to recognize patterns (and without bias!). It is self-learning." From her perspective, AI can help close the translational gap in medicine.[3] Thus, the genetics revolution not only resembles the rapid transition to personal computing in the 1980s, it also relies on technological advances for its success.

Many scientific authorities, including the National Science Foundation, recognize computational data science as a fundamental pillar of emerging science. This shift in epistemologies prompted investment in genomic medicine. In 2015, President Obama announced the Precision Medicine Initiative, a $215 million project that Obama described as using precision medicine to harness advances in genetic research and revolutionize health care. Hoping to participate in the ushering in of a new era characterized by tailored disease prediction, Big Data juggernauts such as Google, Apple, and Amazon have contributed to the project. Functional medicine practitioners and proponents also believe that the future of medicine, grounded in genomic technoscience, is swiftly approaching.

However, as the geneticization of health unfolds within a neoliberal model of bioconsumption, the future of medicine largely depends on consumers' interest. That is, the consumption of informational biology depends on the degree of "biological potential" consumers feel is embedded in their individualized genetic information (Lee 2013). Who is able to act on this biological potential? Dr. Bland asserts that bioconsumers have "[a greater] understanding of the information in the human genome" and are beginning to understand the epigenetic effects of lifestyle and diet on gene expression. Meanwhile, "consumer-facing" DNA testing companies and wellness counseling providers are constantly marketing their services to consumers in new and adaptive ways. For example, during the COVID-19 pandemic, LifeDNA circulated Facebook advertisements inviting potential consumers to find out their susceptibility to COVID-19 by using their existing test results from 23andMe, AncestryDNA, or MyHeritage.

This raises the question of how "biological potential" is harnessed and for what purposes. Bioconsumers must identify and navigate around these genetic testing companies' potential conflicts of interest. Dr. Paul Beaver, co-founder and chief scientific officer of Fitgenes Ltd. and founder and director of 3P Healthcare Pty Ltd., notes that companies are often "primarily vehicles for selling supplements/weight loss shakes." At the same time, a number of wearable devices have emerged for monitoring biometrics and epigenetic responses. These consumer-facing services and devices present novel opportunities for creating health while also emphasizing the dangers of neoliberal bioconsumption.

At the same time, the booming biotech industry is "consumer oriented" in ways that allow the "consumer genetic space" to evolve faster than the "provider genetic space." Dr. Bland explains, "Consumers have access to their genetic information at a faster rate than providers are being trained . . . to provide tailored genomic medicine." Given the accessibility of genomic information and the absence of epigenomic counseling, Patel asserts that bioconsumers must switch from receiving doctor's orders (which he likens to an "owner's manual") to figuring out how to interpret their own genomic data and implement life changes (what Patel compares to a "user's manual"). In Patel's opinion, "Eighty percent of people don't need to see the practitioner, they need to *become* the practitioner because their action steps are going to bring about the solution." As a bioconsumer, I often acted as my own practitioner. As a medical anthropologist, I recognize how my bioconsumptive power and "practitioner" authority are thoroughly dependent on my socioeconomic privilege and cultural capital (Bourdieu 1984).

My physician emailed my genetic profile results to me in July 2019. However, because we were waiting for my other lab results before scheduling our next appointment, I did not speak to him about my genetic profile until mid-August, more than five weeks later. In the meantime, I used my epidemiological research training to scour PubMed and come up with my own interpretation of my DNA results. By the time I spoke to my physician, I had already implemented most of the changes he suggested. A year later, I completed a sixty-hour nutrigenomics course that was designed for physicians. The course provided me with deeper insight into my specific genetic SNPs and allowed me to further tailor my diet and supplementation. My experiences support Patel's assertion that, as bioconsumers of informational biology, patients are "the doctors of the future."

At the same time, I point to how the framework of bioconsumption inherently promotes unequal access to personal genomic data. Science journalist Max Lugavere notes, "Now, thankfully, technology has gotten to a point where it's become cheap enough that each of us can afford to look under the hood of our biology, so to speak. What that offers is the chance to circumnavigate various flaws that we might have in our genome."

I disagree. I would not have been able to act as my own doctor if I did not have the financial resources to pay for the test out of pocket, the educational background to research and interpret the results, and the structural conditions necessary for implementing the lifestyle interventions suggested in the test results. I furthermore argue that economic capital and cultural capital (i.e., education) are nailed together in our social structure since, more often than not, economic capital facilitates educational achievement. Thus, relative privilege-disadvantage shapes individuals' access to and interpretation of informational biology.[4]

Critics of the Human Genome Project would argue that access to genomic information is of little consequence since most of the matter in human DNA was poorly understood and was dismissed as "dark matter" or "junk DNA." The $3.8 billion project revealed that humans have approximately twenty-two thousand to twenty-three thousand genes—approximately half the number of genes as a single grain of rice. Furthermore, gene variants that actually cause disease, as opposed to those that are associated with disease risk, are very rare (Dobbs 2018, 248).

Functional medicine proponents agree that "true genetic diseases" are rare. Dr. Dimitris Tsoukalas, president of the European Institute of Nutritional Medicine, explains that only one in twenty-five hundred individuals are born with a congenital, genetically inherited disease. As founder and CEO of Metabolic Healing Inc. Michael McEvoy further indicates, "Science is very good at identifying . . . diseases that are due to what's called haploinsufficiency of a gene," that is, when a gene is mutated or deleted, insufficient "gene products" (RNA and proteins) are made. This situation leads to monogenetic congenital diseases, which are diseases caused by a single gene and present at birth.[5]

However, from the perspective of functional medicine, critics of genomic medicine often fail to consider the value of *epi*genomic therapeutic approaches. Dr. Tsoukalas argues, "What we do after our birth, which is epigenetics, influences and changes our health." In contrast, chronic disease results from ongoing gene-environment interaction over time. As Dr. O'Bryan puts it, "We've learned it's important to know what your genes are—it's really important—but your genes don't determine whether you get a disease or not. Your genes determine whether you're vulnerable to getting a disease or not." Similarly, Dr. Szyf explains that the true risk factor is not the gene, but the environment that activates the gene. "The [genetic] risks are very small. Therefore, we should focus on the big risks. And the big risks are probably, in the end, environmental." This emphasis on the role of epigenetic "after-birth factors" in driving chronic disease figures into my concept of nested ecologies and challenges existing understandings of genetics. In essence, the concept of nested ecologies dovetails with a paradigm shift in anthropology: instead of debating whether our genes or our environment contribute more to human biocultural diversity, researchers are now asking how genome, epigenome, and environment interact (Sobo 2020).

## EPIGENETICS

Epigenetics is the process by which the environment shapes the epigenome, thus regulating gene expression and influencing genotype (Sobo 2020). The word "epigenetics" combines the Greek word "epi," which means "above," with "genetics." From the perspective of functional medicine, the genome is brought to life through the "epi," not vice versa. Dr. Szyf asserts, "The DNA sequence cannot explain the mystery of development." Describing research that dates to the 1940s, Dr. Szyf explains that each individual possesses one set of DNA, and yet this DNA gives rise to "millions of different cells that have different forms and shapes." These different forms and shapes are referred to in genetics as "phenotypes." Dr. Szyf continues, "There must be something between DNA and the phenotype that takes the DNA and gives different interpretations in different contexts." That "something" is epigenetics.

From an anthropological perspective, Thayer and Non assert that epigenetics, "the study of heritable chemical modifications to DNA," can enrich research since epigenetics marks change in response to many of the social, cultural, political, economic, or ecological processes anthropologists study (2015, 722; Borghol et al. 2012). Thus, epigenetic processes can provide a biological explanation for how environmental experiences such as migration, trauma, food insecurity (Maupin and Brewis 2014), paternal investment (Mattison, Scelza, and Blumenfeld 2014), and social inequalities become embodied (Lock 2015; Niewohner 2011). Furthermore, epigenetics could be leveraged to better understand racial inequalities in health (Kuwaza and Sweet 2009). The increased emphasis on epigenetics marks a transition from genetics to postgenomics and the discovery of a new social body (see Lock 2012; 2017).

## MECHANISMS

Functional medicine practitioners make sense of epigenetic complexity by viewing individual patients through the lens of systems biology. Dr. David Quig, a nutritional biochemist, states on the *FxMed* podcast, "In order to truly know what's going on, you have to consider also substrate levels and very, very important epigenetic factors, including nutritional deficiencies, the co-factors, environmental toxicants, oxidative stress, and even drugs that the patients might be taking." Dr. Fitzgerald agrees: "You need to think about [the] whole person being in [their] environment, so their nutritional status and their toxin exposures and the medications they've been on and their mental [and] emotional . . . stress response—the whole kit and caboodle—can have an influence on [the epigenetic] pathway." In their view, epigenetics extends far beyond how proteins and enzymes are coded for by different SNPs.

Thus, from the perspective of functionalized medicine, a personalized systems biology approach must inform any genomic therapy. Nakayama points out that there are approximately eight hundred known SNPs, meaning each individual can have hundreds. SNPs cannot be treated in isolation since individual SNPs may have contradictory effects. Nakayama characterizes an individual's genomic profile as their potential backdrop, but emphasizes that it is the clinician's job to evaluate their *expressive genotype*, including their signs, symptoms, diagnoses, and triggers. Knowing a patient's genomic profile is not enough to know what is the proper treatment for them.

At the same time, "the proper treatment" for a single patient is in constant flux. For this reason, Dr. Bland recommends using genomic information to decide which biomarkers need the most vigilance, then using quarterly lab testing to "titrate" nutrition and supplementation. That is, genetic information helps practitioners identify which biological molecules to monitor in their patients' blood and urine and how to adjust patients' diet and supplement regimen to bring lab values into the optimum range. Some functional medicine practitioners use metabolic testing to gain insight into what is happening in the body in real time. Extending Dr. Naviaux's analogy of the body as a clockwork mechanism,[6] Dr. Quig continues, "It's sort of like hyper-focused mini-metabolomics really, pulling it all together, what's really happening genetically and epigenetically." This metabolic approach is primarily focused on how nutrition can be optimized for each individual's biological uniqueness.

At the same time, functional medicine practitioners critique how the food industry "hijacks" our biology with noxious epigenetic effects. Using the example of how calorie-rich foods cause a spike in dopamine and likewise stimulate certain genes, Dr. Lynch comments, "Food science—they've got it dialed in for a reason. They want you to spike your dopamine so you're addicted to that food . . . . TVs, commercials, the smell of food . . . . That's epigenetics." In essence, genes are far from static, but are instead constantly turned "on" and "off" by common experiences and circumstances.

## ANALOGIES

Functional medicine practitioners have provided numerous analogies to describe the *epi*(genome). Dr. Randy Jirtle, professor of *epi*genetics at North Carolina State University and senior scientist at the University of Wisconsin, offers an analogy that draws from his background in computer science. "I think of the DNA as being like the hardware of your computer. So then the epigenome is the software that tells the genes when, where, and how to work." Then, extending Dr. Szyf's comments regarding phenotypes, Dr. Jirtle explains that although human beings have one set of DNA, they have 260 different cell types because "every computer is running a different software program, doing a different job, but the hardware, i.e., the DNA, is the same in every situation."[7]

Other functional medicine interlocutors have also offered technological analogies to explain epigenetics. For example, Dr. Sinclair likens genetics and epigenetics to digital and analog information. "There really [are] just two main types of information in our body that we get from our parents. The first is genetic." Describing the static, unchanging nature of the four types of bases found in a DNA molecule (adenine [A], cytosine [C], guanine [G], and thymine [T]), Dr. Sinclair describes genetic information as "digital." Pausing to reflect on how his analogy may be unintelligible to young viewers, he jokes, "It's like the music that is on a DVD—those things we used to use to store movies." Then, referring to how physical changes in the chromatin determine whether genes are expressed or silenced, Dr. Sinclair emphasizes that the epigenome is an "analog" system because it is constantly changing and adapting. "We have an analog version of information, the epigenome, which determines which genes in the DNA are turned on and off." While the DVD in Dr. Sinclair's analogy represents genetic information, the epigenome is the reader of the information.

Another analogy equates genetics and epigenetics to large and fine-tuning knobs. Dr. Bland explains, "We have this big tuning knob called our 'genome.' Then we have a fine-tuning knob called our 'epigenome,' which are marks that we put on our genome from experiences that we have that regulate how our genome is going to be expressed." On the topic of genetic expression, Dr. Bland notes, "We really can't change our genes, but we can change aspects of our genetic marking that we call 'epigenomic' that then pattern how our genes are going to express themselves." With these words, Dr. Bland builds upon Dr. Jirtle and Dr. Sinclair's explanations by explicitly addressing individuals' ability to influence genetic expression by harnessing the power of epigenetics.

Other analogies range from equating genetics to industrial manufacturing and epigenetics to varying renditions of a script. Nessa Carey writes, "We talk about DNA as if it's a template, like a mold for a car part in a factory. . . . Unless something goes wrong in the process, out pop thousands of identical car parts." Given what we have recently learned about epigenetics, however, Carey asserts that the industrial manufacturing analogy is insufficient for describing genetic expression. After comparing different movie versions of Shakespeare's *Romeo and Juliet*, Carey concludes, "Identical starting points, different outcomes. That's what happens when cells read the genetic code that's in DNA. The same script can result in different productions" (2012, 1).

In a similar vein, McEvoy describes epigenetics in syntactic terms. He likens the process of epigenetics to "punctuation marks in the sentence." He explains, "If a sentence didn't have punctuation marks and then it was just a bunch of letters in a sequence, it would be much more difficult to read." In this analogy, the process of epigenetics creates spaces between letters so that sentences (i.e., genes) can be read and understood. The "punctuation" McEvoy describes is determined by a complex dance between external and internal factors. According to McEvoy, external factors include "diet, lifestyle, toxins, stress and even emotions." These external factors influence "actual intricate biochemical and biological processes that are involved in suppressing or expressing certain genes." These internal mechanisms include acetylation, DNA methylation, and histone modification.

Indeed, a great deal of functional medicine discourse revolves around the biological mechanisms that affect epigenetic changes. Genes are turned on and off through the attachment and detachment of different chemical groups—processes known as methylation, acetylation, and other forms of histone modification (phosphorylation, ubiquitylation, and sumoylation). When these processes go awry, disease follows. McEvoy indicates, "Problems in DNA acetylation, problems in histone modification, [and] problems in methylation of DNA are intricately tied in many different disease processes." Of these, insufficient DNA methylation is the predominant mechanism presented in functional medicine discourse with regard to disease etiology—so much so that Dr. Lynch simply states, "The primary job for methylation is to control gene expression." As such, DNA methylation is considered by many functional medicine practitioners to be an important cause, mechanism, and consequence of disease.

Dr. Fitzgerald documents the role of DNA methylation in Alzheimer's disease (Qazi et al. 2017), hypertension (Demura and Saijoh 2017), major depressive disorder (Aberg et al. 2018), and atherosclerosis (Dunn et al. 2014). Due to its combined influence and influenceability, DNA methylation has emerged as a primary tool for optimizing epigenetic expression. Dr. Fitzgerald explains that DNA methylation can be improved using dietary and lifestyle interventions. "Methylation adaptogens" such as green tea and rosemary can be harnessed to help functional medicine practitioners regulate patients' methylation status, thus potentially minimizing disease while extending both healthspan and life span.

Dr. Fitzgerald's interest in methylation is inspired by the 2003 agouti mice experiment by Dr. Rob Waterland and Dr. Jirtle. This study was described in *Are You What Your Mother Ate?*, a 2017 documentary, as the most widely cited study in the history of science. The experiment showed supplementing methyl donors in the maternal diet during pregnancy could not only change the coat color of the offspring, but also determine the offspring's tendency for obesity. In the documentary, Dr. Jirtle describes how when the agouti protein is expressed, the mouse's coat is yellow, and, at the same time, "the agouti mouse doesn't realize that it's full. It literally eats itself into obesity, diabetes, and cancer." The experiment was so effective because genes are most susceptible to "deregulating and programming" during the earliest stages of gestational development. Dr. Jirtle explains why his study has been so fascinating to members of the scientific community: "What this means is that, at least in animal models, [the] fetal origins of adult disease susceptibility were for the first time demonstrated to be due to changes in the epigenome" (*Are You What Your Mother Ate?* 2017). This study transformed the way we view diseases and ushered in the era of "environmental epigenomics."

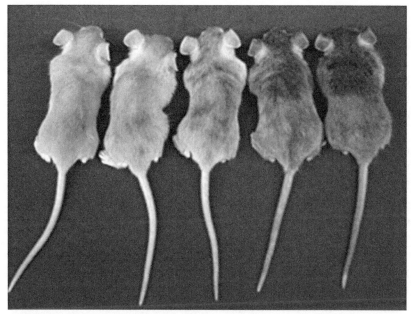

*Agouti mice. Photo demonstrating how maternal BPA exposure shifts offspring coat color distribution toward yellow. This figure originally appeared in Dana C. Dolinoy, Dale Huang, and Randy L. Jirtle, "Maternal nutrient supplementation counteracts bisphenol A-induced DNA hypomethylation in early development," Proceedings of the National Academies of Science 104(32): 13056–13061, doi: 10.1073/pnas.0703739104. Copyright (2007) National Academy of Sciences, U.S.A. Full-color image hosted at https:// tinyurl.com/Nested-Ecologies-Images.*

Given the conclusive results of animal models, the question is: Can "nongenetic, transgenerational and fetal origins of disease" be established in humans?[8] To answer this question, Dr. Fitzgerald turned to Laura Schulz's 2010 study on the Dutch Hunger Winter of 1944–1945. The Dutch Hunger Winter was a bitterly cold period in Western Europe, following four years of brutal war. Dutch people burned their furniture in order to stay warm. Meanwhile, a German blockade placed devastating restrictions on food availability for the Dutch. At the most challenging point, the population was struggling to survive on approximately 30 percent of their normal calorie intake, and people ate grass and tulip bulbs to eschew starvation (see Carey 2012, 2). These circumstances created a remarkable epidemiological study population in that all survivors of the Dutch Hunger Winter simultaneously suffered from one discrete period of malnutrition.

Using retrospective analysis, Schulz observes that, on one hand, mothers who were malnourished toward the end of their pregnancy were more likely to give birth to low-body-weight babies. Over the course of their lives, these offspring had lower rates of obesity when compared to the rest of the population. On the other hand, women who experienced starvation toward the beginning of their pregnancies gave birth to normal-weight babies. These babies experienced a higher rate of obesity and other health problems during their lives. Carey notes that "[e]ven though these individuals had seemed perfectly healthy at birth, something had happened to their development in the womb that affected them for decades after. . . . Events that take place in the first three months of development, a stage when the fetus is really very small, can affect an individual for the rest of their life" (2012, 4). Perhaps even more intriguing, the lifelong effects for individuals born during and shortly after the Dutch Hunger Winter were also present in the next generation.

While the Dutch Hunger Winter is perhaps the most prominent example, other studies have also established the intergenerational effects of food availability. Dr. Fitzgerald describes a study by Kaati et al. (2002) that demonstrated grandparents' experience with low food availability during prepuberty was correlated with low cardiovascular disease mortality. Meanwhile, a surfeit of food during prepuberty correlated with increased diabetes mortality for grandchildren (Bygren et al. 2014). Furthermore, studies on the Chinese famine of 1959–1961 found that the mother's exposure to famine during gestation was associated with her child developing dyslipidemia and cognitive impairment later in life (Xin et al. 2019; Wang et al. 2016). In another example, paternal exposure to cold temperatures increased brown adipose tissue formation in offspring (Sun et al. 2018). According to Dr. Fitzgerald, all these examples signal transgenerational, nongenetic origins of health and disease.[9]

The transgenerational effects of hunger and famine can be explained by adaptations to fetuses' metabolisms adapted while in utero. Anticipating an external environment of nutritional scarcity, the fetuses developed a slower metabolism, giving them a survival advantage. Dr. Lynch explains, "These women who were pregnant at the time did not have adequate food. . . . That made the genes in the developing infant say, 'Hey, there's not much food coming in here. I need to be thrifty. I need to hold on to this nutrition as much as I can and not burn it. I need to conserve it.'" However, after birth, offspring faced a nutritional environment that was discordant with the one to which they were adapted in utero. These individuals' metabolisms were conserving every calorie when it was no longer necessary to do so. In

Dr. Lynch's telling, offspring grew into adults who simply walk over to the refrigerator and are faced with a constant supply of processed, calorie-dense food. This mismatch led to obesity, dyslipidemia, and cardiovascular disease, among other diseases.

Other epigenetic studies have examined the effects of adverse childhood experiences (ACEs). For example, Rachel Yehuda et al. have conducted research on intergenerational transmission of trauma among the offspring of Holocaust survivors (see Mayer 2016, 119; Yehuda et al. 2016). Speaking on the topic of how adversity in early life can influence DNA methylation over the course of one's life, Dr. Szyf describes a study he did on children who lived through a 1998 ice storm in Quebec (see Cao-Lei et al. 2015). While the ice storm only lasted a few days, families were without electricity for up to six weeks. As a cohort, the children suffered from pronounced changes in their DNA methylation. Dr. Szyf explains, "We know . . . what happened was because of adversity. It wasn't because they carried bad genes." Due to a random occurrence (living in Quebec during a devastating ice storm), children were epigenetically "damaged" in different ways. Dr. Szyf's observations lead me to wonder what will be the long-term epigenetic effects of extended shelter-in-place due to COVID-19.

At the same time, findings like Dr. Szyf's are relevant for everyday life in the absence of natural disasters and pandemic viruses. Dr. Rollin McCraty, director of research at the HeartMath Institute, notes, "Childhood adversity and loneliness . . . cause rapid changes in the way the DNA expresses." Niki Gratrix, co-founder of Optimum Health Clinic, explains how emotional trauma is passed down intergenerationally: "If a father has been emotionally traumatized, it changes the epigenetic expression of genes and it actually affects the RNA expression of sperm." In lab experiments with mice, the progeny have the same epigenetic expression of the traumatized father. In essence, our emotional traumas are inherited by our children and are potentially passed down for many generations.

Given the intergenerational transmission of epigenetic marks, epigenetics serves as a mechanism by which environmental information shapes evolutionary change. At the same time, however, anthropologists Zaneta Thayer and Amy Non (2015) suggest "healthy skepticism," noting the risk of a neo-reductionist framework that overemphasizes molecular pathways at the expense of historical and socioeconomic contexts. In this vein, Margaret Lock writes, "Although the contribution of environments, social and physical, to human development, health, and illness, are now well recognized, there is a distinct danger that the molecular endpoints that these variables bring about, and very little else, will receive due attention" (2013, 292). Thus, the best epigenetic studies will provide a rich sociocultural context within which to interpret data.

In this vein, Conching and Thayer (2019) argue for the theory of historical trauma as a way to understand why historically subjugated populations—despite their unique histories, environments, and lifestyles—consistently experience poorer health outcomes compared to the general population. They furthermore suggest that historical trauma unfolds via epigenetic mechanisms. First, personal exposure to trauma is more common among populations that have experienced historical trauma, and this personal exposure can induce epigenetic modifications that contribute to poor health. Second, intergenerational epigenetic modifications occur resulting from parental and grandparental exposures. Conching and Thayer's explanation of how epigenetic mechanisms may produce historical trauma is significant since epigenetic effects are not necessarily permanent, and thus, the high prevalence of poor health among historically disadvantaged communities could be reduced by improvements in environmental conditions.

Issues of subjugation and disadvantage are overlooked when functional medicine practitioners and proponents emphasize the importance of individuals' choices for ensuring the best possible epigenetic expression in future generations. Sayer Ji, founder of *GreenMedInfo*, emphasizes that current choices, such as drinking alcohol and smoking cigarettes, can have a negative effect on offspring. In this same vein, Dr. William Li describes how sperm can be affected by toxic chemicals such as bisphenol A, diethyl phthalate, and cadmium. He writes, "Noxious chemicals such as benzene (in petroleum), perchloroethylene (used in dry cleaning), and cigarette smoke that a mother may be exposed to during pregnancy can leave their marks on the fetus's DNA, which will persist in the child for the rest of its life" (2019, 62). While these functional medicine interlocutors' assertions are informed by recent discoveries in epigenetics, I am wary of how individuals' present-day decisions are communally moralized due to their potential impact on the lives of future generations.[10]

This leads me to an important implication of epigenetics: new linkages between "behaviors" and (extrapolated) "risks." As an ethnographer whose work up until now has focused on reproduction, I am acutely aware of how moralizing tendencies can place an unequal burden on the shoulders of women. I argue that, in an era of booming epigenetic research, future parents—especially mothers—are subject to an emerging moral regime (see Richardson et al. 2014; Faircloth 2017; Harman and Cappellini 2015). For example, when describing translational epigenetics as an "amazing, emerging field that is just starting to blossom," Dr. Lynch simultaneously indicates that "[w]hen a woman is pregnant, we think that if we give the right prenatals and the right nutrients, we are going to impact that child's life—and we are, absolutely. What you might not understand is we are also impacting that child's children as well—your grandchildren."[11] In my prior research, I analyzed meritocracies regarding particular birthing practices (see Vega 2018). Given the central importance of epigenetics in functional medicine, I am hyper-attuned to how epigenetic research can undergird meritocratic pregnancies while neglecting broader political economic factors that shape and constrain maternal choice, biology, and behavior (Lock 2005).

Michelle Pentecost (2018), a physician and anthropologist, examines the developmental origins of health and disease (DOHaD) and epigenetic knowledge as "biosocial" objects embedded in global discourses. Pentecost partnered with Fiona Ross, a social scientist and nurse, to document how "the first thousand days" (conception to two years) are cast as a time frame for intervention (Pentecost and Ross 2019). In the process, they signal how South African nutrition policy foregrounds categories of persons while obscuring social conditions and how questions are framed according to particular knowledge horizons (what they call a "knowledge effect"). In a 2020 article, Pentecost and Maurizio Meloni, a social theorist and a science and technology studies scholar, frame DOHaD as a "theoretical spyglass into postgenomic biology." They argue that DOHaD frameworks make novel assertions to justify fragmented claims about preconception and explore the epistemic and political implications of these claims.

Functional medicine offers a number of claims that, following Pentecost and Meloni, must be examined for the epistemic and political implications. For example, Dr. Szyf believes "the new science of epigenetics" can develop early detection tools to identify children who are at risk and can benefit from epigenetic interventions.[12] However, instead of exploring social determinants of risk, he indicates, "I am hoping that one day we . . . will be able to develop DNA methylation diagnostics. That we can—maybe at the placenta, maybe in the cord blood, maybe later—find babies that . . . are at risk." While Dr. Szyf acknowledges that a variety of potential challenges during pregnancy can place the developing fetus at risk for negative epigenetic effects, he frames these as individual tragedies that mothers face—not acts of structural violence (see Farmer et al. 2006). Given the nature of these individual tragedies, this is the question for Dr. Szyf: "How can we intervene very early to prevent that risk from manifesting itself?" In this view, the risk of individual babies is tied to the traumatic experiences of their individual mothers; thus, the earliest possible opportunity for risk prevention is in the womb.[13] Dr. Szyf continues, "We need to think about the kinds of intervention—behavioral intervention—some sort of an enrichment environment that will send the opposite signals to what was sent." Unfortunately, this focus on behavioral intervention obscures the need for structural change.

Furthermore, I argue that while epigenetic approaches offer actionable insight for prevention, they can also hyperbolize "risk" in ways that revise understandings of biological permeability and subject women to increased scrutiny (see Pentecost and Meloni 2020; Rose 1998). The notion of a "zero trimester"—an extended phase of life starting at menarche when a woman's "poor choices" (e.g., drinking alcohol, using drugs) could cause potential harm if she accidentally or intentionally becomes pregnant—already extends public health surveillance to all of women's reproductive years (see Waggoner 2017). When the notion of a zero trimester is combined with emerging epigenetic research, the "choices" of parents (especially mothers) are characterized as of utmost importance since parents' present-day "choices" determine who their children become. That is, the conditions that a mother faces during pregnancy not only determine the health of the child, but also her pre-pregnancy "choices" prefigure her future children's identities.[14]

At the same time, I must acknowledge that epigenetic factors give rise to powerful physiological effects. According to functional medicine practitioners and proponents, epigenetics plays the primary role in determining our health status at any given point in time—more so than our genes themselves. Kresser concurs, "I think one of the biggest mistakes we made . . . is not understanding the deep connection between human beings and our environment. That if we change the environment, we are changing ourselves." By way of example, Nakayama indicates that SNPs, like MTHFR and COMT, have a low probability of disease, except when there is an environment that triggers them into expression. In essence, functional medicine providers privilege the *epi*(genome) over the (epi)*genome*. This perspective reiterates the importance of nested ecologies—how external ecologies shape internal ecologies.

Furthermore, epigenetics is more easily modified than genetics since, as Matt Riemann, founder and CEO of the Ultimate Human Foundation, clarifies, "[o]ur epigenetics are our environment and our lifestyle, the foods we eat, the way we move our body, the people that we hang out with, the things we think." As such, epigenetics are prime targets for functional medicine intervention. Thus, instead of considering the genome in a way that silences epigenetic factors (see Dobbs 2018), functional medicine practitioners embrace the e(m)p(t)i-ness of the genome by emphasizing the biosocial "epi-ness" of genetic expression. Furthermore, this approach allows functional medicine practitioners to maximize individuals' diet and supplementation based on their single nucleotide polymorphisms (SNPs), thus prompting epigenetic changes and preventing polygenetic chronic diseases.

This action-oriented approach to the human genome is premised on a (re)definition of SNPs. Dr. Yael Joffe refers to SNPs as "spinning changes." They are not errors or mistakes; however, they do change something within the body, and therapeutic approaches must also change to meet the unique *strengths* and *needs* of every individual's genomic profile. McEvoy explains, "We have to appreciate that all genetic SNPs represent a potential limitation in one sense, but a benefit in another sense." By way of example, he describes how the MTHFR C677T allele is known for predisposing individuals to different kinds of cancer and hyperhomocysteinemia, but for individuals who have inherited Lynch syndrome, this SNP can actually protect against cancer. McEvoy then turns to the APOE gene. The APOE-4 SNP is associated with increased Alzheimer's incidence, while APOE-3 is neutral and APOE-2 confers greater longevity. McEvoy indicates, "While it's true that individuals that [have two copies of APOE-4 have the highest risk] for developing Alzheimer's, they also have the ability to protect themselves from pathogens in the environment." In essence, functional medicine practitioners reject binary approaches that cast SNPs as inherently harmful by pointing to how every SNP confers some benefit from an evolutionary perspective.

This approach serves as a corrective to how certain SNPs have been mediatized and portrayed as determinants of disease. For example, Ji notes that although we associate BRCA with increased risk for breast cancer, there are many variants of BRCA, including some that actually protect against breast cancer. While the SNPs with the most deleterious effects are the ones that have garnered the greatest media attention, functional medicine practitioners are drawing attention to how SNPs can also code for wellness.

At the same time, functional medicine practitioners acknowledge that epigenetics is an emerging science and we are just beginning to scratch the surface. Dr. Lynch asserts, "Epigenetics—modifying genetic expression to improve your life and health—is a cutting-edge aspect of medicine that most practitioners don't understand" (Lynch 2020, 9). At the same time, he affirms that individuals can transcend their inherited tendencies to disease by using the right tools. "Health issues that had puzzled my clients for years suddenly made sense when they discovered through our work together that their SNPs had at least partly created those issues. Problems that had seemed overwhelming—even dooming—became manageable as clients learned that they could use diet and lifestyle to reshape their genes' behavior" (Lynch 2020, 3).

Given the malleability of genetic expression, functional medicine practitioners are adding epigenetics to their preventative medicine toolkits. For these practitioners, genomic information is no longer about the relative risk of disease occurrence, but rather about identifying actionable change for disease resiliency. Dr. Ritamarie Loscalzo, chiropractor and clinical nutritionist, notes that genetics tell patients what may happen in their future, allowing them to adapt their lifestyle now and prevent negative downstream effects. Dr. Loscalzo reframes the distinction between monogenetic congenital diseases and polygenetic chronic diseases in a slightly new way: "There are very few genes where the genetics outweigh the epigenetics." From this perspective, knowledge regarding individuals' genomes is empowering instead of defeating.[15]

From the perspective of functional medicine, genomic testing can guide personalized approaches for reducing pressure on the "weakest link" in your "genetic chain." Turning to the APOE-4 SNP, Dr. O'Bryan explains the statistics: "If you have two 4s—you got one from your mother, you got one from your father—[the likelihood that you will develop Alzheimer's] is 90 percent by the age of sixty-five." Resisting fatalism, he continues, "The stats are accurate, but all of the people these statistics are based on are people who didn't change their lifestyle. They didn't change their environment. They didn't know." Dr. O'Bryan explains to his patients that the APOE-4 genotype simply means if the patient were to become highly inflamed, the inflammation will begin to affect the patient's brain before other parts of the body. Thus, the key to preventing Alzheimer's in people with the APOE-4 geneotype is reducing inflammation in the body.

Using this epigenetic approach, Dr. O'Bryan works to reframe notions of "risk" among his APOE-4 patients. He describes an archetypal exchange with a patient with the APOE-4 genotype: "When patients come back, and their tests show they're an APOE-4 . . . I say, 'Mrs. Patient, [these results are] not good, but it's really good news because now we know where to focus our attention.'" With these words, Dr. O'Bryan reconfigures personal genomic risk as an opportunity for prevention. In his archetypal exchange, he then goes on to explain, "Now the APOE-4 means that you're genetically vulnerable, and that's the deck of cards you got. You can't change that. But now you're going to [ask], 'Is my lifestyle throwing gasoline on the fire?'" Dr. O'Bryan counsels his APOE-4 patients about how lifestyle can have powerful epigenetic effects. He explains to patients, "When [inflammatory biomarkers] come down, as far as we know, you're not at risk of Alzheimer's." This statement represents a paradigm shift in genetics. While genetic risk has previously been considered lifelong (and perhaps increasing with age), an epigenetic approach suggests that genetic risk only manifests under certain conditions.

In essence, the science of epigenetics supports functional medicine's conceptualization of disease (including chronic disease) as conjunctural and therefore reversible. By embracing epigenetics, functional medicine reiterates its rejection of the conventional notion of chronic disease as permanent and degenerative. In this vein, neurologist Dr. David Perlmutter emphasizes that the APOE-4 gene marker is not a determinant, especially given the brain's amazing degree of neuroplasticity and neurogenesis. Neuroplasticity is the brain's ability to make new connections between nerve cells based on outside stimuli. Neurogenesis is the ability of the brain to generate new brain cells throughout the entire life span. In order to promote neurogenesis among his patients, Dr. Perlmutter focuses on increasing BDNF activity using exercise and turmeric, among other epigenetic interventions.[16] His actions recall Ji's comments about SNPs that code for wellness since Dr. Perlmutter aims to offset the detrimental effects of certain SNPs by amplifying the positive effects of other SNPs.

However, while protective SNPs can be "upregulated" to produce positive outcomes, negative epigenetic effects can likewise unleash detrimental outcomes. Dr. Bland clarifies this point by noting how professional football players who have suffered multiple concussions are more likely to develop dementia later in life. He compares these injuries to "bruising of the brain." However, contrary to bruises that are visible on the human body, "[t]his particular injury has a replicative sequence over time that doesn't get better—in fact, it gets worse. These people don't get dementia immediately. Their brains become more fungiform over the course of twenty or thirty years—post even their careers as football players." He clarifies that the only possible underlying mechanism by which this can occur is epigenetic change of gene expression. Explaining the etiology, he says, "We have a mechanical signal called 'concussive energy in injury' being translated into progressive gene expression change of alarm in the brain in which the collateral damage is the neuron itself, which leads, ultimately, to neuronal depletion, and dementia." The dementia is progressive and continues on in the absence of the original stimulus since "[y]ou've reset gene expression in a new pattern of homeostasis—which is the homeostasis of degeneration." In essence, just as epigenetic influences can prevent neurological degeneration, they can also be the cause.

Epigenetics, then, has transformed how functional medicine practitioners treat "disease." According to Kresser, genome testing is the most helpful for patients with complex chronic multisystem illness—for example, tick-borne and mold-related illnesses, chronic inflammatory response syndrome, autoimmune diseases, and chronic viral activity. He explains that it can be difficult to identify the best lever for initial intervention in these cases, especially since these complexly ill patients may not be able to tolerate treatments that start in the wrong place. Genetic profiling, the process of determining an individual's DNA characteristics, can help practitioners identify the first domino that needs to fall in a sequential healing approach.

Furthermore, genetic profiling can help functional medicine practitioners determine what medications are right for each patient's genetics. Dr. Bryan Glick focuses on the importance of CYP450 testing for preemptively determining how drugs and supplements may not only be ineffective, but may also cause harmful side effects. According to Dr. Glick, this type of testing "cracks open" the question of why some patients get side effects and why others respond well to medication. If providers do not understand how certain medications are contraindicated for a particular patient's CYP450 profile, they may decide that more aggressive treatment (for example, surgery) is needed when, in fact, the patient simply needed the correct medication for their genes.

A patient's CYP450 profile can also guide dosing. On one hand, if the patient is a fast metabolizer for a particular drug, they may require a dose that is multiple times higher than the general guideline. Lacking this information can be detrimental—for example, if a doctor suspects that a patient is addicted to pain medication when, in actuality, the patient is simply a fast metabolizer. On the other hand, slow metabolizers need a fraction of the generally recommended dose, and failure to take their CYP450 metabolism into account can have disastrous results, including overdose and death.

Functional medicine providers have reframed cancer as an epi(genetic) phenomenon, thus begging the question: How can "lifestyle" changes among cancer patients extend life span and produce better outcomes? Dr. Servan-Schreiber is an example of someone who used lifestyle to live a longer, happier life. When I read his book, *Anticancer: A New Way of Life*, I did not focus on the fact that he eventually died of a malignant brain tumor, but instead on the fact that his passing occurred nearly twenty years after his initial cancer diagnosis. In the second edition, Dr. Servan-Schreiber acknowledged that his eventual death may be due to cancer, but he insists that he did not regret changing his way of life because his nonconventional approach to cancer significantly extended his life and improved his quality of life. His focus was not on *how he would die*, but instead on *how he would live*.

Due to their epigenetic approach, functional medicine practitioners problematize the genetic basis for cancer. In this vein, Dr. Servan-Schreiber wrote, "If cancer was transmitted essentially through genes, the cancer rate among adopted children would be the same as that among their biological—not their adoptive—parents." He turned to a study published in the *New England Journal of Medicine* that analyzed more than a thousand adopted children in Denmark (see Sorenson et al. 1988). The study found that the genes of biological parents who died before fifty had no influence over the adoptee's cancer risk. In contrast, adoptees had a fivefold increase in rate of mortality if their adoptive parent died from cancer before age fifty. Since adoptive parents pass on habits but not genes, Dr. Servan-Schreiber asserted that "[t]his study shows that lifestyle is fundamentally involved in vulnerability to cancer." He provided further evidence from a study demonstrating that genetic factors make a minor contribution to cancer susceptibility among identical twins (see Lichtenstein et al. 2000). He concluded, "All research on cancer concurs: Genetic factors contribute to at most 15 percent of mortalities from cancer." In essence, the epigenetic approach unseats prior notions of genetic fatality and focuses on prevention.

The epigenetic approach thus poses new opportunities for therapeutic intervention. Dr. Szyf argues that even genes that are described as "causing cancer"—for example, BRCA1—still need to be turned "on" to be expressed. In his view, "a good epigenetic strategy" can overcome an individual's risk for developing particular diseases. Recent advances have rendered epigenetic strategies feasible. This is not a novel concept to Dr. Szyf. Two decades ago, his lab proposed that DNA methylation is a prime target for cancer treatment. "When I was a graduate student, I looked at cancer and I said, 'The problem in cancer is that these cells are expressing a different genetic program than they should. Skin cells should remain in the skin, they should not metastasize to the lung. So something is going on with the way the DNA is working that changes the program.'" Referring to present-day debates regarding genetic editing, Dr. Szyf acknowledges, "Yes, you can change a program by changing the DNA, genetics. But, if DNA methylation indeed controls the way genes work, it stands to reason that it changes in cancer." McEvoy elaborates, "Cancer is a primary example of how DNA methylation gone bad is found in different regions of certain cell types that express cancer activity." Thus, upregulating methylation is a primary strategy for preventing cancer in functional medicine.

Methylation, along with other bodily processes acting together in a biological system, can be optimized through diet. Dr. Fitzgerald cites multiple sources when documenting the epigenetic effects of food on cancer—for example, parsley, garlic, turmeric, green tea, soybean, tomatoes, red grapes, milk thistle, and cruciferous vegetables. She notes one study that states that "[v]itamins A and C . . . have recently been shown to intensify erasure of epigenetic memory in naive embryonic stem cells. . . . Vitamin A and C cosupplementation synergistically enhances reprogramming of different cells to the naïve state, but overuse may exaggerate instability of imprinted genes" (Hore 2017).[17] Focus on nutrition and supplementation is consistent with the idea that disease does *not* result from the deficiency of a synthetic chemical. In Ji's words, "Cancer is not the result of the lack of chemotherapy." Instead, the functional medicine approach opens up the possibility of effecting epigenetic, "anti-cancer" change through alternative and complementary therapies. In theoretical biologist Dr. Josh Mitteldorf's view, learning to "reprogram our epigenetics" will produce benefits for disease prevention that equal or surpass past medical breakthroughs such as sanitation, vaccines, and antibiotics.

Despite the documented impact of diet, functional medicine practitioners do not propose using nutrigenomics in lieu of existing cancer treatments. Instead, epi(genomics) can be harnessed to both improve and evaluate outcomes from mainstream treatments like chemotherapy. Dr. Haase describes how epi(genomics) can be used in real time to see if cancer treatment is effective or not. "Liquid biopsies" (isolating cell-free DNA floating in blood to do a full genetic sequencing) were introduced in 2015 as a revolutionary tool in cancer therapy (see Karachaliou et al. 2015). From these biopsies, providers can obtain a copy-number instability (CNI) score. Dr. Haase explains, "This is very closely correlated with the degree of tumor load present in the body and can therefore be used to reliably predict who is responding well to the therapy." Emphasizing the transformative impact of this epi(genetic) technology on cancer care, Dr. Haase analogizes the use of genomic biomarkers in cancer treatment to checking for viral load in the treatment of HIV.

While I appreciate the merits of this epi(genomic) approach, I simultaneously argue that it (epi)geneticizes cancer without signaling the effects of social inequality on biology. Functional medicine practitioners often neglect structural inequality when they focus on either emotions or biology. This leads functional medicine practitioners to emphasize lifestyle and diet changes, instead of exposing social determinants of health (how, for example, class, "race," and gender inequality lead to disparate health outcomes) and arguing for social justice. For example, Dr. Lynch explains that methylation can be influenced by an individual's "choices" and behaviors. In so doing, he analogized genes to children in need of supervision: "Imagine your kids in your home having free access to sugar, the TV, and no sleep at night. . . . You have chaos." Explaining how this analogy applies to epigenetics, Dr.

Lynch continues, "If [you have an MTHFR SNP and] you're eating a ton of protein, you have high oxidative stress." This approach renders individuals responsible for managing their genetic expression through their behaviors and dietary choices.

I argue that the epigenetics of cancer underlines the need for health care equity. A July 2020 study found that among more than forty thousand medical insurance policies from commercial and public payers, none provided coverage for liquid biopsies at the start of 2016. By mid-2019, the coverage rate had increased to 38 percent (Douglas and Gray 2020). While the study describes a rapid increase in coverage, unequal access to this epi(genomic) technology means more privileged patients will be "empowered" by their informational biology when treating cancer while less privileged patients are "blindly" treated with chemotherapy.

At the same time, cancer treatment can be too expensive even for those who are insured. In their 2017 article in the *Journal of Clinical Oncology*, Olszewski et al. document a substantial financial barrier to accessing orally administered anticancer therapy and argue for urgent attention from policymakers. Individuals who are uninsured may be barred from accessing cancer treatments entirely. Thus, cancer serves as an example of how promising therapies and technologies privilege socioeconomically "empowered" bioconsumers, while potentially excluding less privileged "others."

Furthermore, epigenetics provides a molecular biological framework for assessing how structural inequalities manifest in individuals' bodies. The disadvantaged do not possess the financial resources needed to pursue an "epigenetic strategy" based on modifying "lifestyle factors." Thus, they are stripped of the overlapping potentials for preventing cancer, extending life span, and improving quality of life. Those who get cancer are more likely to have been exposed to environmental toxicants (read: poor and minority individuals), thus pointing to the importance of environmental justice (see Ward et al. 2004).[18] Adding insult to injury, not only are socioeconomically disadvantaged individuals more likely to develop cancer, cancer patients are up to five times more likely to go bankrupt than people without cancer (see Ramsey et al. 2013). Thus, an epi(genetic) approach to cancer emphasizes the embodied effects of intersectional privilege-disadvantage.

The epigenetics of cancer also lays bare the need for social justice in food access. Harking back to Dr. Fitzgerald's comments, nutrition has direct epi(genomic) effects that can reduce cancer risk. However, we live in a society in which citizens have unequal access to quality nutrition. Food access is shaped by intersecting axes of inequality, including class, race, and gender. While food systems affect everyone, the harshest consequences fall to the most socioeconomically and physically vulnerable individuals. Despite pressing issues of social inequality, functional medicine interlocutors describe epigenetics (read: behaviors) as determining who we are.

Meanwhile, recent advances in the field of epigenetics have prompted medical anthropologists to evaluate the "remaking of local biologies in an epigenetic time" (see Meloni 2014). Lock (2005, 2013) has critiqued the field of epigenetics for its reductionist tendencies. At the same time, Jörg Niewöhner, referring specifically to Dr. Szyf's lab, argues that epigenetic researchers are the first group of molecular biologists to appreciate the notion of local biology. He writes, "Trying to incorporate 'social life' into molecular analyses makes immediately plausible that even something seemingly hardwired such as gene expression may be connected in significant ways to local cultural practices" (2011, 16). If molecular biology can demonstrate how genetic expression is shaped by local culture, it could become very easy for biologists to also accept the anthropological argument that "genotypes are rendered meaningful in a cultural universe" (Shook et al. 2019, 44).

In essence, the study of epigenetics opens the door to intellectual exchange between the fields of molecular biology and medical anthropology. Meloni argues that epigenetics asks questions that only make sense given a local biologies approach. While these questions would have been impossible for molecular biologists to imagine in the early 1990s when Lock introduced the concept, these scientists are now asking, for example: "Do the poor have different patterns of methylation than the rich?" (Meloni 2014, 2). Such questions, in turn, prompt medical anthropologists to ask if epigenetics is the molecular translation of local biologies or whether it is a development to which local biologies can bring a serious critique (Meloni 2014). This type of exchange between molecular biology and medical anthropology is valuable because, as Shook et al. write, "culture and epigenetics are very much a part of the human condition, and their roles are significant parts of the complete story of human evolution" (2019, 45).

I agree with Lock that the epigenetic view is reductionist. External factors do not produce biological changes and influence health outcomes by acting upon genetic expression alone. Assuming that this is true would not only be false from a social science perspective (since it represents the geneticization of social life), but also from a biological perspective (since it accepts that health and disease exclusively manifest through [epi]genetic mechanisms).

At the same time, I find "local biologies," with their primary emphasis on culture and social factors, insufficient for describing environment/human entanglements. Recognizing the need for additional conceptual tools and responding to current molecular biological research on epigenetics, Niewöhner and Lock (2018) offer "situated biologies" as a potential middle ground in debates that cast biology as either local or universal.[19] While the concept of situated biologies is an outgrowth of local biologies, it also builds upon Niewöhner's 2011 reconceptualization of the body as the "embedded body."

I appreciate Niewöhner and Lock's portrayal of the body as embedded, situated, and entangled. However, given my observations of functional medicine discourse, I offer nested ecologies as a way for thinking about how multiple external factors simultaneously occurring outside the body (political, economic, social, and physical) influence an individual's internal ecology via systems biology. At the same time, I use the concept of nested ecologies to critique how functional medicine interlocutors epigeneticize individuals by locating the underlying causes of disease in "behaviors."

I will provide examples to elucidate my critique. Dr. Fitzgerald describes how Mark and Scott Kelly, identical twins, were deemed "no longer identical" while Scott spent a year living on the International Space Station and Mark remained on Earth as the control subject (NASA 2018). Carey writes, "Whenever two genetically identical individuals are non-identical in some way we can measure, this is called epigenetics" (2012, 6). Both Scott's consumption of folate and the length of his telomeres increased significantly while in space. Meanwhile, Mark's folate and telomeres remained stable. Scott's epigenetic changes returned to baseline upon his return to Earth. By pointing to the epigenetic underpinnings of Mark and Scott's divergent biology, Dr. Fitzgerald emphasizes how epigenetics creates individuals.

Springboarding from outcomes like those of Mark and Scott Kelly, functional medicine interlocutors argue that twin studies allow us to imagine the disparate outcomes that would result if individuals made different choices throughout their life. In interviews, both Dr. Lynch and Riemann emphasize how twin studies provide "takeaway" lessons for singleton viewers. As Riemann indicates, "Our genes plus our environment and lifestyle equal our phenotype, which is who we are when we look in the mirror and how we think when we look in the mirror." Dr. Lynch elaborates, "How many twins do you know that are identical in personality and their actions? They might look the same initially but as they age they're gonna start looking different, right?" Almost as if responding to Dr. Lynch, Riemann explains, "Identical twins have the exact same genetic makeup, yet over time they become very, very different people because of their environments and their lifestyles, the food they eat, the jobs they do, the people they hang out with, the environments and climates they choose to live in." Dr. Lynch concurs, "It's their choices, which they have chosen to do that are affecting their genes. . . .

It's the power of the epigenome which is controlling how their genes are expressed. . . . Your choices matter in life." According to functional medicine interlocutors, twins studies demonstrate how individuals with the same genetic makeup can become very different people due to epigenetic effects.

Indeed, according to emerging research, choices can determine one's biological age, independent of one's chronological age. Knowing this, Dr. Fitzgerald rhetorically asks, "Can we turn back the clock?" As if in response, Dr. Josh Mitteldorf writes in an email newsletter, "In the next decade, researchers will acknowledge that aging is not an inevitable deterioration of the body. It is driven by an epigenetic program." Dr. Mitteldorf's optimism is based on recent research findings.

Fahy et al. used a protocol intended to regenerate the thymus to successfully reverse epigenetic aging and immunosenescent trends in humans. Their study, which produced a "mean epigenetic age approximately 1.5 years less than baseline after 1 year of treatment (−2.5-year change compared to no treatment at the end of the study)," has gained high visibility in functional medicine discourse (Fahy et al. 2019). For example, shortly after the study results from Fahy et al. were released, Dr. Fitzgerald mentioned the study in her webinar. Their study design is based on Steven Horvath's research on the relationship between methylation and aging (see Horvath 2013) and the assertion that "epigenetic 'clocks' can now surpass chronological age in accuracy for estimating biological age" (Fahy et al. 2019, e13028) According to the Fahy study, "[o]ne of the lessons that we can draw from the study is that aging is not necessarily something that is beyond our control. In fact, it seems that aging is largely controlled by biological processes that we may be able to influence" (Pullano 2019). I signal that while biological age can be epigenetically influenced, the ability to do so is directly tied to privilege.

As the Fahy study came to life in functional medicine and public discourse, a research industry began to emerge around epigenetic clocks. I began receiving emails regarding the study from Life Extension (a supplement company) and Zymo Research (a company that provides products and services for cellular biology, epigenetics, and microbiome research). I was intrigued by the Zymo Research advertisement for their Human DNAge Epigenetic Clock Service. According to the website, their service has potential applications in arthritis, allergies, diabetes, circadian rhythms, fertility, and forensics research.

After reading the information posted on the company's website, I received an email from Zymo Research describing their DNAge Epigenetic Aging Clock Service. "We utilize our proprietary SWARM® (Simplified

Whole-panel Amplification Reaction Method) technology to analyze DNA methylation patterns of these aging-related loci." DNA methylation is so intimately tied to the aging process that Dr. Sinclair indicates to *Health Theory* viewers that his lab "reads the methyls" bound to DNA when determining biological age. "What we've discovered over the last twenty years is that certain types of enzymes help package the DNA and help with the DNA repair. . . . Without those . . . we basically will age more rapidly. [Methyls] accumulate as you get older in very predictable ways." Using the approach Dr. Sinclair describes, Zymo Research's Epigenetic Clock reports determine DNAge® (DNA methylation age) and ΔAge (the difference between DNAge® and chronological age).

Zymo Research markets its test as a source of actionable knowledge since "[d]ifferential DNA methylation has been observed between diseases such as HIV and controls, and is modifiable by environmental factors such as diet, exercise, and drugs."[20] Dr. Sinclair concurs, "What is really exciting is that we've discovered that you can make them more active to make sure the DNA is packaged correctly and the repair is very efficient. There are ways you can do that." Offering exercise, diet, and intermittent fasting as examples, Dr. Sinclair argues that certain behaviors render enzymes that "control our body" more active and in the process "make us healthier." From a functional medicine perspective, an individual's health is not genetically determined—instead, it is largely under the individual's control.

"Modifiable treatment targets" are so important from a functional medicine perspective that they even take precedence over epigenetic testing. Dr. Quig describes his usual interaction with colleagues who seek him out for consultation. He asks them to "tell me about their stress level. Tell me about their exposures." The last thing he tends to ask is, "Do you have any genetic data for this individual?" Similarly, Dr. George Slavich, associate professor of psychiatry and behavioral sciences at UCLA, suggests that his practitioner colleagues focus on modifiable treatment targets for immune system health. These modifiable treatment targets include developing a good diet, reducing psychological and emotional stress, living an active lifestyle, and maintaining good sleep hygiene.[21]

From the perspective of functional medicine, the science of epigenetics is so conclusive regarding the importance of lifestyle that it has rendered genetic testing an optional, albeit useful, source of biological evidence to support the provider's treatment decisions. Instead of performing genomic testing on each and every patient, practitioners recruit epigenetic science to legitimize "lifestyle medicine." Lambert expresses her appreciation for emerging science on epigenetics since it "provides some legitimacy to what many people have known for a long time: that your environment, your lifestyle, all these things matter."

Here, I must point out that, according to functional medicine discourse, modifiable factors do not include structural factors such as class, "race," and gender inequality. Instead, common modifiable factors are predicated on the assumption of a minimum of middle-class privilege. For example, the idea of intermittent fasting—restricting food consumption to a limited number of hours per day in order to promote "anti-aging"—is likely only attractive to those who are not facing food insecurity. Sobo and Loustaunau (2010) offer a similar critique when they explore the connection between stress and hypertension and signal that social structure and poverty contribute to disease susceptibility and risks (see Dressler 1990; Wyatt et al. 2003; Mays, Cochran, and Barnes 2007).

While epigenetic clock testing and interventions may constitute the next wave of epigenetic anti-aging strategies in functional medicine, telomere length has been studied extensively by functional medicine researchers as an indicator of biological age. Dr. Tsoukalas explains, "At the end of [chromosomes], we have the telomeres, which is the last part that protects the chromosome. In Greek it's called 'telos,' last, and part, 'meros.'" According to Dr. Prescott and Dr. Logan, "[t]elomeres are like plastic caps on the end of shoelaces, except in this case their function is not to prevent cotton laces from fraying" (2017, 85). They explain that our "ancestral past and future self in the form of DNA strands" are protected by our telomeres. Each time our DNA replicates, telomeres shorten slightly. Dr. Tsoukalas asserts, "The shorter our telomeres, the older we are at the biological level." Telomeres shrink by an average of 1.5 percent per year, and, in the process, DNA becomes increasingly unstable, thus leaving aging individuals susceptible to disease and mortality.

The aging process, however, is highly variable. According to Dr. Tsoukalas, telomeres may shorten as a result of stress, overwork, and overlapping viral infections. Describing the consequences of long-term stress on telomeres, Dr. Prescott and Dr. Logan write, "Serious forms of trauma and adversity in early life have been linked to shorter telomeres much later on, even at mid-life and beyond. The shortening can be kicked into higher gear by the total environment in which we live, and the way we live" (2017, 86). They go on to identify exposure to synthetic chemicals, excessive alcohol, smoking, processed foods, and poor sleep as factors that accelerate telomere erosion. Given the impact of these multiple factors on the aging process,

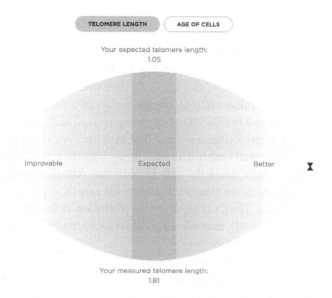

*Screenshot of my TeloYears lab results. These telomere length test results were reported around my thirty-second birthday. My reported biological age was twenty-seven. Full-color image hosted at https://tinyurl.com/Nested-Ecologies-Images.*

telomeres are referred to as "the documentarians of life and lifestyle" (Prescott and Logan 2017, 85).

Telomere length has become a modifiable target from the perspective of functional medicine since increases in telomerase can relengthen telomeres. Describing a recent study conducted with his research team, Dr. Tsoukalas said, "Our patients that . . . took supplements that covered their deficiency in minerals and vitamins and . . . also ate the correct food . . . had longer telomeres. Actually, they had 13 percent longer telomeres . . . than the average population." Dr. Tsoukalas indicated that, similar to epigenetic clocks, "lifestyle, diet, handling of stress . . . and also exercise, can activate telomerase and help the body [lengthen telomeres]. But in order for the body to be able to again build the telomeres, it needs to . . . have antioxidants." Dr. Prescott and Dr. Logan expand upon Dr. Tsoukalas's nutrition-oriented approach. "It has also been shown that emotional intelligence and optimism are associated with longer immune cell telomere length. . . . Mindfulness—appreciation for the present moment and viewing the environment with a child-like sense of wonder—is also linked to longer telomeres" (2017, 86). In addition to relaxation, Dr. William Li also suggests regular exercise to increase telomerase and, therefore, telomere length (see Li 2019, 70).

## EFFECTS

I point to unequal access to the resources that potentiate modifiable targets and lead to epigenetic change. In so doing, I acknowledge my own privilege and argue that functional medicine's well-intentioned emphasis on proper nutrition and mindfulness fails to engage the social structures that determine food access and the likelihood of feeling relaxed and optimistic.[22] For example, Dr. Raphael Kellman writes, "The keys are your many genes, and the song is your overall health. The pianist, my friends, is you!" (2018, 61). Dr. Kellman's analogy places the individual in the ultimate seat of power. I argue that individuals are able to influence their genetic expression *if given the correct resources*. Thus, I critique the neoliberal logics that underpin this individualistic approach, thus allowing debates surrounding epigenetics to sidestep the role of social inequality.

In a similar fashion, many functional medicine interlocutors have argued that increases in chronic disease are owed to changes in behavior, not genetic changes occurring across the population. Dr. Patrick Gentempo, the founder of Creating Wellness, states, "Our genes are not what changed in the past thirty, fifty, or one thousand, two thousand years. It's not a genetic issue. It is an epigenetic issue." Citing data from the *New England Journal of Medicine*, Dr. Tsoukalas indicates, "Ninety percent die from nontransmittable diseases. These are diseases that are mainly related to our lifestyle, to our diet, to our stress factors, to the lack of water, to the lack of exercise—to all these things that . . . should be there but they are not there anymore."[23] In the absence of health-supporting resources, chronic disease proliferates. Chronic disease can, then, predispose individuals to transmissible disease—94 percent of COVID-19 deaths occurred in those with comorbid health conditions (CDC 2021). Dr. Tracy Gaudet, director of Patient Centered Care at the Veterans Health Administration, describes this as the fatal cost of being unhealthy.

Providing greater tangibility to their claims, functional medicine interlocutors offer diabetes and autoimmunity as examples. Dr. Jason Fung, a nephrologist, asserts, "The genetics is a sideshow, because genetics can explain the difference in risk between individuals. . . . However, it does not explain the increase in type 2 diabetes in an entire population, for example." Since type 2 diabetes has skyrocketed in the last few decades, Dr. Fung concludes, "This is clearly an environmental problem." For him, genetic information, while useful, is secondary to environmental factors that affect us all. Similarly, Patel indicates that the increase in autoimmune disease is not due to a rapid change in genetics, but rather to a rapid change in environment.

In response to these comments regarding the epigenetics of disease, I highlight the importance of critical analysis regarding choice, along with environment and lifestyle.

## RETHINKING EPI(GENOMIC) "LIFESTYLE CHOICES": THE ENVIRONMENTAL EFFECTS OF SOCIOGENOMICS

I argue that people often live in environments and under circumstances that are not of their own choosing. Instead, the way in which people organize their day, their work activities, their ability to access resources, their engagement with different types of knowledge (Bateson 2000), and even what people believe and how they think are all shaped by structural axes of social inequality. I turn to specific instances that demonstrate how lifestyle factors and environment (both physical and social) are emphasized in functional medicine discourse. Functional medicine practitioners assert that the way that we experience the world around us, including how we interact with others, has powerful epigenetic effects. While this may be true, many functional medicine practitioners fail to note how structural factors often predetermine individuals' experiences.

Instead, when describing lifestyle as a determinant, many functional medicine interlocutors have tended to emphasize the importance of perception. To make this argument, Dr. Bland describes Loma Linda, California, the "anomalous Blue Zone." While other "Blue Zones"—places with high concentrations of centenarians—are described as places where communities continue to follow a "traditional lifestyle,"[24] Loma Linda is strikingly exceptional because it is not located in a non-Western, less industrialized region. According to Dr. Bland, "Loma Linda, California . . . is a metropolitan LA area that happens to be an island in the sea of industrialized America. Right? So, why is that a [Blue] Zone?" This Blue Zone evinces and resists multiple, overlapping binaries in functional medicine discourse: healthy vs. unhealthy, traditional vs. modern, and Western vs. non-Western. Dr. Bland explains that centenarians in Loma Linda are members of a Seventh-day Adventist community who drink the same water, breathe the same air, and live along the same freeways as residents living in contiguous areas; therefore, their increased longevity is not due to reduced environmental toxins and a "traditional, non-Western" way of life.

The longevity of Seventh-day Adventists in Loma Linda has powerful implications for functional medicine. Dr. Bland asks, "Can we adjust to manufacture a gene expression pattern that will live a hundred years of healthy living by thinking, acting, and believing the right things?" According to functional medicine, the answer to this question is an unequivocal "yes." Riemann asserts, "Our minds are extremely powerful in the conversation about genetic expression. It's the way we perceive our environment, not necessarily the environment itself, that actually causes our result and our response from our brain and the chemicals that are produced from that encounter." In this view, it is up to individuals to achieve greater longevity by changing their thoughts, actions, and beliefs, even in the presence of environmental injustice.[25]

Instead of referring to "perception," other functional medicine interlocutors have pointed to how experiences are mediated by our "emotions." Dr. Lynch closes the perceptual gap among genes, hormones, and neurotransmitters by indicating that shifting emotions or reactions to external stimuli can "turn on" genes. Dr. McCraty echoes the instantaneity of epigenetics effects, asserting that "the minute we get into a loving state or appreciative state vs. a frustration state, we're having instantaneous communications with, and changes at, the level of the DNA." He indicates that epigenetic change can occur at a much faster rate than hormonal fluctuations. From this perspective, the quickest and most effective ways to shape genetic expression are by managing stress, reducing anxiety, and fostering gratitude.

As a person who has recovered from numerous chronic diseases, I consider these practices an important part of my healing journey. I take seriously the power of the mind in shaping health outcomes. Each day, I spend fifteen minutes developing a sense of serene determination, reminding myself of my body's innate capacity for recovery, and, if necessary, framing a loving response to interpersonal conflict. This daily practice has helped me tremendously. Thus, I appreciate the intention behind Dr. Bland and Riemann's arguments about the epigenetic effects of thought processes.

Furthermore, I appreciate functional medicine's emphasis on what Dr. Bland calls "our psychosocial environment." In his view, our experiences stem from our observations of the world, which include "the relationships we have, the joy of living, a sense of attribution, the feeling of purpose, [and] locus [of] control." These variables modulate how our genes—especially the 98 percent of the human genome that is called "dark matter"—are expressed at the molecular level. From a medical anthropology perspective, Dr. Bland's relational approach is to be commended. However, this approach does not consider how unequal power dynamics in relationships are intersectionally determined (Crenshaw 2014) nor how "the joy of living" unfolds within historical, political, and socioeconomic contexts (Goldstein 2003). With respect to "locus of control," I argue that individuals' ability to feel and believe that they, as opposed to external forces, have control over the outcomes in their lives is instantiated by having at least the minimum requirements for survival and potentiated by increasing capital. One's needs for "purpose" and "attribution" are superseded by the need to survive in situations of extreme scarcity.

I must flag the dangerous potential slippage embedded in arguments that link epigenetic processes to thoughts and emotions. An inordinate focus on perception, thoughts, and beliefs can lapse into noxious assumptions that biological outcomes fully depend on the patient's "mental strength."[26] For example, Riemann states, "It's actually our perception of our environment and our lifestyle, which is dictated by our mind, that determines which genes are switched on or off at a given moment in time." Comments like these can be interpreted as suggesting that those suffering from chronic illness shoulder the burden of intersecting inequalities while "thinking their way" to good health. In so doing, this focus neglects the role of social structure in shaping thoughts, actions, and beliefs. While individuals can change their thoughts, actions, and beliefs for the better (e.g., "personal growth"), there are limits to the benefits these changes can provide in the absence of environmental and social justice. I am wary of how well-intentioned functional medicine experts, focused on the effects of emotional well-being on health, may unwittingly run the risk of deemphasizing structural inequality.

When functional medicine practitioners and health educators speak about lifestyle as a "choice," they seem unaware of how their assertions are situated within their own middle- and upper-class lives (Haraway 1988). Riemann supplied the potentially most striking example of "structural myopia" during my ethnographic research period. He asserted, "We can choose what food we put in our mouth. We can choose when we move our body and how we move it. We can choose who we hang out with. We can choose how much sleep we get and how we think about things around us. . . . We get to choose where we live. We get to choose everything." In his view, "we" get to choose all the things that are controlling our gene expression and health status at any given moment in time.

I strongly disagree. The type of food that people eat is shaped by where they live, what they have access to, what foods cost, and what they can afford. Furthermore, people have different degrees of education in nutrition, which is related to economic capital and is a form of cultural capital (Bourdieu 1984). Who we hang out with—our social network—is also a form of capital. To make this clear, I'll offer the following example: It is unlikely that there are many minorities from inner-city backgrounds in the Yale Corinthian Yacht Club.

Similarly, when and how people move their bodies depends on their work schedules, their neighborhoods, and whether they have access to a gym or the internet. As a graduate student, I taught "Health and Life" workshops to Guatemalan refugees living in Oakland, California. My impoverished students were eager to exercise their bodies, but their cramped living spaces were in notoriously violent neighborhoods, and they did not have access to parks, public spaces, gyms, or the internet.[27] My job was to teach them how to do challenging exercises using only their bodies and approximately fifteen square feet of floor space.

Riemann's claim that we choose where we live furthermore signals his privileged myopia. People buy their way into neighborhoods; thus, their entry is predicated on economic capital. Many neighborhoods continue to be racially segregated. I am a professor living in one of the poorest counties in the United States. When I moved to McAllen, I bought a home in a middle-class neighborhood. As a person of brown skin, I have been stopped on multiple occasions while walking my dog by white neighbors. They greet me and then ask if I am a dog walker, explaining that they are seeking dog-walking services. This example shows how "race" intersects with socioeconomic privilege, and how, as a female professor of color, I am "out of place" in my own neighborhood.

My point is, "we" do *not* get to choose "everything" that affects our health status unless "we" are privileged in multiple ways. My critique is not a personal affront to Riemann. Instead, I argue that in order for inequity to be remedied, inequity must first be acknowledged. I desire a world in which everyone has the "locus of control" over the epigenetic factors shaping their health, but society will not move closer to realizing my hope if people do not call out social injustice where it exists. My ethnographic observations suggest that many functional medicine practitioners and proponents do not consider fighting for social justice as a part of their work, or they simply do not know where to begin. If the latter is true, I would suggest that functional medicine practitioners and health educators recognize how their own perspectives and choices are framed by their relative socioeconomic power. This type of hyper-self-reflexivity (Kapoor 2004) would help reorient functional medicine's current conversation regarding positive "perspective" and correct "choices" toward issues of social justice.

In the absence of hyper-self-reflexivity, functional medicine practitioners and proponents may actively adjust to patients' financial needs without confronting the fact that their patient population is likewise relatively privileged. For example, some functional medicine practitioners guide their patients away from genetic profiling when they believe the patient's money can be better used to implement lifestyle and dietary changes. Patel suggests that bioconsumers "handle all the basics first before you dive deeper into your genomics because you want to be as well as possible for as little cost as possible." In a similar vein, Kresser asserts that most people should start with lifestyle and diet. That is, only those who are complexly ill need a genomic therapeutic approach, including epigenetic counseling, a customized diet, and supplementation protocol. Dr. Lynch agrees, "Genetic testing, while useful, is casting blinders on people because they're forgetting the basics in life. . . . Pay attention to your genetics, absolutely, but do not forget that the basics and the fundamentals in your life are . . . actually more important than the SNPs you are finding." The "basics and fundamentals" he describes resemble Riemann's list of "choices."

I argue that what is considered "basic" from a functional medicine perspective can be difficult for many to achieve when seen through the lens of social inequality. Kresser asserts, "The causes [of most disease] are, of course, poor diet, lack of physical activity, lack of sleep, not managing stress, lack of social connection, lack of pleasure [and] fun—all the things that are so crucial for human beings." From Dr. Szyf's perspective, poor lifestyle habits can make anyone ill, regardless of their genes. "If you become overweight, and you don't exercise, your chances of getting disease, whatever genes you have, are very high." These descriptions run the risk of inadvertently blaming victims. Furthermore, they conceal insidious relationships between poor diets and lifestyles and socioeconomic poverty. Given the prevalence of "food deserts" (Walker, Keane, and Burke 2010; Beaulac, Kristjansson, and Cummins 2009) and troubling food insecurity, I suggest both readers and functional medicine interlocutors acknowledge the striking overlap between "poor diets" and "diets of the poor."

Essentially, I argue that by suggesting that managing emotions is the key to improved health among disadvantaged populations,[28] the functional medicine proponents reveal what I call "structural myopia." I use this analogy to describe how an individuals' view is situated within their own intersectional experience vis-à-vis social structure, leaving them blind to others' experiences and, at times, the structure in general (Haraway 1988; Crenshaw 2014). This inattention to structure could lead to public health programs focused on teaching stress management to the poor instead of providing increased social support to alleviate the causes of stress in the first place. It would place the onus on disadvantaged individuals to reduce the anxiety caused by social inequality instead of championing universal responsibility for creating a more just society. In my perspective, overemphasis on emotional inputs can be just as myopic with regard to structural inequality as overemphasis on biological factors.

It is crucial that I simultaneously (re)emphasize the good intent behind many of my informants' comments when diagnosing "structural myopia" in functional medicine. Functional medicine practitioners who use epigenetic approaches in their clinical practice hope to prevent devastating chronic disease before it occurs. For example, Dr. Joffe views genomic health information as an opportunity to shape changes in behavior through relatively simple changes to individuals' dinner plates. Likewise, Dr. Sabbagh asks, "If I am genetically prone to getting Alzheimer's, can I create an intervention program that will buffer, mitigate, or offset that genetic risk?" He has seen positive outcomes using "lifestyle programs" rooted in "precision health" and suggests this approach will also prove useful for diabetes, heart disease, and cancer.[29] "Lifestyle programs" are meant to be "empowering" since, instead of succumbing to their "genetic fate," individuals can proactively prevent diseases caused by industrialized "lifestyles."[30] Despite these good intentions, many Americans simply lack the necessary resources to participate in functional medicine.[31] Privilege-disadvantage plays a determining role in access to epigenetic therapies. This reality signals the effects of social inequality on genetic expression.

## SOCIOGENOMICS: THE (EPI)GENETICIZATION OF SOCIAL LIFE

The term "sociogenomics" is used by functional medicine interlocutors to describe how the quality of individuals' social connections can produce epigenetic effects. Kresser states, "If we don't have social connection, that's going to impact every different aspect of our health." Kresser's summation is supported by the work of anthropologists and molecular biologists. Kay Martin, a bioevolutionary and sociocultural anthropologist, coined the term "social DNA" to describe the phenotypic expression of epigenetic rules based on social group formation and kinship. She points to how *Homo sapiens* "are the product of gene-culture coevolution spanning at least five to seven million years" (2018, 27). She describes extended evolutionary synthesis (EES), a theory that frames "heredity as a developmental process influenced not only by genes, but by an organism's cumulative interaction with its chemical, natural, and social environments" (35). Her work simultaneously points to how organisms flexibly modify their genetic phenotype in response to rapid environmental change, and, at the same time, how social factors figure into epigenesis as a form of non-random evolution.

Meanwhile, the "reawakening" of molecular biologists' interest in genomics has led to new insights into social epigenetics. Dr. Szyf explains, "The attention to epigenetics . . . changed around 2004. If you look at the PubMed citations, you see an inflection in the curve—an exponential inflection—where genetics is kind of stable and epigenetics is going up." In 2004, Dr. Szyf's team launched the field of social epigenetics by providing the first set of evidence that the social environment in early life can influence DNA methylation. He continues, "[A] paper from our group that showed . . . that [rat] maternal care can change DNA methylation in the children. That was the first glimpse into social epigenetics." Twelve years later, social epigenetics studies continue to astound. Dr. Bland describes a 2016 study that demonstrated how two genes are epigenetically modified by methylation in the wolf's genome to produce the dog's docility (see Janowitz et al. 2016).

These animal studies have set the stage for human social genomics—what Dr. Slavich calls "the science of community." He argues that human interaction is as important as diet and exercise for determining health. While other presenters at the Interpreting Your Genetics Summit signaled that "alcohol consumption, smoking, sedentary lifestyle, poor diet, and psychological stress" can lead to "poor health outcomes," Dr. Slavich emphasized how these can be the result of "poor connections with those around us." He suggested that social factors are even more determining than biological factors and emphasized that low levels of stress and high levels of social connection are more protective than not smoking, eating a good diet, and exercising regularly. Dr. Slavich's argument is supported by the work of Steve Cole, professor of medicine and psychiatry and behavioral sciences at UCLA School of Medicine and author of "Social Regulation of Human Gene Expression" (2009). Cole has also demonstrated that HIV-positive gay men with less social support are more likely to develop AIDS, children with asthma who perceive the social world as frightening are more likely to struggle with inflammation, and people with more social ties get fewer colds.

Furthermore, Dr. Slavich explained that the hardest life events (those with the worst impacts) are those that threaten close social interactions (e.g., getting divorced) since these may damage one's sense of social self and social safety. Dr. Deanna Minich, a certified nutritionist, describes one specific epigenetic mechanism by which these experiences of "targeted rejection" can unleash an inflammatory response: "When we are isolated from supportive tribes, we can actually drive up inflammatory cytokines and markers. Things like IL6 and TNF-alpha could go up." In turn, Dr. Slavich indicated that inflammation "is the common underlying biological pathway for cancer, cardiovascular disease, and depression." Extending Dr. Slavich's thought, Dr. Davis describes inflammation as "the monster" driving diabetes and "so many other chronic diseases we see in society today." The impact of inflammation can be cumulative since those with sustained inflammation are at risk for accumulating multiple diagnoses over time.

In contrast, positive social interactions can confer protective effects. Yale psychiatrist Joan Kaufman, along with a team of researchers, found that a single monthly experience of loving connection with a trusted adult counteracted about 80 percent of the combined effects of severe abuse in fifty-seven school-aged children who had been removed from their home because of abuse (Kaufman et al. 2004). These findings reframe the nature-nurture controversy as a false dichotomy. Carey explains, "We are finally starting to unravel the missing link between nature and nurture; how our environment talks to us and alters us, sometimes forever" (2012, 7). Expanding on how phenotypic expression of genes is influenced by social learning and culture, Kay Martin asserts, "Those who maintain that the human saga has been directed either by the genome or by culture alone are only half right. It is their interface—their complex, synergistic, and dynamic interaction—that accounts for the origins and trajectory of our genus" (2018, 12). I agree with both Carey and Martin, but suggest an increased emphasis on how *social inequalities* differentially shape the effects of "nature" and "nurture" on individuals' bodies.

Although "sociogeonomics" is not usually used by functional medicine interlocutors in this way, I suggest that the term be expanded to include the epigenetic effect of social inequality. Just as functional medicine interlocutors concur that environmental toxins can effect long-term epigenetic consequences, I point to how *social inequality* exacts lasting biosocial, epigenetic effects. By also embracing the epigenetic consequences of social inequalities, functional medicine practitioners and proponents would embrace the full essence of nested ecologies.

I further argue that in addition to its numerous biological and social implications, epigenetics has implications for epidemiology and medical anthropology. Specifically, functional medicine experts recruit epigenetic science to critique epidemiological study designs. Dr. Bland indicates that current epidemiological studies are innately flawed because they assume all study subjects share a common underlying etiology when, in fact, very different (epi)genomic responses can lead to the same health outcome. Similarly, Dr. Beaver reframes disease labels as merely identifiers for different symptoms.[32] He argues these "symptoms" can be caused by diverse underlying drivers of immune dysfunction, including inflammation, oxidative stress, methylation, and vitamin D metabolism. Potential underlying drivers are linked to individuals' genetic profile. At the same time, individuals with the same upstream causes of ill health can have very different downstream manifestations. In either case, personalized lifestyle adaptations can be made to optimize health.

~ *Interlude* ~

# A "VAMPIRE" NO MORE

After spending thirteen years hiding from the sun, I was fed up with hav-ing to cover my skin with long sleeves, a hat, sunscreen, sunglasses—every kind of protection—just to go outside. There were so many activities I missed doing that involved being in the sun and exposed to heat—so many experiences I missed out on because I couldn't uncover myself, not even for a few minutes. I always had two EpiPens on me—one as a backup in case the other one failed—plus oral antihistamines. Preventing a reaction became a way of life, but, despite my best efforts, I had hives regularly.

I read Dr. Amy Myers's books, *The Autoimmune Solution* and *The Thyroid Connection*, which familiarized me with her functional approach to the immune system. Meanwhile, I printed and read everything Alison Vickery posted on her website about histamine intolerance. Vickery's posts were enough to fill a four-inch binder, and among them was a post about the link between histamine intolerance and small intestine bacterial overgrowth (SIBO). Hoping to learn more about how SIBO can contribute to histamine intolerance issues, I attended Dr. Myers's free SIBO webinar. The webinar helped to clarify my understanding of how certain gut microbiota can, in fact, produce histamine. When these bacteria invade the small intestine, they become the most common cause of histamine intolerance. Further-more, SIBO is often the underlying cause of IBS, a diagnosis I had had since age fourteen.

Although I gleaned some valuable information from the webinar, most of the event was, essentially, promotional material for Dr. Myers's SIBO Breakthrough Program, a $379 online course including three supplements and a protein powder. To save money, I decided to proceed without the program. I researched SIBO further and integrated antimicrobial supple-ments, probiotics, and binders into my self-designed personal protocol. At the same time, I began eliminating everything in my life that could be causing my immune system to overreact. This included many foods that, to the average person, seem harmless.

For a few months, I layered together three diets to create my own personal therapeutic approach: the low-histamine diet, SIBO diet, and Autoimmune Paleo diet. The low-histamine diet eliminates foods high in histamine, such as fermented foods (cheese, wine, prosciutto, yogurt, sauerkraut, vinegar), shellfish, ripened fruits, some fruits regardless of ripeness (strawberries, papaya, tomatoes, citrus fruits), anything canned or ready-made, leftovers, and black and green tea, among others. The SIBO diet limits fruits to one cup per day, while eliminating juices and dried fruit. It also limits the total consumption of grains, legumes, and starchy vegetables to one cup per day. The Autoimmune Paleo diet eliminates grains, legumes, dairy products, eggs, nuts and seeds, coffee, chocolate, nightshade vegetables, certain spices, all processed foods, refined sugars and alternative sweeteners, emulsifiers, and food thickeners.

As you might imagine, following this diet was hard—very hard. I was committed to a month of perfect adherence, but after several weeks, I had an apple pie à la mode during a date night with Rikin. He reminded me I was violating my therapeutic dietary plan. At first I resisted, then I cried. I was starving, cranky, and resentful about all of my temporary restrictions. After a brief tantrum, I got back on the horse and recommitted to a month of perfect adherence. I was back at day one. My next attempt was successful, but the process caused me to quickly drop ten pounds from my already slender frame. After thirty days, famished and underweight, I began the process of slowly reintroducing foods back into my diet.

At the same time, I was aware of how my genome made it more difficult for me to detoxify everyday xenobiotics. Not only did I need to eliminate foods that could potentially trigger my immune system, I also needed to purge my life of toxic chemicals. I went through our house and began identifying every product that was not given the "green light" by the Environmental Working Group, a nonprofit organization that conducts research on toxic chemicals in common consumer items like cosmetics and household cleaners. This included so many things—cleaning supplies, hand soap, dish soap, body wash, shampoo, lotion, sunscreen, makeup, skincare, fragrance. . . . The list goes on and on. It was as if my overlapping histamine intolerance and autoimmunity made me allergic to everything, the world, and my life.

Before my initial visit to the immunologist in San Antonio, I was instructed to stop taking antihistamines for five days. This would allow the antihistamines to leave my body and make me more reactive to skin prick tests in the doctor's office. I was unable to complete the requirement. On day two, I began having hives. On day three, the hives covered my entire body and were unbearable, making it impossible for me to sleep and even threatening my airway. Rikin had to administer epinephrine to me in the middle of the night. By the time we got to the doctor's office on day five, the immunologist was unable to obtain any diagnostic information from prick tests.

Hearing how the 10 mg of Zyrtec I had been taking per day for the last three years was now insufficient for keeping my symptoms in check, the immunologist decided to prescribe three different antihistamines—five pills per day. Initially, I took them. After a few days, however, I thought, "What the heck am I doing?" I refused to become more and more dependent on drugs to manage my symptoms. I returned to my 10 mg of Zyrtec per day, but I knew there had to be another way. Since I was removing everything that could be a potential contributor to my histamine intolerance, I was hopeful I could quit taking antihistamines. At the same time, I knew this would be difficult.

I read in *The Health Professional's Guide to Food Allergies and Intolerances*, by Dr. Janice Vickerstaff Joneja, that antihistamines can cause rebound symptoms and, essentially, dependence. Even though I was taking an over-the-counter medication at a dose that is considered normal for many people, I knew I needed to come off it. So I decided to quit cold turkey.

The experience echoed my attempt to stop taking antihistamines before visiting the immunologist. On the second day, hives began creeping across my skin like a patchwork quilt. On the night of the third day, I was in bed, unable to sleep. Every inch of my body was crawling, itching, and screaming. I broke down and took the antihistamine. My symptoms disappeared in under fifteen minutes.

Similar to my "falling off the wagon" with my elimination diets, my failure sparked a renewed determination. I was pissed. I needed to break my dependence on antihistamines. There was just nothing else to it. I started again with day one. Again, on the third night, I was in the grips of anaphylaxis. Unable to sleep, I waited, and waited. I began trembling uncontrollably. My airway began to swell, so I focused all my attention on breathing slowly and shallowly. Rikin was worried. "This has already gone too far! I either need to use the EpiPen on you or I need to take you to the emergency room!" I whispered to him, "Lower your voice. If I get anxious, I am going to have a worse reaction." I slowly walked over to the shower and turned the cold water on high. Cold showers have always helped calm my allergic reactions, and this night was no different. At first, immersion in cold water made me tremble more violently, but it also helped me focus. With fewer hives and a more stable airway, I returned to bed.

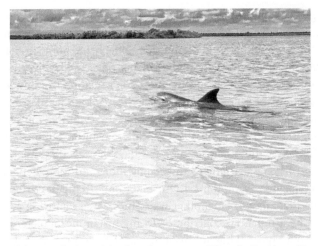

*Dolphins in the Sian Kaʼan biosphere reserve. Photo by Rosalynn Vega.*

Days four and five were progressively worse. During the day, I made sure to avoid histaminergic activities like exercise. During the night, my reactions worsened, and I needed all of my focus in order to breathe and calm my trembling. Rikin was constantly concerned about me. He tried to coax me into taking antihistamines by saying, "Maybe this is something you have to do in steps? Maybe you can just do three days this time, and next time it will be three and a half days. Then after that you can try a few more hours. Then you can just continue adding on a few hours each time." I was not convinced. (Have I mentioned I am stubborn?) I equated my experience of quitting antihistamines with going through a narcotics withdrawal. I needed to bite the bullet and make it all the way through.

Then, on the morning of day six, I woke up with no symptoms. None. It was as if a light switch had been turned off. I had broken through an invisible glass. With some trepidation, I began experimenting with going outside and exposing myself to the sun and heat. Nothing happened. Rikin and I went to the beach at South Padre Island. I was fine. Over time, I became more and more daring, but I still carried my EpiPens with me just in case.

Over the following months, I mailed stool specimens for direct-to-consumer lab testing. The results showed pathogenic bacteria and a slight amount of rare yeast. To correct these imbalances in my gut microbiome, I added bacteriophage, plant-based enzymes, caprylic acid, and tailored probiotics to my supplement protocol. While the idea of swallowing bacteriophages—capsules filled with an active virus that targets pathogenic bacteria—seemed hard to stomach at first, I decided to place my faith in "science" and proceed with my treatment plan. Combining my dietary intervention with targeted supplements produced marvelous results. The IBS symptoms I had been struggling with for more than twenty years vanished—almost as if by miracle.

A few months later, I traveled to Tulum, Quintana Roo. When I arrived at my hotel, I was handed a number of tour pamphlets, including an advertisement for a small boat tour through the Sian Ka'an biosphere reserve. Prior to this visit, I would have discarded the Sian Ka'an pamphlet immediately without even considering the tour. A full day without shade, in the middle of a body of water, with no access to emergency health services, was an unthinkable risk. This time, I looked through the glossy photos for all of the different tours and considered all of them equally. I asked the receptionist, a young French expatriate, which tour she thought was best. She told me she had gone on the Sian Ka'an exploration with her family, and it was perhaps the best tour she had ever experienced.

Several days later, I was out on the water in the biosphere reserve. The sun was high in the sky and its searing rays were beating down on us. The tour guide and boat driver were both well prepared with high UPF rash guards, Buffs, baseball caps, and sunglasses. The six tourists on the boat, myself included, were less prepared. Initially, I tried to use an umbrella or a straw hat, but the wind made it impossible to use both. The skin of my fairer boat mates burned and turned tomato red. My skin quickly deepened in color from golden tan to peanut brown. But nothing else happened!

There was so much of the world I couldn't see or explore when I was allergic to the sun and heat. That day, I saw dolphins, manatees, turtles, alligators, and numerous species of birds in their natural habitat, from just a few meters away. I could not have been more grateful to have overcome my allergies.

CHAPTER 4

# THE POLITICAL ECOLOGY OF "HUMAN" MICROBIOLOGY

I am large, I contain multitudes.
WALT WHITMAN, "SONG OF MYSELF"

Emerging discourse on the human microbiome offers medical anthropologists novel opportunities for theoretical interrogation, methodological exploration, and applied intervention. Sharp (2019) points to anthropology's long-standing concern with human-animal interdependencies and, specifically, to medical anthropologists' sustained attention to nonhuman species as pathogens, vectors, and reservoirs of disease. At the same time, she critiques medical anthropology for being slow to engage contemporary theorizing about interspecies entanglements. Fuentes (2019) similarly indicates that innovative research questions in medical anthropology involving multispecies approaches are primed to produce both theoretical and methodological insights regarding the Anthropocene—the period during which human activity is considered the dominant influence on the environment—and the processes, patterns, and constructs of health. For their part, Brown and Nading (2019) write, "Conditions of the Anthropocene force us to develop new tools to think about human animal entanglement" (5). In their view, human animal health—how animals are implicated in health, well-being, and pathogenicity—prompts us to revisit theorizations of ecology, biopolitics, and care, thus moving beyond traditional boundaries of medical anthropology as a discipline.

In this chapter, I ask not only what studying the microbiome offers to anthropology, but also what anthropology offers to studies of the microbiome. How can we theorize the primacy of the gut in functional medicine and in emerging science at large? If a paradigm shift is underway, what role do social, political, economic factors play? Who are the beneficiaries and what are the costs of "gut science"?

## MICROBIAL EPIGENETICS

In order to bring medical anthropology critiques to bear on functional medicine discourse regarding the microbiome, I must first engage functional medicine descriptions of the multiple ways microbes effect epigenetic change on human genes (henceforth referred to as "microbial epigenetics"). Dr. Kellman characterizes the microbiome—the totality of microbes living within and on us—as "so powerful, it affects even the expression of your genes" (2018, 11). Similarly, Dr. Zach Bush, internist, endocrinologist, and hospice care specialist, states, "We are starting to see the truth that bacteria and fungi are governing human genomics and human health." Thus, the microbiome influences how our genes are expressed and how our bodies function—what Dr. Bland describes as "the major breakthrough of the last decade."

According to functional medicine interlocutors, the science of microbial epigenetics will transform our understandings of human physiology in the coming decade. Dr. Datis Kharrazian, a research scientist, professor, and clinician, writes, "The discoveries of the microbiome will help us understand how our genes combined with diet, lifestyle, and environmental factors impact chronic disease." Dr. Bush indicates that researchers at the University of California, San Diego, and the University of California, Los Angeles, have recently discovered that the ion channels on the surface of bacteria are very similar to the ion channels in human neurons. As a result of this emerging research, he says, "we are watching human biology be redefined every day." Ion exchange is just one of the examples he shares for how microbes interact with human cells.

Nutritional consultant Donna Gates offers an example of microbial epigenetics. "Lipopolysaccharides from gram-negative bacteria can cause leaky gut, fever, blood clotting, etc. Their genes upregulate our virulence genes. This causes inflammation, thus having a harmful effect on the immune system." In turn, Dr. Kellman clarifies, "Changing your diet, lifestyle, and stress levels very quickly alters the composition and behavior of your microbiome." Thus, microbes and human genes share a cyclical relationship since epigenetic factors can also shape the behavior of our microbes.

Functional medicine interlocutors furthermore argue that bacteria can be beneficial to human hosts by complementing or offsetting genomic effects. Referring to SNPs, Dr. Yousef Elyaman, founder of Absolute Health, says, "For every one of these [human] genes, there is a bacteria that could be living inside of us that can actually do the same thing." Thus, if an individual is at a genetic "disadvantage"—for example, a decreased ability to metabolize certain nutrients or produce particular neurotransmitters due to an "unfavorable" SNP—those effects can be offset by gut bacteria that are able to do the work of metabolizing those same nutrients and producing needed neurotransmitters.[1]

Functional medicine discourse (re)frames humans as transitional organisms—that is, beings undergoing constant change. It furthermore challenges anthropogenic perspectives by positioning microbes as protagonists acting upon comparatively passive humans. Dr. Bush asserts that "there is so much non-human life in the invisible world that is in and around you that's actually changing who you are minute to minute, second to second, through your genetics." According to Dr. Kellman, most of our biochemistry comes from our bacteria since "the microbiome has far more genes than you do, by a factor of one hundred and fifty to one" (2018, 11).

Throwing into question the dichotimization of "our bacteria" and "us," functional medicine interlocutors suggest that our microbiomes shape and determine who we are. Dr. Mayer describes how transferring gut microbiota from an "extrovert" mouse to a "timid" mouse causes the timid one to behave in a more gregarious manner. Similarly, transferring stool from an obese mouse to a lean mouse causes the lean mouse to develop a voracious appetite and eat to obesity. Microbiologist Kiran Krishnan rendered findings like these relevant to humans. He asserts, "No two individuals in the world have the same microbiome, not even identical twins." While identical twins share the same DNA, their microbiomes can be up to 30 percent different. Krishnan continues, "That means they have 30 trillion organism difference within the microbiome." From the perspective of functional medicine, dissimilarity between microbiomes potentially explains disparate health outcomes, physiological differences, and distinct worldviews found in twin studies.[2]

Thus, functional medicine interlocutors suggest that the microbiome is what constitutes the bioindividual. Nakayama signals that protocols don't work "because they don't take into account the 'omics' and microbiome of the bioindividual." Likewise, Gates says, "You can't talk about personalized genomics without looking at their microbial genetics. It is a two-way street. . . . Ninety-eight percent of what determines how our body runs is determined by the gut microbiome." Many functional medicine practitioners agree that functional medicine should primarily focus on the gut even before considering genetics. "Personalized medicine" locates biological uniqueness in an individual's microbiome.

By focusing on how microbes epigenetically influence human genes, functional medicine rejects genetic determinism. Functional medicine interlocutors indicate how changes in our microbiome alter the genetic expression of human genes, thus potentiating new states of health. Dr. Kellman calls this "profoundly empowering" since "[i]nstead of being stuck with the dictates of your inherited human genes, you have the power to transform your *microbial* gene pool—by altering your microbiome" (2018, 69). Kellman argues that by shaping their microbiomes, individuals can influence their biochemistry, cognition, mood, and, ultimately, the state of their health.

I embrace the transformative potential of microbial epigenetics; however, extending my argument from chapter 3, I emphasize how "empowerment" to effect epigenetic change is buttressed by socioeconomic privilege. In so doing, I am building upon Amber Benezra's work on how social determinants effect microbiota (see Benezra 2020) and Jamie Lorimer's assertion that "[t]he beneficiaries of this modernized microbial future are unevenly distributed in space and across social groups" (2017, 5).

The primary way that functional medicine practitioners manipulate the microbiome—and therefore the epigenetic effects of the microbiome on human genes—is through food. Dr. William Li writes, "[Epigenetic change] allows DNA to react to environmental and lifestyle exposures, including diet, by amplifying helpful genes and blocking detrimental ones" (2019, 56). Responding to Dr. Li, Dr. Hyman signals that thinking of food as information, not just calories, is a frame shift. He explains that food is "not just energy, but instructions that regulate your stem cells, and your DNA, and your microbiome, and your immune system, and angiogenesis." Dr. Bland explains that while food may not be of utmost concern in the emergency medicine situations for which conventional medicine is best adapted, "[i]n terms of the pattern of emergence of chronic disease, [foods] are the most important things. They watch over our genes 24/7, 365." From a functional medicine perspective, food exhibits a "low signal strength" in the short term, but it is primary in shaping our long-term well-being.

Thus, some functional medicine practitioners have focused on the relationship between diet and aging when describing the microbial epigenetic effects of food. Dr. Li writes, "A good diet, quality sleep, regular exercise, and other healthy activities can protect your telomeres" (2019, 56). Dr. Marvin Edeas, physician and microbiome researcher, goes so far as to assert, "Tell me what you eat, I can tell you how you live and the quality of your lifestyle." From a functional medicine perspective, examining an individual's diet is a good predictor of their longevity.

Furthermore, functional medicine interlocutors argue that what we eat not only shapes our health, but can also have lasting effects on future generations. Ji explains that billions of years of biological information, encoded within our cells, is either activated or remains latent depending on the types of food we ingest. Thus, functional medicine interlocutors recast conventional biomedical understandings of genetic inheritance by positioning food as an epigenetic inheritance system, thus disrupting Euro-American notions of time by signaling how the past is embedded within the present.

Similarly, functional medicine interlocutors argue that our actions in the present are embedded in future (micro)biologies. Dr. William Li writes, "Scientists from Stanford, Harvard, and Princeton studying diet and microbiome have shown that, if we're not careful, the way we eat can actually force the extinction of some gut bacteria, which can impact on the health of future generations" (2019, 47). Dr. Li describes a study in which mice were switched from a plant-based diet to a high-fat, low-fiber diet. The diversity of their gut bacteria suffered greatly. When they returned to a plant-based diet, only some of that diversity was recovered. Dr. Li identifies this persistent defect as a "scar" left on the microbiome. "The microbiome scar became larger over generations when the researchers began breeding the mice and exposing each generation of mice to the high-fat, low-fiber Western-style diet." Generations of eating an unhealthy high-fat, low-fiber diet caused healthy gut microbes to become extinct. Health-protecting microbes could not be regenerated, even after reexposure to a healthier plant-based diet. According to Dr. Li, these recent findings emphasize the important, permanent effects of diet in determining our health and shaping our identities.

As the field of nutrigenomics booms, functional medicine interlocutors express excitement about what they see as emerging scientific understandings on how the gut microbiome produces lasting change in the body through the effects of microRNA on "junk DNA." Dr. Bush likewise explains, "Only 1 percent of your genome . . . will ultimately go on to make an RNA and a protein. The other 99 percent we thought was junk. We called it 'junk DNA.'" This term reflects the extreme degree of ignorance in genetics at the time of the Human Genome Project regarding the true function of this DNA. Dr. Bland explains, "We really are starting to recognize that what used to be called 'junk DNA' is actually, to a great extent, the antennae that are out there receiving information from the outside environment, to then translate that to the genome or to the coding portions of the genes." "Junk DNA" produces microRNA, which act as a communication network and control the genetic expression of different genes in the body.

In this view, microRNA are both a form of epigenetic potential and interspecies communication. Humans excrete microRNA through saliva, urine, breast milk, and feces. If these end up in our soil, it can influence the genetics of plants. Dr. Bush explains, "The microRNA can go into the nucleus of another species and change the behavior of the genes within that species. So we are finding a trans-species genetic plasticity happening across the ecosystem." The microRNA of non-human species can also change the behavior of human DNA. Describing bacterial microRNA, Dr. Achacoso says, "Those can actually fuse directly with our cells, and when they do they actually affect us and direct our genes epigenetically." Krishnan elaborates on Dr. Achacoso's explanation: "Bacteria control our genes by producing microRNA that then sit at the promotor regions of our genes and interfere with how a gene is being expressed. [MicroRNA] can change the structure of the protein that genes produce or change the enzymes that produce proteins." That is, while individual genes are responsible for making particular proteins and enzymes necessary for different metabolic activities, microRNA from bacteria can control human genes by changing the type of proteins and enzymes that genes are making.

From the perspective of some functional medicine practitioners and proponents, we are now living in a post-genomic era (see Lock 2017). Dismissing genetic determinism, Ji notes that "[bacteria] help to orchestrate the complexity of our being." Since only 0.05 percent of all disease is due to congenital monogenetic inheritance, Ji opines that RNA, not DNA, is clearly the future. As readers might imagine, the primary way functional medicine practitioners envision shifting microRNA is through diet. Dr. Achacoso indicates, "Food, for example, has been shown to put out microRNAs that control our epigenome. . . . Things that we eat . . . communicate with us at that [epigenomic] level." Dr. Tsoukalas concurs: "We [know] that microRNAs are present mostly in the vegetable foods. They produce . . . very important epigenetic reactions with[in] our genome." While functional medicine practitioners have always emphasized the primacy of diet, they increasingly point to emerging scientific evidence of how food modulates our genetic response.

At the same time, functional medicine proponents argue that an "ancestral diet," influenced by region, culture, and "tradition," can produce intergenerational effects.[3] Ji notes, "When you think about grandma's recipes, a pinch of this spice here and cooking a certain food a certain way, this information that's embedded in those formulas is as valuable and meaningful and impactful to your life and your body as the genes you inherit." He reframes cultural traditions in culinary practices as epigenetic inheritance systems. As a child, I deemed daycare food—for example, tater tots, hot dogs, and hamburgers—inedible because they were not Popo's home cooking, so I can appreciate the idea of an ancestral diet. However, as an anthropologist, I am wary of how this notion essentializes culture and romanticizes tradition. During my ethnographic research, I observed how functional medicine proponents inadvertently exoticized non-Western Others, thus reinscribing structures of inequality.

Culture aside, functional medicine proponents indicate that food literally constitutes the human. In chapter 3, I noted that the human genome contains a similar number of genes to a single grain of rice. Functional medicine interlocutors emphasize how microRNA from food acts upon the 99 percent of the human genome that was deemed "junk DNA," thus altering gene expression and making us human. Ji explains, "Basically, we're finding that over the course of evolution we have literally outsourced gene regulation to the plants in our environment." Providing one example, Ji notes that turmeric "upregulates one thousand genes and downregulates another one thousand genes." Thinking of humans as interconnected and interdependent with non-human species presents novel opportunities for therapeutic intervention and anthropological theorization (Sharp 2019).

In the next section, I explore functional medicine discourse regarding how this interdependence unfolds through metabolic processes. In addition to microRNA, microbiota act upon human health through the metabolites they produce—the intermediate or end products of metabolic processes. Dr. Achacoso describes the gut microbiome as a unique organ and ecosystem that "has its own metabolites, it has its own way of generating energy, it has its own particular functions." Metabolites produced by the gut microbiome directly affect the functioning of the rest of the body.

## METABOLITES

Seen from a functional medicine perspective, the microbiome is a bountiful resource. Krishnan notes, "We know that our microbiome produces every form of quinols, so CoQ10, ubiquinol—things that we look for . . . and spend a lot of money for in supplements." Providing carotenoids, antioxidants, beta-carotene, alpha-carotene, astaxanthin, and zeaxanthin as additional examples, Krishnan asserts, "All of these amazingly important micronutrients are produced at high levels in a healthy microbiome." Micronutrients are dietary elements needed by the human body in small amounts to maintain health. He explains, "The beauty of it is all being produced right at the site of absorption, right in the microvilli where things need to be sucked right in." Accordingly, functional medicine providers often aim to support metabolic processes instead of relying on constant supplementation since the microbiome produces micronutrients at the very site where they need to be absorbed.

This perspective recasts existing notions of food, digestion, and nutrition. Dr. Achacoso signals that certain key nutrients are derived primarily or exclusively from microbiota. These nutrients include thiamine, riboflavin, biotin, pantothenic acid, folate, vitamin B12, vitamin K, short-chain fatty acids, natural antibiotics, and neurotransmitters (see Kellman 2018, 95). According to emerging science on the microbiome, it is not the nutrients in food, but instead the metabolites that microbiota produce from the nutrients in food that confer beneficial effects for the human body. To make this distinction clear, Dr. Achacoso describes how a friend, a mitochondria researcher, decided to test the standing hypothesis that polyphenols in red wine are responsible for its beneficial health effects. The research found an absence of polyphenols from red wine in the bloodstream. As a result, Dr. Achacoso explains, "it's suspected the gut microbiota [are] actually generating some . . . unidentified metabolite that's actually inducing the beneficial effect to the body." Without the proper gut microbiota for beneficial metabolic processes, consuming "healthy" and "nutritious" foods would not produce the same effect.

In essence, metabolites have captured the attention and imagination of functional medicine practitioners. This "scientific imaginary" (see DelVecchio Good 2010; Smelik 2010; and Miller 2013) has led functional medicine practitioners and health educators to describe microbiota in anthropomorphic and agentive ways. Dr. Achacoso explains, "[Microbiota] actually preprocess everything that you eat." Dr. Li analogizes the "preprocessing" of fiber to "giving a sculptor a block of wood and saying, 'Do something with it!'" In his analogy, "the bacteria, our gut microbiome, take up that block of wood and start making sculptures." The sculptures in Dr. Li's analogy are vitamins, hormones, and neurotransmitters.

Functional medicine discourse on metabolites emphasizes the agency of microbiota in ways that cast microorganisms as being in control of our bodies. Dr. Gail Cresci of the Lerner Research Institute indicates, "We know that the gut microbiota prefer fermentable fiber. . . . The microbiota possess the enzymes and metabolic machinery to digest these fibers. And as a result, they produce beneficial byproducts such as vitamins, short-chain fatty acids." These short-chain fatty acids prevent potentially pathogenic strains of bacteria from behaving in pathogenic ways. Dr. Cresci explains that butyrate, a particularly well-studied short-chain fatty acid, is able to preserve immune function that would potentially be disrupted by pathogenic bacteria. "That preservation of the immune function is linked with more rapid clearance of the pathogenic bacteria as well as a quicker resolution of the good composition of the elimination of the gut dysbiosis." In essence, certain microbiota protect human hosts from potential "invaders."

From the functional medicine perspective, beneficial microbiota also affect a myriad of other functions in the body. Dr. Cresci notes that butyrate regulates inflammation, preserves the intestinal barrier, facilitates the migration of immune cells, and helps to decrease reactive oxygen species in our body—highly reactive chemical compounds that can cause damage to normal physiology. Through histone deacetylation, butyrate modifies the structure of human DNA, thus changing gene expression. Dr. William Li adds, "[Short-chain fatty acids] are anti-inflammatory. They boost our immune system, they help regulate our blood sugar, they lower our cholesterol, they suppress cancer risk, and they prevent blood vessels from [supplying blood to] cancer [tumors] as well." Dr. Cresci expands on this comment, describing how, through the clinical replacement of butyrate transporters, butyrate is capable of destroying cancer cells. Evincing the theme of anthropomorphization and agentification, Dr. Cresci describes the elimination of cancer cells by butyrate as "Batman against the evil."

Thus, when the gut microbiome produces deficient levels of beneficial metabolites, individuals are more susceptible to diseases. Kresser points to "studies where they found that people with autoimmune disease often have lower levels of butyrate, which makes sense. That means that our gut bacteria might actually impact our susceptibility to autoimmune disease." By examining the metabolome—the totality of metabolites in the body, and the metabolic reactions they produce—functional medicine providers may be able to detect and correct imbalances, thus preventing or reversing disease processes. Providing two examples, Dr. Achacoso suggests that metabolic information can be proved useful "if a patient has higher levels of DHPPA, a compound that is found [at higher levels] in autistic kids, or has high levels of arabinose, which is an indicator that the patient may be having intestinal candidiasis." Functional medicine practitioners attempt to correct imbalances through multiple means, including intervening on intermicrobial communication.

Functional medicine interlocutors describe anthromorphized, agentive microbiota as "talking to one another." While current studies correlate the presence or absence of specific bacterial strains to particular diseases, Dr.

Bush suspects that what is really determining human health is "what these bacteria are saying to each other." He explains that one species of bacteria may behave a certain way when isolated in a petri dish, but its behavior changes entirely when it is exposed to another species of bacteria.

Dr. Bush's suppositions speak to anthropological concerns regarding the potential for "post-paleo" microbiopolitics more broadly (see Lorimer 2019; Paxson 2008). In this vein, Wolf-Meyer asks: What are the politics of the microbes themselves? He writes, "Politics would seem to be much more micro than we have been led to believe, and accounting for the motives of our symbionts seems to be increasingly necessary as we shepherd our internal colonies, who may be at war among themselves and with us as well." (2017, 6)

As if responding to Wolf-Meyer, functional medicine researchers describe bacteria as strategizing within their own genus regarding how to interact with bacteria of other genera. For example, listeria, pathogenic, food-borne bacteria that can cause disease in the body, communicate among themselves in order to make group-wide decisions on when to attack. Through a process called "quorum sensing," listeria excrete a chemical signature that only microbes within their same species can read, thus informing each other of their concentration. At low concentrations, listeria are benign and do not express their toxin-producing genes. Mimicking the "dialogue" he imagines among listeria, Krishnan says, "If we start expressing now, we're going to alert the immune system. We're not strong enough to cause any problems, and we're just going to be suppressed." Then, imagining how listeria whisper among themselves as they reach higher concentrations, Krishnan mimics, "Hey, we're at a billion now. We're at ten billion. We're at one hundred billion." After reaching a particular threshold, listeria synchronize their gene expression to begin producing toxins.

While Krishnan portrays listeria as scheming criminals, he describes certain environmental bacteria as the gut microbiome's police. "Certain microbes, like *Bacillus* endospore, for example . . . have the capability of reading all the bacteria signatures and figuring out who's there, who's there at too high concentrations, and who's there at low concentrations." In Krishnan's example, *Bacillus* endospores produce up to twenty-five different types of antibiotics to kill overgrowths of harmful bacteria. At the same time, *Bacillus* endospores produce prebiotics to regrow helpful bacteria that are undergrown. Gates extends Krishnan's anthropomorphizing descriptions of bacteria when she describes *Lactobacillus plantarum* as "leaders." According to Gates, these microbes provide the instructions for other bacteria, telling them what to do. To my ethnographic ear, Krishnan's analogy of bacterial "criminals" and "police" and Gates's description of *Lactobacillus plantarum* as "leaders" are reminiscent of Dr. Cresci's "Batman against the evil." These descriptions suggest that while bacteria may be at war with themselves, as long as "good" bacteria outnumber the "bad," they are not at war with their human hosts.

Krishnan goes on to describe not only how bacteria communicate with each other, but also how they communicate with "our" cells.[4] Krishnan explains, "This is something called inter-kingdom communication." To explain how awe-inspiring inter-kingdom communication truly is, Krishnan provides the following analogy: "If a dog spoke English, we would be fascinated. That would be the most famous dog in the world. Maybe the most famous organism in the world." Returning to the microbiome, Krishnan explains that bacteria speak the language of human cells through the metabolites they produce.

In sum, functional medicine proponents frame gut bacteria metabolites as a vast communication system within the body. Dr. Kharrazian emphasizes that this signaling system has "a powerful impact on the brain, the immune system, the cardiovascular system, etc." Dr. Hazen concurs, "What we are now finding is that many of these compounds [metabolites made by the microbiome] have effects on our bodies. They play a role in the control of blood pressure, heart disease, diabetes risk, obesity. It's really astounding." According to these functional medicine providers, emerging science on gut bacteria metabolites is the major breakthrough of the last decade.[5]

Functional medicine interlocutors refer to this emerging science as "metabolomics." According to Dr. Achacoso, humans have more than four thousand clinically significant metabolites in their bodies, and this number is increasing due to exposure to environmental toxins. He chose to study the metabolome because, while "the genes can tell us what can happen . . . the metabolome tells us what is happening now." Metabolic information provides functional medicine clinicians with what they see as practical, actionable insight regarding how to treat patients in real time.

In the future, functional medicine researchers hope to "listen in" on intermicrobial communication and perhaps even sway the conversation through clinical therapies. Krishnan asks, "How do we interpret some of this speaking among bacteria? Can we use quorum sensing for the good? Can we take bacteria language and cause that to effect changes within the microbiome?" These questions point to the goal of guiding inter-kingdom conversations toward human health across different bodily systems.

## THE GUT-BRAIN CONNECTION: DISRUPTING MIND/ BODY AND SOCIAL/BIOLOGICAL BINARIES

When discussing intermicrobial communication across the human body, functional medicine practitioners describe the gut as the "second brain." Speaking on *Autoimmune Secrets*, Dr. Bush observes that this terminology has gained popularity over the last decade and that emerging microbiome research has rendered this description even "more radical." While the gut has always been the focus of functional medicine therapies, functional medicine interlocutors are turning to microbiome science to support their view of gut microbiota as the "forgotten organ."

This framework problematizes existing notions of human intelligence to such a degree that Dr. George Papanicolaou, a doctor of osteopathic medicine, suggests that the gut is the *first* brain. Providing evolutionary evidence to support his assertion, Dr. Papanicolaou explains that the gut preexisted our cerebrum. The latter—which he refers to as the "second brain"—only developed after the incorporation of mitochondria into the human body. While Krishnan indicates that designations of "first" and "second" are debatable, functional medicine practitioners agree that the brain contains "a powerful intelligence of its own" (Kellman 2018, 20).

Comparisons between the gut and the brain are not only qualitative, but also quantitative. Functional medicine interlocutors tend to describe the weight of the gut microbiome as equal to or greater than the brain. Dr. Sarkis Mazmanian, professor of microbiology at Caltech, indicates that the bacterial cells contained in the human body weigh as much as "the brain itself." Krishnan elaborates, "If you take the full load of microbes within the gut, it weighs about two and a half pounds. When you look at the brain, it's about two and a half pounds." Over the course of my ethnographic research, I encountered similar, weight-based comparisons offered by Dr. William Li and Dr. Mayer.[6]

While the gut microbiome has a similar weight to the brain, the gut may have greater sensory capacity than the brain. Dr. Mayer writes, "Since taste and olfactory receptors are located throughout the GI tract rather than only in the mouth and nose, their original names—'taste' and 'smell'—have become somewhat obsolete" (2016, 61). He furthermore indicates that the sensory network of the gut is distributed over its entire surface area, which, he explains, "is two hundred times larger than the surface area of your skin—about the size of a basketball court" (2016, 65). From this perspective, the gut is the site of our most intimate interaction with the outside world. We "taste" and "smell" as we absorb molecules and nutrients into our very being.

The enteric nervous system is also described by functional medicine interlocutors as more comprehensive than the central nervous system. Dr. Neil Nedley, internist and author, explains, "If we were to scrape all of the nerves off of the gut . . . they would weigh four times the amount of the entire spinal cord." Dr. Mayer similarly describes the enteric nervous system as a network extending from the esophagus to the rectum and consisting of "one thousand times more cells than exist in your brain and spinal cord" (2016, 93). These descriptions portray the gut as a comprehensive sensory network that processes massive amounts of information.

In fact, the enteric nervous system is so comprehensive that it can operate independently of the first brain. This allows people to swallow and digest food even when their limbs are paralyzed. Krishnan further explains that the gut is unique because it is the only part of the body that "can perpetuate without the brain being involved." Every other organ in the human body requires brain signals to function. In contrast, the brain seems to depend on vital information from the gut (Mayer 2016). Seen from this perspective, the enteric nervous system predominates over the central nervous system.

However, in practice, the gut and the brain usually do not operate independently—rather, they operate interdependently. Dr. Maya Shetreat notes that microbes are "in constant communication with all of the other systems of the body. With the brain, it controls how we feel, how we think, how we remember and learn, and how we sleep." Dr. Mayer refers to the influence the gut has on the brain as "the gut-brain connection." He writes, "Twenty-four hours a day, seven days a week, our GI tract, enteric nervous system, and brain are in constant communication" (2016, 57). While human thoughts were once considered to be seated in the brain, functional medicine interlocutors argue that they result from ongoing conversation between the gut and the brain. This recent discovery led Dr. Kellman to propose a "new brain," represented by the following formula (see Kellman 2018, 4):

The New Brain = Brain + Microbiome + Gut

In this vein, Krishnan explains, "As it turns out, the bacteria within the gut have a direct connection to the brain. It's a two-way system." Dr. Kellman concurs, "The brain-gut axis is a two-way street on which information is continually flowing in both directions" (2018, 79). Extending Dr. Kellman's description, Dr. Papanicolaou refers to recent research and asserts that the "vagus nerve is a superhighway from the gut to the brain." The vagus nerve is the primary physiological structure connecting the gut to the brain.

While functional medicine interlocutors emphasize that the gut and the brain are in constant communication, they suggest that the gut dominates the conversation. Dr. O'Bryan emphasizes, "For every message from the brain going down to the gut, there are nine messages from the gut going back up to the brain, and those messages are coming from the microbiota, the bacteria in your gut." For Dr. Kellman, however, the imbalance is even more extreme. He writes, "This conversation is surprisingly lopsided, because most of it—by a factor of 40 to 1—is initiated by the microbiome" (2018, 103). According to functional medicine interlocutors, the gut is the primary command center controlling the human body.

Functional medicine interlocutors' assertions about the gut's communicative dominance are supported by microbiome science. Krishnan explains, "Bacteria within your gut can actually produce chemicals like neurotransmitters, peptides, things that could influence your thought and the way you react to the world around you." Providing specific examples, Dr. William Li writes, "Some gut bacteria . . . have endocrine or hormonal functions and can even produce and release brain neurotransmitters such as oxytocin, serotonin, GABA, and dopamine. These chemicals are active brain signals that profoundly influence our mood" (2019, 36). Dr. Amy Myers writes, "What many people don't realize is that 95% of your neurotransmitters are produced in the gut." These research findings inform the functional medicine view of the gut as thinking and feeling (see Wilson 2015)—a paradigm shift regarding the purpose of the gut in the human body.

This paradigm shift is furthermore supported by intestinal anatomy. Dr. Mayer explains, "The lining of your gut is studded with a huge number of endocrine cells, specialized cells that contain up to twenty different types of hormones that can be released into the blood stream if called upon" (2016, 12). Characterizing the gut as the primary endocrine organ, Dr. Mayer continues, "If you could clump all these endocrine cells together into one mass, it would be greater than all your other endocrine organs—your gonads, thyroid gland, pituitary gland, and adrenal glands—combined" (2016, 12). Due to the gut's powerful hormone-producing capability, the brain may seek "help" from the gut when it detects that a certain hormone is deficient. Krishnan anthropomorphizes the brain and gut when he describes how the brain tells the gut bacteria: "Hey, we need more of this hormone or more of that hormone." In playing its role in endocrine health, the gut is responsive to the needs of the brain.

Functional medicine interlocutors argue that conventional medicine's pharmaceutical approach to neurological disorders produces limited benefits because it ignores the powerful role of the gut. Dr. Mazmanian explains, "The antidepressant Prozac is given to people orally, but only about 1 percent of it gets into the brain to increase levels of serotonin . . . . Even then, we have no way of directing those drugs to the regions of the brain where they are needed the most." Dr. Mazmanian compares the serotonin-deficient brain to a car low on oil. In his analogy, taking antidepressants are akin to pouring oil all over the engine and hoping that some of the oil makes its way through the oil cap. From Dr. Mazmanian's perspective, conventional medicine will have to embrace the power of the gut microbiome in order to overcome obstacles in crossing the blood-brain barrier and treating neurological disorders. "The future of medicine may include the concept of drugs from bugs, meaning that someday, you and I may go to the doctor and be prescribed a pill with live bacteria inside of it as the remedy." These *encephalobiotics*—or biotics for your brain (see Prescott and Logan 2017, 223)—would change the gut, indirectly treating neurological disorders by directly targeting the microbiome.

At present, serotonin is the preeminent hormone in gut-brain discourse for functional medicine interlocutors. Dr. Rodger Murphree, a chiropractor, explains, "You have more serotonin receptors in your intestinal tract than you do in your brain." Dr. Kellman, Dr. Bush, and Dr. Mayer estimate that 90 to 95 percent of serotonin is made in the gut.

Functional medicine interlocutors likely emphasize serotonin in gut-brain discourse because it is an appropriate therapeutic target for functional medicine intervention. Serotonin levels are very responsive to dietary changes. Dr. Mayer indicates, "Serotonin-containing cells [in the gut] are influenced by what we eat, and by the signals that the brain sends to them, informing them about our emotional state" (2016, 23). Dr. Mayer describes how a serotonin-lowering diet has been shown to increase the likelihood of depression in at-risk individuals, including those with a family history of depression. This relationship between diet and serotonin led Dr. Murphree to refer to the "standard American diet" as the "SAD diet." This clever description is both an acronym and a play on words. By prescribing a serotonin-boosting diet, functional medicine practitioners are often able to improve patients' mood without medications.

Functional medicine practitioners may also focus on serotonin because it serves as a clear example of systems biology in action. Neurotransmitters shape both gut and brain health. To explain this concept, Dr. Murphree offers as an example the relationship between irritable bowel syndrome and anxiety or depression. When serotonin is depleted, individuals are more likely to experience anxiety or depression. At the same time, irritable bowel syndrome may occur because serotonin controls gut motility.

Functional medicine practitioners argue that acknowledging this relationship represents a major paradigm shift in how patients are treated. Before seeking his help, Dr. Murphree's patients are often told by conventional doctors "that their low moods are due to not enough Lexapro, Celexa, or Prozac." This treatment approach essentially pins low serotonin on an antidepressant deficiency; however, Dr. Murphree asserts that "no one has a Prozac deficiency." Similarly, when patients are diagnosed with IBS, Dr. Murphree notes that conventional medical practitioners prescribe "Linzess and other medications that have potential side effects." Dr. Murphree is critical of this disease approach since, in his view, "IBS is not a disease." In contrast to pharmaceuticalized approaches to neurological and gastrointestinal issues, functional medicine therapies aim to create a healthy gut microbiome.

In his book, Dr. Kellman describes a 2007 study in which researchers induced stress in rat pups by separating them from their mothers. They then used probiotics to normalize the rat pups' cortisol response. In a similar study, mice bred to be anxious were calmed when given the right bacteria. He writes, "This demonstrates how the microbiome modulates the stress response and how it can modulate genetic inheritance" (2018, 117). In the same vein, Dr. O'Bryan and Dr. Mazmanian emphasize associations between a disordered microbiome and neurological disorders such as depression, anxiety, schizophrenia, and bipolar disorder. Given these associations, functional medicine practitioners often recommend probiotics with proven efficacy in improving psychiatric disorder-related behaviors. I recognize the positive intent behind this endeavor, but I am wary of how this approach may inadvertently normalize trauma and suffering by supplying a medicalized (instead of social) intervention. Psychiatric disorder-related behaviors often arise from a mix of biological, social, cultural, and economic causes (Luhrmann and Marrow 2016). While manipulating the microbiome with probiotics may help to alleviate some of the symptoms, casting a dysbiotic microbiome as the singular cause of the disorder flattens a multi-dimensional problem, obfuscates other contributing factors, and creates a missed opportunity for addressing socioeconomic inequalities.

What Dr. Kellman's literature review reiterates, however, is how gut disturbances can prefigure troubled mental health according to emerging science. Dr. Brogan extends this principle to humans, using the example of gluten. She references the large literature on the role of processed wheat and mental health, rejecting assumptions that gluten-free is just a fad that has been adopted by individuals hoping to lose weight or concerned about gut disturbances. Dr. Brogan explains, "We've had very high quality research, including what's called crossover trials, where they expose people to capsules full of gluten and they develop psychiatric symptoms like depression, and when they take them off it and give them something like rice, it goes away. When they put them back on it, it comes back." The case-crossover study design Dr. Brogan describes creates a causal relationship between gluten and psychiatric symptoms according to epidemiological criteria for causality.

This gut-focused approach also applies to the aging brain. Dr. O'Bryan and Dr. Mazmanian trace Alzheimer's and Parkinson's to a disordered gut microbiome. Dr. Mazmanian explains, "We took mice engineered to have symptoms of Parkinson's and we removed all of their gut bacteria and all of their symptoms were gone. . . . Then we added back certain microbial molecules to these disease-free mice and their symptoms came back." The results of this experiment suggest that certain microbial molecules initiate a cascade of events starting in the gut and producing detrimental results in the brain. Dr. Mazmanian notes that 80 percent of people with Parkinson's also have constipation, and their gut symptoms often precede their neurological symptoms by decades. This finding also suggests that gut disturbances are a useful predictor of neurodegenerative conditions and can thus prompt preventative interventions.

One such preventative intervention involves butyrate, the short-chain fatty acid formerly described by Dr. Cresci, Dr. Li, and Kresser. Dr. Vincent Pedre, clinical instructor of medicine at Mount Sinai School of Medicine, explains, "Butyrate . . . increases your ability to learn and remember and form memories. So, it's basically controlling the plasticity of our brain." Then, speaking to the observations of anthropologist Tobias Rees in *Plastic Reason* (2016), Dr. Pedre continues, "And neuroplasticity, as we know, goes on throughout life. It doesn't end when you are a child." By recommending a butyrate-supporting diet and supplements, functional medicine practitioners can potentially increase brain plasticity, thus preventing neurodegenerative conditions such as Alzheimer's and Parkinson's.

Emerging science regarding the gut-brain connection also has implications for individuals at the opposite end of the life cycle—young children diagnosed with autism. Dr. Mazmanian identifies autism as a neurological condition and explains that one million children in the United States have this disorder. Numbers are on the rise. Based on these statistics, Dr. Mazmanian asserts that "autism may be one of the most pressing social, medical, and economic issues today." He notes that autistic children tend to experience gastrointestinal issues. Their gut dysbiosis can often be linked to Caesarean section birth, childhood antibiotics, and formula feeding. Noting that the gut microbiomes of children with autism are different from those of the general population, Dr. Mazmanian's lab team decided to use fecal transplants from autistic boys to replicate the same altered microbiome in mice. These mice developed dysbiosis, leaky gut, and autism-like symptoms—a finding that prompts me to consider the new politics of microscopic risk (see Wolf-Meyer 2017).

Describing his research, Dr. Mazmanian indicates, "We learned that many of these molecules that are altered in the gut microbiomes of children with autism and in the mice cross the blood-brain barrier and actually change the way neurons and other cells function" (see Gil et al. 2019). In essence, microbial molecules rewire the brain in a way that produces the symptoms of autism. Dr. Mazmanian's study was quickly critiqued for what some have deemed flawed statistical analysis. However, Dr. Mazmanian's contention remains: "Perhaps some sorts of autism aren't diseases of the brain. They may be diseases of the gut." His study furthermore supports other emerging research findings regarding how microbial molecules can affect complex behaviors in animals.

Functional medicine practitioners and, increasingly, conventional doctors agree that the gut shapes "our" personalities.[7] This realization throws into question existing notions of personhood. Dr. Prescott and Dr. Logan write, "It is clear that many characteristics assumed to be inherent in an individual can in reality be determined by the microbial flora of the intestinal tract" (2017, 203). Krishnan indicates, "As it turns out, what makes us human are the microbes that live in and on us. That's 90 percent of who we are."

In the same vein, functional medicine proponents suggest that the gut microbiome largely determines our emotions. As Dr. Mazmanian explains, "The gut is a window into the brain. Molecules not made by us, but made by our microbes, reach our brains, thus affecting our thoughts and emotions, and potentially telling neurons whether to live or die." Dr. Mayer expands, "Your gut microbes are in a prime position to influence your emotions, by generating and modulating signals the gut sends back to the brain. . . . It is the engagement of the gut, and its microbiome, that plays a major role in determining the intensity, duration, and uniqueness of our emotional feelings" (2016, 21, 165). Microbiome research findings suggest that "our" emotional landscape is malleable, and that "we" may experience different thought patterns if "our" gut microbiomes were constituted differently.

The idea that emotions are determined by the gut may not come as a surprise. People have always felt emotion in the gut, which is why we have a plethora of expressions to describe this experience. Dr. Mayer and Dr. Kellman offer multiple examples, including "a knot in your stomach," "a gut-wrenching experience," "butterflies in your stomach," "gut reactions," "gut instincts," "going with your gut," "a sinking feeling in the pit of your stomach," "butterflies in your stomach," and "feeling your stomach 'drop'" (see Mayer 2016, 31; Kellman 2018, 20–21). Dr. Mazmanian unpacks some of these expressions and describes how certain individuals develop stomachaches when they are anxious. Dr. Kellman writes, "The gut is the seat of your primordial emotions—your most basic, deeply felt responses" (2018, 81). In essence, the intestines are a crucial contributor to decision-making processes.

Functional medicine practitioners problematize "choice" by pointing to human-microbe mutualism. Dr. Perlmutter explains, "What you eat, looked at through the lens of your microbes, does affect your behavior and your choices. And, at the same time, those choices that you make affect the health and vitality of your gut microbes." Dr. Prescott and Dr. Logan extend Dr. Perlmutter's comments, writing, "As far-fetched as it may sound, those microbial assemblages may influence your mood and even cravings; thus, they could influence lifestyle choices" (2017, 115). According to functional medicine practitioners, gut dysbiosis can compromise individuals' decision-making ability. Dr. Perlmutter describes a vicious cycle "whereby eating the wrong foods changes the microbiome, it changes your brain, it makes you less able, moving forward, to make the right choices. So you make further bad choices, further damaging your gut bacteria, further changing your brain." Due to the repetition of this vicious cycle, the neuroplastic brain is rewired for disease.

This explanation can be (mis)read as blaming victims for their errant neurobiology and subsequent ill health. I question "lifestyle choices" and "decision-making ability" given the impact of structural inequality on individuals' ability to have a choice. Social, political, and economic factors shape access to food and health care, which in turn shapes biology.[8] Thus, in response to functional medicine's biologized perspective, I offer nested ecologies as a way to simultaneously think about both microbial *and* social assemblages, thus pointing to the role of social, political, and economic factors in shaping the microbiome (see Benezra 2017) and, ultimately, determining health outcomes. This nested perspective is needed because "[t]he beneficiaries of this modernized microbial future are unevenly distributed in space and across social groups" (Lorimer 2017, 5).

Furthermore, distinguishing social, political, and economic factors from biological causes is of consequence because the framing of problems prefigures their perceived solution. For example, Dr. Prescott and Dr. Logan write, "Several studies in humans show clear evidence of gut dysbiosis among users of cocaine. However, a new animal study shows that disturbing the gut microbiome with antibiotics subsequently enhances sensitivity to cocaine reward. In other words, dysbiosis might prime addiction" (2017, 127). These studies suggest that the gut microbiome is the cause of the problem, and, therefore, intervening on the gut microbiome represents an opportunity for treatment and prevention of drug addiction. A biologized problem requires a biologized (and potentially medicalized) solution.

In contrast, a problem caused by structural inequality requires a more equitable social structure for its resolution. I critique descriptions of the gut-brain connection that biologize and medicalize issues such as addiction. Such descriptions eclipse analyses of these issues as symptoms of social injustice. I argue that social problems should not be portrayed as individual problems. They do not emerge from individuated, biologized beings. While there is often a biological element, these issues may also result from social malaise. By viewing people through the lens of nested ecologies, I am not making an either/or argument that pits the biological against the social. Instead, as a medical anthropologist and social epidemiologist, I am disrupting binaries by championing the biopsychosocial approach to health.

At the same time, I aim to bring an anthropological perspective to bear on emerging scientific research regarding how and where the gut and brain are located. Dr. Brogan's team describes a poster (Roberts, Farmer, and Walker 2018) at the November 2018 Society for Neuroscience conference that "called into question the assumption of the brain as a sterile, bacteria-free zone" and, using high-resolution microscope images, "depicted bacteria happily residing in astrocytes, star-shaped brain cells that interact with and support neurons." The bacteria were first discovered by University of Alabama undergraduate researcher Courtney Walker. The presence of Firmicutes, Proteobacteria, and Bacteroidetes—three phyla commonly found in the gut—were later identified by Walker's professor, Rosalinda Roberts, in thirty-four brains. These findings led Dr. Brogan's team to ask, "Perhaps these bacteria traveled from the gut to the brain, climbing up nerves or traversing blood vessels?"

According to researchers, the presence of bacteria in the brain demonstrates a more intimate (and proximate) relationship between the brain and the microbiome than was formerly understood. Dr. John Gray, a psychologist, explains, "What was discovered in 2017 is that for every neuron in the brain there are seven to nine microbes that surround it to make it work. They work synergistically. We didn't know this before—we thought the gut was sterile." Dr. Gray emphasizes that the gut produces microbes that are essential to the functioning of the brain. I argue that, by locating "gut microbes" in the "brain," emerging research challenges existing notions of the body.[9]

Recent findings on the human microbiome are beginning to problematize the Cartesian binary.[10] Dr. Kellman explains, "In the eighteenth century, French philosopher René Descartes contrasted rational thought with 'irrational' emotion, viewing thought, rationality, and intelligence as the essence of being human. But pioneering scientists are now challenging that model of humanity" (2018, 82). Present-day scientists, he asserts, indicate that emotions undergird our ability to think. Dr. Prescott and Dr. Logan state, "The soma-to-mind perspective is critically important." They then add that "[t]here is *no* mind-body dichotomy" (2017, 74). In making these assertions, functional medicine interlocutors are echoing arguments that medical anthropologists have made for decades.

However, I argue that the very terminology they use to describe the "gut-brain connection" reinscribes the very dichotomy they seek to disrupt; that is, the Cartesian binary has seeped into medical terminology to such a degree that practitioners (and the lay public) lack the vocabulary for discussing the "gut" and the "brain" not as two separate entities, but rather as one unified whole. The term "gut-brain connection" does not effectively disrupt this binary approach since the gut and the brain must, by definition, be separate before they can be connected. Anatomical explanations clarify my point: the gut is connected to the brain by the vagus nerve, which passes messages back and forth between these two distinct entities.

I ask, how can we think of the gut as multiply located, including *inside* the brain? How might we consider the brain as multiply located, including *inside* the gut? Moreover, how can we create a new vocabulary to speak about the gut and the brain as one entity? How can we disrupt the synonymization of mind with brain? To answer these questions, I build upon the work of feminist scholar Elizabeth Wilson (2015), who uses the "abdominal migraine" to disrupt the central vs. peripheral nervous system binary and locates emotions in the "minded" gut (and the "gutted" mind).[11] In an effort to propose one unified noun that encapsulates the gut and the brain, I propose the term "gastroencephalon." The gastroencephalon is, in essence, the multiply located mind, or, as Dr. Prescott and Dr. Logan indicate, "the mobile mind" (2017, 4). The gastroencephalon merges the "gut" and "brain," while also indicating the predominant role of the intestines in sensing, feeling, thinking, and decision making.

In a similar vein, reframing the gut stands to disrupt existing notions of "inside" and "outside" with respect to the body. As Ji explains, "When we look at ourselves through this microbial lens, where we 'end' and the living and breathing environment 'begins' is no longer as clear as the boundary of our skin." Dr. LePine describes how he asks patients to imagine themselves drawing a line on their skin with a magic marker. This line starts on the arm, extends up to the shoulder, neck, and chin and continues into the mouth. Dr. LePine notes, "You can go all the way down into your esophagus, stomach, and your intestines, and you are still on the same surface." From a topological vantage point, Dr. LePine asserts, "[t]he skin and the gut are 'outside' of the body, even though the gut is folded in." For this reason, Dr. Lorenzo Drago, professor of clinical microbiology at the University of Milan, explains that when treating atopic dermatitis, he simultaneously recommends probiotics to treat gut dysbiosis, and this approach produces better outcomes. Taken together, these descriptions of the skin and gut illuminate how functional medicine interlocutors are expanding the realm of possibility for locating the interface between human and environment.

## "GERMS": FROM FOES TO FRIENDS

Reframing the gut furthermore challenges the binary of human Self vs. microbial Other. From the perspective of functional medicine, microbes *make us* human. Referencing how the human genome has approximately the same number of genes as an earthworm, Dr. O'Bryan asks, "Why are we the dominant species on the planet?" According to him, the gut microbiome is what distinguishes humans from earthworms and all other animals on the planet. Many functional medicine interlocutors agree with Dr. O'Bryan by attributing the complexity of humanity to microbes.

Time and time again, functional medicine practitioners and health educators have also argued that, by the numbers, people have more bacterial cells than human cells in their bodies. For example, Dr. O'Bryan explains, "You have ten times more cells from the bacteria in your gut than all the [human] cells in your body put together." This ten-to-one ratio is reiterated by Dr. Hyman, Dr. Bush, Dr. Edeas, and Dr. Mayer. As Ji writes, "We are more microbial than human"—a perspective that is echoed by naturopath Dr. John Dempster.

While functional medicine practitioners and health educators agree regarding the ratio of bacterial cells to human cells, estimates comparing the number of bacterial genes to human genes begin to differ. Dr. O'Bryan, Dr. Hyman, and Ji have all stated that bacterial genes outnumber human genes in the body by a factor of one hundred to one. Krishnan notes, "As it turns out, the microbial genes within our body amount to about 3.3 million in total. We've got one hundred and fifty times more bacterial viral DNA in our body than human DNA." Dr. Edeas estimates, "We have two hundred or three hundred more genome from bacteria than cells." Dr. Mayer's estimate is the highest: "The one thousand bacterial species that make up the gut microbiota contain more than 7 million genes—or up to three hundred and sixty bacterial genes for every human gene" (2016, 17). By all accounts, microbial genes far outnumber human genes. That is, microbes not only act upon human genes to produce epigenetic effects, but also "our genes" are almost entirely microbial.

Functional medicine proponents furthermore indicate that the microbiome plays an important role in the functioning of the immune system. Dr. Cresci indicates that the intestinal tract houses 80 percent of our immune function. Krishnan expands on this: "Your immune tissue, 80 percent of which is in your gut . . . is covered with bacteria. So it's up to the immune system, in communication with the bacteria, to figure out who's friend, who's foe, what should they attack, what shouldn't they attack." This portrayal discards prior notions of bacteria as "germs" (i.e., vectors of disease) and instead characterizes microbes as integral to immune defense mechanisms against invaders.

Functional medicine interlocutors emphasize the presence of bacteria everywhere in the body. Krishnan expands upon observations of microbes in the brain: "Contrary to preexisting notions that blood, cerebral spinal fluid, and amniotic fluid, etc. are sterile, they are actually filled with bacteria." Author, television presenter, and podcaster Dr. Rangan Chatterjee explains that these omnipresent "bugs" co-evolved with humans. These realizations have prompted functional medicine practitioners and health educators to recast microbes; the prior background villains of the story are now slipping into the roles of supporting actors and even protagonists.

When anthropomorphizing microbes, functional medicine interlocutors emphasize that nearly all microbes are protective of human health and only a small subset of microbes can cause negative effects under certain conditions. Dr. Stanley Hazen, chair of the Department of Cellular and Molecular Medicine at the Lerner Research Institute and section head of Preventive Cardiology and Rehabilitation at the Heart and Vascular Institute of the Cleveland Clinic, describes the majority of bacteria as "necessary, beneficial, and good." Dr. Mayer clarifies that beneficial microbes "are referred to by scientists as symbionts or commensals" (2016, 94). Krishnan explains that symbiotic or commensal bacteria account for more than 98 percent of microbes found in humans.

Functional medicine proponents suggest that their view of bacteria as beneficial represents another major paradigm shift in medicine. In the past, bacteria were described as ranging from "passive squatters" to "vectors of disease" (Li 2019, 35) to "sinister foes" (Prescott and Logan 2017, 12). According to Mazmanian, "insidious little creatures" was another description from the past. In contrast, bacteria are presently described as "sophisticated" and "healthy" (Li 2019, 35) and "ancient friends" and "silent partners" (Prescott and Logan 2017, 12).

Functional medicine interlocutors argue that humans could not exist without bacteria. Dr Li goes as far as to describe microbes as "nurturing our human cells" (2019, 36). Dr. Kellman writes, "Bacteria enable us to digest our food, maintain our immune system, and cope with stress. They have a dramatic impact on our thyroid, heart, liver, bones, and skin" (2018, 7). Harking back to the gastroencephalon, Dr. Kellman notes that bacteria optimize brain function by facilitating mental clarity, emotional processing, effective learning, and accurate recall. According to microbiome research, microbes determine so much about us, ranging from the growth of abdominal fat to our sexual fitness and social behavior (see Li 2019, 36).

Medical anthropologists are starting to examine the paradigm shift functional medicine practitioners describe. Leslie Sharp (2019) argues that the shift from bacteria-as-pathogen to interspecies entanglement requires more theorization by anthropologists. Cautiously noting that we *may* be on the cusp of a paradigm shift, Wolf-Meyer asks, "Are we seeing an ontological shift in biomedicine away from the molecular and towards the microbial?" (2017, 8) At the same time, he signals that broad application of microbial medicine is subject to economic, institutional, and political forces. What kinds of science and industry are benefiting from this turn toward the microbial (Wolf-Meyer 2017)?

Over the course of my ethnographic research, I noted how fascination with the microbial is beginning to penetrate the realm of bioconsumption. At the Sprouts supermarket checkout counter, I flipped through a health-focused magazine while waiting my turn. The magazine was littered with references to the microbiome. One short article summarized findings from *Nature Medicine* to assert that *Akkermansia muciniphilia*, a type of gut bacteria, regulates weight and type 2 diabetes. What appeared to be a full-length article, "Prebiotics Boost Gut Health by Providing 'Food' for Probiotics," turned out to be "sponsored content" upon further examination. A non-sponsored article was simply titled with a quote: "Hippocrates Said, 'All Disease Begins in the Gut.'" I heard this quote repeated many times before within functional medicine discourse. How did the microbiome penetrate the public imaginary?

First, the public imaginary is influenced by "scientific discovery." As Dr. Li puts it, "Today, the microbiome is recognized as one of the most

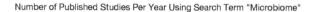

Number of Published Studies Per Year Using Search Term "Microbiome"

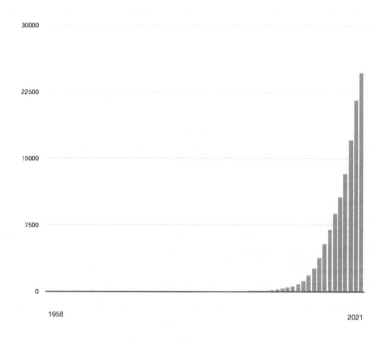

*Bar graph showing the number of studies published each year that match the search term "microbiome." https://pubmed.ncbi.nlm.nih.gov/?term=microbiome&timeline =expanded. Full-color image hosted at https://tinyurl.com/Nested-Ecologies-Images.*

exciting and disruptive areas of medical research" (2019, 39). Dr. Bush concurs that, regardless of the field, medical journals are all acknowledging the link to bacteria. While there were fewer than one hundred new studies on the microbiome every year up until 2002, the number of new articles has exploded in recent years: 10,545 in 2017; 13,133 in 2018; 16,421 in 2019; 20,012 in 2020; and 25,191 in 2021. At the time of this writing in April 2022, current statistics show that new studies on the microbiome are being published at a pace of approximately eighty per day, with nearly thirty thousand new studies projected for publication this year (National Library of Medicine, 2022).

However, public fascination with the microbiome is not merely due to "science learning more." Lorimer (2017) signals how microbiome science is entangled with the political economics of North American biotechnology and biomedicine. For example, the work on the microbiome of the built environment was funded out of US interest in detecting acts of bioterrorism, and the translation of the microbiome for therapeutics is driven by venture capital and the pharmaceutical industry. Referring to Ed Yong's *I Contain Multitudes: The Microbes Within Us and a Grander View of Life*, Lorimer highlights how many of the scientists named in the book advise or hold stock in microbiome companies.

I argue that, as the result of political and economic structures, the microbiome is marketed to bioconsumers in everyday life. In the realm of functional medicine, laboratories and providers similarly situate the gut as a profit-producing site—so much so that I've heard feces referred to as "brown gold."[12] Patients purchase microbiome mapping tests, supplements, and functional medicine consultations when they "buy into" the gut as the root of their health issues.

Second, the bioconsumption of the microbiome is buttressed by "scientific" (social) narratives that reframe the relationship between humans and microbes. Functional medicine practitioners argue that through the process of ingestion, the gut is the body's most intimate point of contact with the outside world, and through digestion, the external world physically constitutes the Self, thus reconfiguring humans as microbial beings (think: nested ecologies). Humans *are* microbes → microbial humans.

In response, medical anthropologists question, sometimes cynically, the degree to which we might identify an emergent animism (see Wolf-Meyer 2017). In this vein, Prescott and Logan describe "family, friends, co-workers, classmates, and strangers" as "teeming with little microbial pets" (2017, 290). Similarly, Dr. Cresci indicates, "I like to tell people, 'You know, you're not just thinking about yourself here when you eat, you have trillions of little pets living inside of you that you should also be considering, that you need to be feeding them, and feeding them properly because they're helping you.'"

Wolf-Meyer (2017) further asks if this depiction of life represents "the final nail in the coffin of humanism." Krishnan says, "We used to think of ourselves as *Homo sapiens sapiens*, this amazing creature that moved up the evolutionary ladder, the food chain, and we're just so awesome." Then, referring to how microbes facilitate digestion, nutrient absorption, and thought processes, Krishnan stresses that "we can barely do anything for ourselves." Dr. Kellman creates an analogy that emphasizes the dependence of humans on microbes: humans are children to microbial parents. He writes, "Like children who don't realize how their parents have smoothed their way behind the scenes, we have depended, from our very first moments as humans, upon bacteria" (2018, 69).

While Wolf-Meyer (2017) would likely remain skeptical if he were given the opportunity to respond to functional medicine interlocutors,

Dr. Prescott and Dr. Logan critique the anthropocentric tendency to see humans as the most important entity. Given that less than 1 percent of combined human and microbial genes are of human origin (Mayer 2016, 17), Dr. Prescott and Dr. Logan write, "Maybe the microbes are the host and we are in their world!" (2017, 115).

## VIRUSES AND BEYOND

In addition to bacteria, the microbiome consists of viruses, yeast, fungi, and other organisms. Describing different types of organisms that constitute the microbiome, Dr. Bush explains, "We have somewhere around three hundred thousand species of parasites. There are over five million species of fungi. . . . There are ten to the thirty-one phages—that's a one with thirty-one zeros after it—it's too large of a number to have ever been named." Functional medicine interlocutors suggest that, like bacteria, all these organisms constitute the human being.

Of these organisms, however, viruses are second to bacteria as the most discussed in functional medicine discourse. Many functional medicine interlocutors explicitly point to how bacteria and viruses co-create human life. Dr. Bush describes how viruses provide humans with needed "genomic updates." According to Krishnan, "It's looking like 99 percent of metabolic function, things that we do on a daily basis that make us human, is coded for by bacterial and viral DNA." In this view, the contribution of viruses is essential to human life.

Bacteriophages (interchangeably referred to as "phages") are a type of virus that infects bacteria and are used by some functional medicine practitioners to target and treat pathogenic bacteria. Ji explains, "Bacteriophages . . . in some ways, oversee the bacterial populations." While he initially indicated that bacteriophages can "kill" some bacteria, he later indicates that a good portion of bacteria are being "digested" by bacteriophages. This subsequent description shifts the portrayal of viruses and bacteria from antagonists to co-evolved members of our internal ecosystem who inhabit different levels of the food chain.

Although certain viruses can be protective to our health, popular notions of viruses as vectors of disease persist. Dr. Edeas humorously describes how many patients react when told they are going to be treated with a virus: "Oh my God, you will [infect] me with virus?" In response to this question, Dr. Edeas tells patients that the bacteriophages he uses for treatment are a "fantastic" type of virus that infects specific pathogenic bacteria but does not infect human cells. The functional medicine approach to bacteriophages turns existing understanding of viruses on its head: while viruses can threaten human health, they can also be effectively used in medical therapies.

Scientists are currently conducting research on using bacteriophages for targeted, therapeutic purposes—what Sharp describes as "enfolding interspecies sensibilities within praxes of care" (2019, 163). Among them are Dr. Paul Turner and Dr. Benjamin Chan at Yale University. Dr. Turner explains, "We are essentially living in a huge ocean of viruses, especially bacteriophages." Average individuals as they go about their days, he says, are "inhaling dust particles just as they're walking on this planet and, undoubtedly, those dust particles have viruses adhered to them, and the majority of them are going to be bacteriophages. . . . You'll see them in water, in the food you eat, especially if you like salads." Dr. Bush provides a few mind-boggling statistics that support Dr. Turner's description: one liter of seawater can contain up to $10^{10}$ viruses, one gram of soil contains $10^9$ viruses, newborn babies' feces contain $10^8$ viruses one week after birth, and there are $10^{15}$ viruses in the adult human body. Given the omnipresence of viruses, Dr. Turner and Dr. Chan have turned to the question of how phage technology can be harnessed for biomedical purposes.

The two go on to describe how their research has produced life-saving results. In one case, a male patient had a long-standing infection that was resistant to standard antibiotic therapy. Dr. Chan indicates, "We deployed [a] phage, in addition to antibiotics, to try and treat his infection. A single application seems to have done the trick, and we were able to clear that infection from him." In another case, a male patient had a graft from an aortic arch replacement that was infected with pseudomonas. Dr. Chan recounts, "After a couple of years, and some debridement and standard treatment, he formed a draining fistula, which was in the upper right, upper left quadrant that was draining pseudomonas." The research team had to receive permission from the FDA to use phage therapy in an emergency situation. Their treatment was successful.

According to functional medicine practitioners, phage therapy could have a broad range of applications in the future—for example, in treating autoimmune diseases. Dr. Fitzgerald describes how two types of bacteria have been shown to trigger rheumatoid arthritis. "It just seemed extraordinary to me that one might be able to turn off [rheumatoid arthritis] potentially, with using phage therapy against these two bacteria." The power of viruses may also be harnessed to treat cancer. For example, Harrington et al. (2019) engineered oncolytic viruses (OVs)—viruses that preferentially replicate in tumor cells—that optimize immune-mediated tumor eradication. In essence, future research may use viruses to produce valuable therapies for a number of diseases.

This potentiality is bolstered by functional medicine's emphasis on how viral DNA constitutes a significant part of the human genome. Dr. Jason Shepherd, a neurobiology researcher, explains, "Viruses and retroviruses copy and paste themselves into . . . the host's genome, and our own DNA is, in fact, riddled with these viral elements." During the course of my ethnographic research, functional medicine interlocutors estimated the percentage of human DNA from viral origins to be between 10 and 50 percent. Building upon how my colleagues in medical anthropology are beginning to explore how humans may be "microbial," my ethnographic observations prompt me to ask how humans may also be reframed as viruses. In extending this question, I am reflecting upon Lorimer's (2019) assertion that "hookworms make us human." Lorimer notes a historical transition from human disentanglement from hookworm to contemporary anxieties about their absence and even restoration of worms and their salutary ecologies. While hookworms are parasites, not viruses, I draw inspiration from Lorimer's work and ask how humans and viruses may be interdependent. How can we think of human-virus entanglements beyond the existing scope of virus as pathogen?

As if speaking to these questions, Ji explains, "On some level, viruses are just pieces of genetic information in search of chromosomes. They are a mechanism of horizontal gene transfer, and information transfer." Then, providing a provocative example, Ji notes that although HIV is widely considered to be "the most horrific virus," this category of virus (i.e., a retrovirus) is responsible for producing parts of the human genome that resulted in essential organs such as the placenta. Dr. Bush likewise describes how the genes of ancestral endogenous retroviruses are expressed by the human placenta and how emerging research is showing that hundreds of millions of HIV-positive individuals are asymptomatic due to their innate immune function. Dr. Shepherd comments, "It turns out that these Bond villains of nature were only masquerading as bad guys and were, in fact, double agents all along." According to functional medicine, humans would never have evolved into the species we are today without endogenous retroviruses.

Furthermore, functional medicine interlocutors credit retroviral DNA with humans' neuroplasticity and encephalization—the evolutionary increase in the brain's complexity and size. Dr. Shepherd says, "We recently made a surprising discovery—that we may have viruses to thank for our own cognition and ability to learn." He describes how the brain undergoes structural changes as we learn and how the ARC gene is essential to the synaptic plasticity that facilitates learning and cognition (see Rees 2016). He continues, "The protein that ARC encodes for looks a lot like the HIV capsid." Upon realizing this structural similarity, Dr. Shepherd's research question became: "Can ARC actually act like a virus?" Through close research and examination, he identified a formerly unknown method of cellular communication: Operating like a virus, ARC can share its own genomic material from cell to cell. His research findings reiterate that as humans, we are, in part, viruses.

In the introduction, I pointed to how social narratives are overlain on viruses, thus eliciting responses ranging from empathy to disgust. In this chapter, I extend that argument to examine how novel narratives are being socially constructed to anthropomorphize bacteria and viruses and cast them in a virtuous light. While bacteria and viruses have always existed and have tended to operate via the same mechanisms, emerging "science" is causing them to transform before our eyes. In essence, my argument is that narratives, not bacteria and viruses, have changed, and, furthermore, "science" is in the business of socially constructing narratives. These "scientific" (social) narratives have a direct impact on the public imaginary and how we conceive of ourselves vis-à-vis the microorganisms that live within us.

## THE HOLOBIONT

Research into the microbiome is transforming our notion of what it means to be human by recasting "individuals" as "superorganisms" including trillions of microbes (Kellman 2018, 7, 68). Krishnan asserts, "We thrived as humans because we were able to pick up organisms from our environment and create this superorganism." Dr. Achacoso states, "We are organisms that are built on networks upon networks of organisms." In the same vein, Ji writes in an email newsletter, "Constituted by at least ten times more bacterial, viral, and fungal cells than actual human cells, we are more accurately described (at least in biological terms) as a 'meta-organism' than a hermetically-sealed-off body isolated from outside life." These explanations give new meaning to the phrase, "the body multiple" (see Mol 2003).

In arguing for a multiplicitous body, functional medicine proponents are advancing holobiont theory—the idea that each "person" consists of a multitude of organisms that work synchronously for the sake of the community.[13] Dr. Kellman writes, "You are not only one human individual—you are *also* a community of bacteria. For you to be happy and healthy, your bacterial community must thrive" (2018, 8). According to Dr. Li, the term "holobiont" describes an organism that functions as an "assemblage" of multiple species in ways that are mutually beneficial. Similarly, Dr. Prescott and Dr. Logan write, "You aren't really one species, but rather an assemblage of different species. These assemblages are referred to as holobionts" (2017, 114). Thinking of humans as an "assemblage" thoroughly reframes existing notions of humans as "individuals."

In essence, human holobionts are, in the words of Dr. Li, "no longer simply human." Dr. Bush concurs, pointing to "this . . . astounding, bizarre reality that we are not human, we are a living ecosystem." Linking holobiont theory to microbiome research, Dr. Li continues, "You are a holobiont because your body is not a singular entity, but rather a highly complex ecosystem including 39 trillion bacteria, mostly good, teeming inside and on your body's surface" (2019, 35). Ji explains that according to holobiont theory, our "fate is and always was inseparably bound to all its symbiotic microbes." Krishnan analogizes humans to "a walking, talking rainforest. . . . Different ecologies within the body have to communicate with one another. We require all of their help in order to be human." According to Dr. Prescott and Dr. Logan, holobiont theory is of enormous consequence to people's sense of "Self" because it frames people as "multi-species ecological units" (2017, 115). In this view, personhood emerges from the union of microbial and human cells. Humanity unfolds through microbes and is therefore framed and potentiated by the microbial lifeworld.

I argue that this ecological turn in functional medicine reflects wider environmental anxieties (see Lorimer 2019). Dr. Hazen notes, "What we eat is actually our largest environmental exposure." From a functional medicine perspective, external ecologies (e.g., food and environmental exposures) are incorporated into the person's body, experience, and identity. These perspectives in functional medicine evince how the gut is being positioned as the site of contestation at the societal level by those who identify environmental contaminants and genetic modification in the food system as a likely cause of chronic disease (e.g., Bayer's $10 billion settlement after its herbicide, Roundup, was linked to non-Hodgkin's lymphoma and the heated debates about the products of the chemical company Monsanto).[14] Concerns about GMOs, of course, extend beyond health and into the realm of intellectual property rights, labor rights, concerns about corporate profit, and a reframing of what "colonization" means with regard to genetics.[15]

In this context, microbes offer "model ecosystems" for liberal hopes and dreams (see Lorimer 2017, referring to Paxson and Helmreich 2014). That is, the idea of the microbiome speaks to the environmentally minded by offering a microenvironmental ethics and by undermining contemporary notions of social Darwinism and offering a social and communitarian model of evolution. Lorimer (2017) writes, "The unmet challenge—as with other liberal dreams of techno-scientific salvation—is to situate the implications of microbiome science within the wider political, economic, and ecological contexts" (6). In making this assertion, Lorimer signals medical anthropology's strength in political ecology, the study of the relationships among political, economic, and social factors with environmental issues and changes.

I agree with Lorimer and hope to contribute to an "anthropology of microbes." Thus, I offer my concept of nested ecologies as a way of simultaneously emphasizing the plurality of both the body's internal and external ecologies. External ecologies include political, economic, social, cultural, and physical factors. Like Matryoshka dolls, there are many layers to nested ecologies. Furthermore, joining Benezra (2017), I hope to explore how bioscience and anthropology might jointly address pressing health problems. Specifically, how might anthropologists continue to leverage ethnographic findings to hold microbiome science accountable for engaging social, political, and economic conditions?

# CHAPTER 5
# THE SOCIAL MICROBIOME

We think of our bodies as stable biological structures that live in the world but are fundamentally separate from it. That we are unitary organisms in the world but passing through it. But what we're learning from the molecular processes that actually keep our bodies running is that we're far more fluid than we realize, and the world passes through us.

DR. STEVE COLE, PROFESSOR OF MEDICINE AND PSYCHIATRY
AND BIOBEHAVIORAL SCIENCES, UCLA SCHOOL OF MEDICINE

Functional medicine and conventional medicine approach nutrition differently with respect to patient care. Dr. Brogan indicates that doctors often receive no more than one hour of nutrition in their four years of medical education before going on to residency, where the subject is completely neglected. Thus, she suggests, "If you ask a conventionally trained doctor . . . they would say, 'It's probably a good idea to eat a healthy diet, but it is no way a causal factor in pathology.'" Her point was reiterated by Dr. William Li, who writes, "Only one in five medical schools in the United States requires medical students to take a nutrition course. On average, medical schools offer a mere nineteen hours of coursework in nutrition" (2019, xviii). Furthermore, doctors lack access to continuing medical education courses on nutrition.

This educational blind spot has set the stage for conventional doctors' unfamiliarity with emerging research on the microbiome. Dr. Mayer writes, "The majority of healthcare providers are neither on top of the rapidly progressing science of the microbiome, nor trained in giving evidence-based nutritional advice" (2017, xi). Dr. LePine asserts, "Most physicians are not even aware that most of your immune system is in your gut." Likewise, doctors are not trained to focus on the effects of the nutritional and physical environment on patients' health. Dr. Prescott indicates, "I completed my training with virtually no knowledge of important things like nutrition and the effect of the whole environment on the health of the whole person. In a world of lifestyle disease, the importance of nutritional and environmental health cannot be emphasized enough, yet orthodox medicine still places little emphasis on them" (2017, 6). Dr. Brogan, Dr. Li, Dr. Mayer, and Dr. Prescott were originally trained in conventional medicine, thus their critiques of medical education are based on their personal experience.

Lack of training has direct consequences for patient care. According to Dr. Li, very few doctors know how to discuss a healthy diet with their patients. He describes a recurrent experience he had with terminally ill patients at a Veterans Administration hospital. He writes, "Then, as they were leaving my office, they would almost invariably turn and ask me: 'Hey, doc, what can I eat so I can help myself?' I didn't have an answer to that question—because I hadn't been educated or trained to deal with it. That struck me as wrong" (2019, xix). With this example, Dr. Li does not characterize doctors' inability to discuss diet with patients as a personal failing of the individual doctors. Instead, he includes himself among doctors who have experienced a terrible "side effect" due to not being trained in nutrition.

Many doctors, especially those who treat patients with chronic diseases like diabetes, obesity, and heart disease, face similar challenges. Dr. Leigh Frame, director for the Integrative Medicine Program at the George Washington University School of Medicine and Health Sciences, emphasizes that doctors "have no training in diet and exercise. [For] exercise, we can refer them pretty easily to a personal trainer and that can be taken care of. . . . But that nutrition knowledge is a little bit harder to get." Patients are generally not offered nutritional guidance by their physicians, and insurance rarely covers visits to a registered dietician. She continues, "It would be great if physicians could have a quick five- to ten-minute chat with their patients and be able to guide them in the right direction."

Nutrition has been neglected in medicine to such a degree that it must be re-embraced as an "emerging science." Dr. Brogan needed "scientific" validation of the importance of nutrition before crossing over to lifestyle-based medicine. She explains, "Science was my religion." In her case, locating scientific evidence allowed her to interrogate the validity of functional medicine through the lens of her medical training.

The "new science of nutrition" that functional medicine interlocutors espouse is built upon microbiome and epigenetic science. Dr. Li explains that this "new science" extends beyond conventional nutrition—which largely focuses on macronutrients such as lipids, proteins, and carbohydrates—by combining food science with life science and revealing the important nutrigenomic effects of diet. In this vein, Dr. Brogan explains, "Food is an informational vector that speaks to and interacts with your genes and governs their expression." Given that food shapes our microbiome, and, thus, our very being at molecular, metabolic, and epigenetic levels, functional medicine interlocutors argue that this "new science" merits both interest and funding.

I argue, however, that portraying nutrition as a "new science" runs the risk of erasing traditional and embodied knowledges.[1] Many traditional medicine doctors and patients, operating outside of biomedicine, have not neglected nutrition and therefore are not in need of a re-discovery. Dr. Brogan acknowledges, "If you were to ask recovered patients, if you were to ask clinicians of any variety from traditional medicine to alternative, holistic, functional medicine . . . they would tell you, 'Actually, [food] is potentially the most critical starting point.'" In response, I call out how embodied and "traditional" knowledge are rendered invisible, only to "emerge" through "scientific discovery" as major advancements in medicine. In some ways, medical embrace of nutrition is a form of "emergent traditionality" (Hobsbawm and Ranger 1992)—a return to traditional knowledge in novel packaging.

## FUNCTIONAL MEDICINE VIEWS FOOD AS MEDICINE

Using the lens of nested ecologies, I underscore the functional medicine perspective that when we ingest the external world, we build our bodies from the nutrients we absorb. Dr. Josh Axe, chiropractor, naturopath, and nurse, has on many occasions repeated, "You are what you eat what they ate." By expanding the popular saying, "You are what you eat," Dr. Axe emphasizes not only that the food you eat is incorporated into your body, but also that the natural environment in which your food grows or the nutritional environment in which it is raised will determine its quality and nutritional value. From a functional medicine perspective, food is a vital conduit, connecting multiple layers of external and internal ecologies.

Functional medicine's focus on nutrition can be traced to its founding father. Dr. Jeffrey Bland was trained in nutrition at the American College of Nutrition, where he is a certified nutrition specialist. He was the director of nutritional research at the Linus Pauling Institute of Science and Medicine in the early 1980s. Following his lead, functional medicine practitioners have truly taken the adage "food is medicine" as a guiding principle. As Dr. Fitzgerald explains, doctors were "forgetting about nutrition as a variable in medicine" at the time of functional medicine's emergence. From her perspective, functional medicine was a "new medicine" that completely shifted the paradigm by recognizing the powerful influence of the individual's diet, including both the micronutrients and macronutrients that are absorbed. Given the numerous successes I have experienced over the course of my recovery, I argue that functional medicine adds value to existing medical techniques. However, I must reiterate that a focus on nutrition is only new from a biomedical perspective.

At times, functional medicine interlocutors do briefly acknowledge traditional knowledge regarding nutrition; however, these conversations focus on the nutritional biologization of "ancestry." The underlying logic is that individual humans' ability to digest and absorb particular nutrients is dependent on the environment in which their ancestors lived and ate. Dr. Liu describes ancestral diets as a "template" for what individuals should eat. "I think when people start looking at their own ancestry and the nutrigenomics, they'll find that there are certain bacteria that probably are going to work a little bit better because they've had exposure to it for tens or even thousands of millennia." Krishnan similarly emphasizes the importance of an ancestral diet, but he furthermore signals the importance of how foods are grown and prepared. From this view, interacting with dirt, avoiding over-sterilization, and consuming diverse foods are basic habits that are of benefit to "our microbial community," thus perpetuating health and wellness.

Functional medicine interlocutors furthermore contend that ancestral diets are important because individuals may be differentially adapted for digesting different foods. Dr. Prescott and Dr. Logan explicate individuals' differential adaptation: "Our gut microbes have always been passed on to our offspring. We can trace several of the key microbial families in our gut today as those inhabiting our common ancestors living a minimum of 15 million years ago" (2017, 113). Providing one specific example, Ji shares that, according to recent metagenomic analysis of genomes from a community of individuals, "certain Japanese have a type of bacteria that borrowed an enzyme from a bacteria that lives on the marine seaweed that their ancestors ate." Ji describes how approximately nine hundred years ago, Japanese people began eating nori seaweed, and this generated a novel ability to consume sulfated polysaccharides in a land-evolved species. In essence, this additional enzyme allowed Japanese individuals to consume several hundred thousand new foods from the sea.

From a functional medicine perspective, this adaptive relationship to food also explains why Chinese individuals reap greater benefits from drinking green tea when compared to non-Chinese counterparts. Dr. Edeas explains that the "Chinese probably have a kind of microbiota who process this green tea." Dr. Edeas's use of the anthropomorphizing word "who" instead of the inanimate word "that" is probably because he is a native French speaker. At the same time, this anthropomorphization foreshadows this chapter's discussion of what I call the "social microbiome." Dr. Edeas goes on to posit, "I believe that the beneficial effects of curcumin in term of cancer prevention is more powerful in the Indian population than maybe other countries like Germany or France." Each of these examples emphasizes how a population's adaptive relationship to food determines the diversity of gut microbiota, thus potentiating the nutritional value of "traditional" ingredients.

In contrast, functional medicine experts characterize the Western diet as pathological. Krishnan describes "universal dysfunctions" in the microbiome of the "typical Westernized person." He indicates, "These universal dysfunctions in the standard American gut are actually the drivers of many of the chronic illnesses that we all are most afraid of and have to deal with on a regular basis." From a functional medicine perspective, Americans are perhaps the only population whose diet is not rooted in traditional cuisine.

"Health foods" in the United States often appropriate ingredients from traditional cuisines around the world. However, according to functional medicine interlocutors, these foods often fail to produce the benefits observed in other populations because they are mismatched to the biology of individual American consumers. Krishnan states, "One of the things about globalization is it's lost upon us what we're really adapted to consume." Referring to the recent coconut craze, Krishnan continues, "How many of us actually live near coconut, natural coconut trees?" Instead of following health food fads, Ji concludes that the "different dietary patterns that come with your cultural inheritance and your particular ancestry may confer life-saving benefits." There may be some truth to these statements. At the same time, I argue that these descriptions of "cultural inheritance" essentialize entire "races" and nationalities without acknowledging diversity and differences within these purportedly unified groups. This approach uses science to reify "race" and misses a valuable opportunity to problematize assumptions about social assemblages (see Roberts 2012).

As I have mentioned, functional medicine portrayals of ancestral diets reinvent "tradition" (Hobsbawm and Ranger 1992) through the scientific making anew of "ancestral knowledge." Dr. Prescott and Dr. Logan assert,

"Cutting edge science is validating the collective knowledge of our ancestors" (2017, 174). They then cite René Dubos, who opined, "From a purely biological point of view, the best environment for the human species may have been the pre-industrial, pre-agricultural world based on the hunting-gathering way of life" (2017, 252). This particular argument romanticizes the past in a way that problematically disregards how the rise of industrialization and agriculture has extended human life span and healthspan.

These two tendencies—essentialization of culture and "race" and the romanticization of the past—have led functional medicine practitioners and health educators to describe diet in binary ways that collapse "ancestral" on to "non-Western" and "modern" on to "Western." Dr. Prescott and Dr. Logan write, "Traditional groups, in relation to European or North American populations, are almost always differentiated by far greater diversity of their intestinal/stool microbiota" (2017, 116–117). They go on to describe how microbial diversity declines in populations that are transitioning from traditional to Western lifestyles and from rural to urban settings. These dichotomizing descriptions are problematic because they create a universalized "non-Western" category. For example, Dr. Prescott and Dr. Logan write, "Whether examining the traditional Mediterranean, Japanese, Nordic, or unique hunter-gatherer diets, these dietary patterns are united in being rich in plants and fiber" (2017, 152). These quotes exemplify an essentialized, binary approach to "cultural" diets and erroneous assumptions that non-Westerners are somehow untouched by the passage of time.

The Mediterranean diet was the most common example I encountered over the course of my ethnographic research. Dr. Mayer describes a vacation to Italy where he observed families strolling in the piazza and learned about how people grow, harvest, and eat their food. He furthermore positions the Mediterranean diet as a potential therapeutic method for the prevention of neurological disease. He writes, "Based on this growing scientific evidence, studies are now underway evaluating the benefits of the Mediterranean diet for slowing the progression of Alzheimer's and Parkinson's disease, or for the improved pharmacologic treatment of depression" (2016, xii). Dr. Mayer's portrayal of the Mediterranean diet as a nutritional panacea for neurological issues contradicts assertions that individuals should eat the "ancestral diet" for which they are microbially adapted. However, it is a perfect example of how functional medicine interlocutors romanticize the diets of "Other" cultures and imagine that these "Others" continue to live life as if frozen in an idealized past. Furthermore, like many functional medicine interlocutors, he describes how "scientific evidence" reconfigures a particular "traditional," non-Western diet as an emerging approach to healing.

## THE HYGIENE HYPOTHESIS: ANTI-BIOS?

This return to the past relates to functional medicine notions of *anti-bios*— that which threatens life (see Prescott and Logan 2017). The scientific validation of germ theory by Louis Pasteur between 1960 and 1964 ushered in a new era focused on good hygiene to prevent the spread of disease. However, functional medicine interlocutors contrast our modern-day hygiene practices with the *techniques du corps* of our "ancestors" (see Mauss [1934] 2010). Dr. O'Bryan cites recent studies to support his assertion: "Children need to play in the dirt." He continues, "If you think of how our ancestors lived, they were always foraging in dirt. They were walking around in dirt. It's so foreign to even think about that now today, but it's so critically important." From a functional medicine perspective, interaction with dirt is a question of how humans were biologically designed.

However, an entire industry has unfolded in stark contrast to this perspective. Over time, scientists have created more effective methods for detecting and killing bacteria, and increased hygiene has gone hand in hand with increased technology. According to functional medicine interlocutors, this hyper-focus on hygiene has resulted in "a landscape where *all microbes* are marketed as germs" (Prescott and Logan 2017, 120). Indicating how marketing shapes consumers' habits, Krishnan says, "They'll say it kills 99.9 percent of bacteria. What has gotten into the psyche of the average American consumer or the Western consumer is that we need to sanitize and sterilize our environment. That includes our own body." By linking beliefs about hygiene to socially ingrained bodily practices, functional medicine interlocutors signal how marketing shapes habitus (Mauss [1934] 2010).

Hygiene habitus affects every area of life. Dr. Chatterjee notes, "We have got to the point where we think all bacteria are bad, so we want to kill them. We use antibacterial soaps; we just try and get rid of microbes as much as possible." Dr. O'Bryan expands, "We clean everything. We sterilize. We've got antibacterial soaps, antibacterial laundry detergents, antibacterial everything." While functional medicine interlocutors agree that antibiotics are necessary under certain circumstances, they also point to the consequences of antibiotic overuse.

Functional medicine practitioners and proponents subscribe to the "hygiene hypothesis." This hypothesis upends prior definitions of "hygiene" as essential for maintaining health by maintaining that greater cleanliness actually increases the likelihood of disease. Citing a recent study, Dr. O'Bryan explains that children who grow up in homes where dishes are washed by hand are 40 percent less likely to have allergies than children who grow up in families that use dishwashers. The same is true for children who are born into a household with a dog (Wayne County Health Environment Allergy and Asthma Longitudinal Study 2015). In essence, early childhood exposure to particular microorganisms contribute to the development of the immune system—what Dr. O'Bryan compares to "doing bicep exercises for the bacteria in your gut." In contrast, Krishnan explains what happens when individuals are not properly exposed to microbes: "Our immune system becomes more and more naïve. When the immune system is naïve, it attacks everything it sees." By most accounts, we are living in the cleanest environment ever in history. According to the hygiene hypothesis, this is detrimental to our health.

From the perspective of functional medicine, excessive hygiene contributes to the recent explosion of autoimmune diseases and allergies. Krishnan indicates that a naïve immune system may begin attacking benign "invaders" such as peanut protein, dairy, and ragweed pollen. "It can be as severe as an autoimmune disease. It starts attacking your own intestinal cells. It starts attacking your own joints. It starts attacking your own brain tissue. It causes severe chronic diseases." In this vein, Dr. O'Bryan advises, "Wash your dishes clean, of course. But . . . the science tells us . . . that the more sterile you are, the more at risk you are of developing allergic diseases, which includes autoimmune diseases." In addition to allergies and autoimmunity, functional medicine interlocutors critically opine that excessive hygiene can lead to a broad range of health issues, including asthma, skin disorders, and brain dysfunction. According to a 2021 study by Yeoh et al., gut microbiota composition reflects disease severity in COVID-19 patients.

Thus, from a functional medicine perspective, excessive hygiene is a form of anti-bios—a threat to life itself. At the same time, the concept of anti-bios extends beyond hygiene and includes a broad range of substances and behaviors. When asked why microbiomes are so much less diverse in the developed world, Dr. Kellman points to antibiotics and cesarean section. He then adds, "Other key factors include a diet full of processed foods and artificial sweeteners; increased exposure to toxins and industrial chemicals; and higher levels of stress, particularly the stress that can result from isolation and loss of community" (2018, 112). According to Dr. Prescott and Dr. Logan, anti-bios includes an ultra-hygienic environment, foods and beverages that damage the gut microbiome, overuse of antibiotics, antimicrobials in our personal products, heavily chlorinated water, environmental pollutants, medications, and artificial sweeteners and emulsifiers (2017, 87). They extend anti-bios from material conditions to social values. "Humans need a living wage, anything less is anti-bios" (2017, 257). I wholeheartedly agree.

While each of these forms of anti-bios threatens well-being, antibiotics have garnered the most public attention. Nonetheless, Dr. Chatterjee asserts that many of his conventionally trained medical colleagues are not aware of the consequences of overprescribing antibiotics. At the same time, parents often ask for antibiotics because they have been "schooled" into thinking that symptoms like fever and ear pain require antibiotics. By requesting antibiotics, parents are trying to do what is best for their children, and by supplying prescriptions for antibiotics, doctors are trying to do whatever they can to help.

The "schooling" to which Dr. Chatterjee refers can be traced to a 1970s view of the body as a battleground. In order to explain this historicized view, Dr. Mayer compares the treatment of infectious disease to that of cancer. He writes, "Physicians took a scorched-earth approach to rid the body of disease, using toxic chemicals, deadly radiation, and surgical interventions to attack cancer cells with increasing force" (2016, 6). With respect to broad-spectrum antibiotics, Dr. Mayer describes how this strategy kills or cripples many species of bacteria in an attempt to wipe out disease-causing bacteria. He continues, "For decades, the mechanistic, militaristic disease model set the agenda for medical research: As long as you could fix the affected machine part, we thought, the problem would be solved; there was no need to understand its ultimate cause" (2016, 6). In the process, the collateral damage of broad-spectrum antibiotics was rendered an acceptable risk. Thus, from a functional medicine perspective, antibiotic resistance is not a problem that is coincidentally emerging in our present era.

Instead, the culture of ultra-hygiene, combined with decades of physicians overprescribing antibiotics, has caused harmful health effects in multiple ways. Dr. Cresci notes, "Antibiotics kill pathogenic bacteria, but they also kill the good bacteria and the good gut microbiota as well." The bacteria that survive broad-spectrum antibiotics may mutate into antibiotic-resistant "superbugs." Krishnan explains, "One of the things that people just don't realize, any time we use antimicrobial products, what we're doing is selecting for more virulent and more pathogenic and more harmful organisms." Furthermore, Dr. Cresci's research reveals how antibiotics decrease the production of short-chain fatty acids, and how this, in turn, renders host cells more susceptible to invasion by pathogenic bacteria. All these instances lead to gut dysbiosis that, from a functional medicine perspective, sets the stage for chronic disease. However, according to Dr. Cresci, it was not until the 1980s and 1990s that physicians began to realize, "Oh my gosh, all of these broad-spectrum antibiotics, they have negative effects. The bacteria, the pathogenic bacteria are adapting to them. They're genetically modifying

202 | NESTED ECOLOGIES

themselves to survive it." To date, we continue to lack new antibiotics for containing drug-resistant infections (World Health Organization 2020).

I can provide a personal example of the iatrogenic potential of antibiotics. At an advanced stage in my recovery, I tested positive for *Clostridium difficile*, one of the pathogenic bacterial strains that Dr. Cresci has researched.[2] *Clostridium difficile* infections can be fatal and occur after use of antibiotic medications or treatment in a health care facility. This is the first layer of iatrogenesis—if I had not been treated with antibiotics in the past, I likely would not have a *Clostridium difficile* infection today. Alarmed, I asked my functional medicine provider what I should do about the infection. Before responding, he asked if I had been experiencing symptoms related to a *Clostridium difficile* infection. I confirmed I was symptom free. He went on to tell me *Clostridium difficile* can be deadly, but it can also be harmless—the difference lies in the constitution of the microbiome. The rest of the microbial "community" determines the behavior of *Clostridium difficile*. He assured me since I was not experiencing any symptoms, there was no cause for worry.

This experience ended with one layer of iatrogenesis. If, however, I had consulted a doctor who decided to treat my *Clostridium difficile* infection with antibiotics, the treatment would have killed *Clostridium difficile* bacteria and other members of my microbial community that protect me from the potentially fatal effects of *Clostridium difficile*. Dr. Cresci's research suggests, in this hypothetical scenario, that I would be more vulnerable to pathogenic bacteria invading my cells in the future, including by antibiotic-resistant *Clostridium difficile*. This scenario signals the potential for second and third layers of iatrogenesis.

For functional medicine practitioners, the potential for iatrogenesis figures prominently into a cost-benefit analysis regarding antibiotics. Dr. Chatterjee notes, "Antibiotics are life saving for sure, but at a cost. . . . What we need to tease out is, can we use the best of them in the right situation and mitigate some of the downside?" In clinic, Dr. Chatterjee sees cases of toddlers who have already had six courses of antibiotics. In order to address the "cultural norm" of antibiotic overuse, Dr. Chatterjee suggests frank conversations between parents and doctors that weigh the risks against the benefits. Dr. Chatterjee indicates that in order to demonstrate that he has the child's best interest at heart, he tells parents, "Look, if this was my child, I don't think I'd use an antibiotic for this." In his experience, parents are more receptive to this empathetic phrasing. This example demonstrates how antibiotic overuse and, conversely, its proper use, are socially constructed and socially maintained at a communicative level.

At the physical level, microbiome health and, conversely, dysbiosis, are also socially created and maintained. Krishnan recalls a microbiome conference where emerging research was presented on the effect of one person's antibiotic treatment on the rest of the household. In the study, when one individual took an antibiotic, other members of the same household experienced the same disruption to their microbiomes without taking the antibiotic. This applied to intimate and nonintimate partners alike. Krishnan notes, "They could measure this even up to six months after the one individual was done."

In essence, functional medicine interlocutors view antibiotic overuse as a societal problem with detrimental effects. Dr. Bush notes, "If we use and steep ourselves in antibiotics, we are going to die quicker. And that is exactly what we are seeing—with every single antibiotic exposure you have in your life, your life expectancy goes down." Dr. Bush's assertions apply to prescription antibiotics and alcohol-based hand sanitizers alike. Harking back to my concept of the microbial human, he continues, "We sterilize down to a state where we can't be human because we've lost the ecosystem itself. And we are suffering chronic disease for that." Viewing chemical sterilization as a threat highlights the interconnectedness of external and internal ecologies and thus reiterates my notion of nested ecologies.

As an alternative to antibiotics, functional medicine practitioners and researchers are turning to phage therapy,[3] diet, and supplements. Dr. Edeas explains, "We have a huge problem with antibiotic resistance. One of the strategies to combat resistance is to use microbiota and to reduce the resistance. We need . . . phages who can control this kind of bad bacteria." For her part, Dr. Cresci describes how she reacted to the 1990s discovery of antibiotic resistance by using nutrition and probiotics "as a way to modify the self, the host, [and] to modifying their immune function to fight off these bacteria." She has been using "immune nutrition" to prepare patients for surgery so they will be more resistant to pathogenic bacteria during and after the procedure.

## INTERVENING ON THE MICROBIOME TO TREAT CHRONIC DISEASE

According to functional medicine, seemingly unrelated diseases can all be linked to one singular etiological process.[4] To elucidate how webs of disease often begin in the gut, Krishnan explains that gut dysbiosis results in disrupted gut mucosa, which, in turn, disrupts the immune response and leads to dysfunction of the gut barrier. He notes that this process "eventually allows for the leaking in of toxins, food particles, viral particles, and so on that create chronic inflammation in the body." Expanding on Krishnan's explanation, Dr. Li and Dr. Hyman both indicate that dysbiosis is linked to an enormous range of diseases (see Li 2019, 50). These include asthma, psoriasis, multiple sclerosis, chronic fatigue syndrome, cavities, dementia, autism, Alzheimer's, Parkinson's, schizophrenia, depression, cancers, polycystic ovarian syndrome, nonalcoholic fatty liver disease, obesity, diabetes, atherosclerosis, heart failure, autoimmune diseases, irritable bowel syndrome, inflammatory bowel disease, Crohn's disease, colitis, celiac disease, and anxiety.

The widespread effects of dysbiosis have led many functional medicine interlocutors to assert that virtually all chronic diseases are linked to a disordered microbiome. From this perspective, dysbiosis is the root cause for millions of suffering Americans—people that Dr. Prescott and Dr. Logan refer to as "the walking wounded." They write, "It would seem that something about the way we are living is disordered" (2017, 8). This comment suggests that the "wounds" of dysbiosis are potentially preventable through diet.

In this landscape, microbiome testing companies have emerged to capitalize on the link between diet and health. These companies employ physicians and scientists who provide personalized diet recommendations based on bioconsumers' mailed-in stool samples. As a subscriber to one such company's email newsletter, I received regular updates on company-sponsored microbiome research. Conflicts of interests embedded in company-sponsored science are ripe for anthropological critique.

At the same time, these potential conflicts of interest are not lost on providers. Dr. Prescott and Dr. Logan, comparing science to NASCAR, write, "Perhaps those standing at the podium of 'science' should wear the corporate-emblazoned fire-suit. Why not display their backers' names, the patents they hold, the financial investments in their own work?" (2017, 258). They assert that this type of disclosure would allow bioconsumers to know "exactly the brand of science" they are being sold. For now, company sponsorships are often hard to detect. Meanwhile, biotech companies are incentivized to invest in microbiome research since, according to Dr. LePine, "[Poop] is brown gold." His description points to how the microbiome is a detailed source of three things: information about the body's functioning, health-protective potential, and lucrative earnings.

Since functional medicine interlocutors consider pharmaceuticals insufficient for creating health, manipulating the microbiome through diet has become a prime endeavor for functional medicine practitioners and bioconsumers. Dr. Li asks, "How can we do a better job at preventing disease, before we have to cure it?" (2019, xvii). Food is the functional medicine answer to this question. Dr. Prescott and Dr. Logan describe a study by their good friend and colleague Dr. Felice Jacka demonstrating that improving the quality of patients' diets had a greater impact on alleviating major depressive disorder than belonging to a social support group (Prescott and Logan 2017, 161). Dr. Kellman (2017) describes how, after treatment of their microbiomes, virtually all his patients have recovered from their chronic diseases. The diagnoses that he has successfully helped reverse range from gastrointestinal concerns to fatigue, Lyme disease, and neurological disorders. Over the course of my ethnographic research, many functional medicine practitioners described how patients suffering from a range of conventional diagnoses are able to recover their health through microbiome interventions.

Dr. LePine provides two compelling examples. The first example occurred when Dr. LePine was training at a Veterans Affairs hospital. A male patient was admitted in a coma due to hepatic encephalopathy. They treated him with neomycin (an antibiotic), laxatives, and probiotics. Dr. LePine explains, "Within twenty-four hours, the patient emerged from the coma like a complete Lazarus." He compares it to "a miracle" because the patient "woke up from the dead." The experience caused Dr. LePine to realize the power of the gut and to heed the relationship between the gut and the brain.[5]

In a second example, a female Alzheimer's patient traveled from Canada to work with Dr. LePine. After conducting a complete workup on the patient, he found that she had "mercury, oral bacteria, gut bacteria, gluten issues, herpes simplex, [and the] APOE-4 genotype." He began treating all her health issues by making changes to her diet. As a result, the woman recovered her ability to talk and drive on her own. Within a matter of months, her husband said, "I have my wife back." Dr. LePine concludes the story by suggesting that a lot of people who struggle with brain fog are actually suffering from a less extreme version of what happened to this patient—bacteria-producing compounds with psychoactive and inflammatory properties.

In response to Dr. LePine's successful treatment stories, Dr. Hyman describes how he manipulated his own microbiome with extraordinary results. "Last year, I developed colitis. . . . I checked my stool and I had really low levels of *Akkermansia*." He explains that *Akkermansia* is an intestinal bacterium that is supportive of human health. The absence of *Akkermansia*, Dr. Hyman indicates, "has been linked to autoimmune disease, it's been linked to poor response to immunotherapy for cancer, it's been linked to cardiometabolic disease and diabetes." Dr. Hyman decided to repopulate his gut primarily through diet. He recounts, "I started to research it and created this cocktail of cranberry, pomegranate, green tea, acacia fiber, some probiotics, [and] other prebiotics. . . . Literally, within three weeks I went from full-blown colitis to completely normal—perfect." This experience served as a "wake-up call" for him with regard to the importance of diet over and above supplementation with probiotics.

However, when an individual's microbiome is damaged beyond repair, functional medicine practitioners turn to fecal microbiota transplantation (FMT). Analogizing the ecosystem of the microbiome inside the body to a rainforest, Dr. LePine explains that "some people's ecosystems are so disturbed and so messed up, it's like napalm has hit your rainforest." Inserting a bit of humor into his explanation, he continues, "What you need to do is 'repoopulate' the microbiome, and you can't do that with just probiotics." Dr. Li describes FMT in more technical terms: "A procedure known as fecal microbial transplantation (FMT) has been developed to treat dysbiosis by replacing unhealthy bacteria with beneficial gut bacteria from the stool of a healthy donor" (2017, 50). As Dr. Li's description suggests, functional medicine practitioners often compare a stool transplant to an organ transplant.

Given its curative effects, stool transplant may be selected by functional medicine practitioners as their treatment of choice for patients with particular pathologies. For example, Dr. Peter Konturek, professor of gastroenterology at University of Erlangen, director of Thuringia Clinic's Department of Medicine, and an expert on FMT, uses FMT to treat *Clostridium difficile* infections, the most common infectious disease in German hospitals. After three years of using the FMT method, Dr. Konturek considers the procedure to be very effective. He notes, "In severe forms of *Clostridium difficile*, we have even [seen a] significant increase in survival of patients." Furthermore, Dr. Hyman mentions a recent study in which, "children with autism who got stool transplants had a marked improvement up to two years out from just replacing the gut microbiome." Based on early randomized studies, FMT also has potential indications for the treatment of IBS, ulcerative colitis, and gout.

Fecal microbiota transplantation is yet another example of how "ancient" practices—even those that are potentially considered repulsive and barbaric—may be rendered "emergent" medical interventions when they are validated by "science." Dr. Konturek signals that while FMT seems bizarre, it is actually derived from healing practices in ancient China. In his view, the "breakthrough" of present-day FMT is how scientists can "check the effectivity of transplantation by sequencing the gut microbiome in the patient before and after this procedure," thus providing, "evidence that this fecal transplantation is really working." In essence, what science has done is to validate a preexisting practice—the breakthrough is the validation, not the technique. The example of FMT problematizes overlapping binaries that collapse "science" with "modernity" on the one hand and (presumed non-scientific) "knowledge" with "antiquity" on the other.

While FMT is currently a therapy of last resort, it may inspire preventative therapies in the future. According to Dr. Yousef Elyaman, the future of medicine will include manipulating the microbiome. Dr. Prescott and Dr. Logan write, "Vaccines derived from innocuous soil-based microbes . . . may soon be applied as preventatives in mental disorders via the immune system" (2017, 63). Meanwhile, Dr. Kellman writes, "I know that our new era of 'microbiome medicine' can radically transform our treatment of both body and brain" (2018, 5). While the future remains to be seen, functional medicine practitioners jointly believe that intervening upon the microbiome is a powerful way to reverse disease and promote health. Their belief is reflected in my notion of nested ecologies.

## BRINGING NESTED ECOLOGIES TO BEAR ON PLANETARY DILEMMAS: EMBRACING THE GAIA 2.0

According to functional medicine, health is created through the unity and balance of both internal and external ecosystems. Thus, I developed the concept of nested ecologies as a heuristic tool for understanding how each individual body's unique "ecology" is situated within economic, political, social, cultural, and physical environments. This heuristic extends to the microbiome. My concept encapsulates Dr. Prescott and Dr. Logan's description of the body as a habitat for bacteria. They write, "The microbiome is defined as the microbes (and their genetic material) found in various ecological niches, such as the human gut or skin" (2017, 7–8)—what I call the "internal ecology." The concept of nested ecologies furthermore incorporates Dr. Kellman's assertion that "we are not impermeable—we are constantly exchanging bacteria with the plants, animals, and humans in our environment—even with the soil and sediment of our planet" (2018, 8). I call this the "external ecology." Pointing to the connection between internal and external ecologies, Ji refers to herbalist Paul Schulick, who aptly named the interstitial layer of microbial communities within the soil and our gut a "life bridge" (Schulick, Newmark, and Sarnat 2002). In his email newsletter, Ji writes, "This bridge can be visualized both 'spatially' as a physiological bridge that connects our bodies via microbes directly to the Earth, forming an inseparable whole (the holobiont), and 'temporally,' by bridging the gap between the present and the ancient past." While I appreciate Schulick's analogy of a bridge, I prefer to describe the relationship between internal and external ecologies as "nested" because this disrupts binary notions of "person" and "the environment" as separate entities.

The nested relationship I describe is rooted in practical realities—realities that Dr. Chatterjee was made aware of during a "mind-blowing" conversation with a farmer. The farmer showed Dr. Chatterjee scientific measurements demonstrating that the microbiome of soil determines the nutrient density of plants. Farmers have always known that the quality of the soil determines the quality of the harvest—only now scientific tools are emerging to quantify this relationship. This is yet another example of how empirical knowledge is rendered "novel" through scientific validation. The conversation caused Dr. Chatterjee to realize that as a doctor, he had been neglecting how the external ecology of the soil's microbiome shapes human health. Many functional medicine practitioners have had a similar realization. My hope for the future is that functional medicine practitioners advocate for change in our food system as an integral part of their work as doctors and healers.[6]

For now, the majority of functional medicine practitioners are not fighting to transform the health-damaging practices of Big Ag. Instead, they are implementing changes in their own lives. Dr. Chatterjee indicates that if he is able to optimize the microbes in his garden by composting, "[t]he food that's growing out of that fertile soil is going to be more nutrient dense. It's going to nourish my microbiome when I eat it. It's going to nourish my children's microbiome when they eat it." Since Dr. Chatterjee is unable to check the nutrient density of produce in the supermarket, his solution is to grow his own. His description of "nourishing the microbiome" by ensuring soil health gives new meaning to Dr. Hyman's analogy of the gut microbiome as an internal garden. In Dr. Hyman's analogy, the garden can either be filled with toxins, weeds, and poisonous plants, or it can be a flourishing and rich garden. The concept of nested biologies highlights the link between Dr. Chatterjee's backyard garden and Dr. Hyman's internal garden.

Similarly, Dr. Minich explains how she is implementing her desire to enrich her gut microbiome with soil. "Sometimes I'll go out in the garden and I maybe won't clean something probably as well as I would have, as if I bought something from the store." Dr. Daphne Miller supports Dr. Minich's ecological habitus, explaining that "the microbiome of our soil . . . circles back to our own internal environments." (By using the term "ecological habitus," I am referring to how functional medicine discourse socially ingrains new ways of interacting with the ecological environment.) Dr. Minich is reinforcing the nested relationship of her microbiome to that of the soil, thus literally incorporating the outside world into her own body. As someone who has focused on improving microbiome health as part of my health journey, I acknowledge that functional medicine's recommended ecological habitus has produced positive health outcomes. At the same time, as a medical anthropologist, I signal how functional medicine practitioners' microbially optimized gardens are markers of privilege since growing organic vegetables requires multiple resources: land, education, and time.

Furthermore, by pointing to how functional medicine practitioners and the majority of their patients are able to control their health through nutrition, I suggest that our lifeworlds are becoming more individualistic. How might we view control over one's own health as evidence of the public's loss of trust in authority? While I focus primarily on functional medicine providers in this chapter, over the course of my ethnographic research, I observed how patient-client-consumers purchase their authority as experts on their own biological processes, which, in turn, restructures the power dynamics of patient-provider interactions.[7] In essence, I argue that capitalism prefigures and positions certain individual bodies for "achieving" health through the consumption of the "right" kinds of foods, products, dirt, and germs.

In contrast, changing the detrimental practices of Big Ag would ensure that broad sectors of society have access to nutrient-dense produce. Dr. Miller describes how the rise of monoculture and agricultural chemicals over traditional farming methods has reduced the diversity of nutrients in our soil and thus our diet. Dr. Prescott and Dr. Logan further explain, "The loss of crop and dietary diversity translates into loss of microbial diversity in the gut. . . . Many scientists are concerned that the health-protective properties of fruits and vegetables are being eroded" (2017, 158). Dr. Michael Ash is an osteopath, naturopath, and nutritional therapist specializing in the mucosal immune system. "If the soils continue to be depleted as they are," he says, "there's just no way that we can compensate through medicine, supplements, and behavioral patterns for the nutrients that those soils have been devoid of." Given the connections functional medicine practitioners make between soil depletion and poor health, I argue that the pursuit of systemic change in agriculture should be considered a medical enterprise.

My argument is supported by Gaia 2.0 (see Lenton and Latour 2018). Before I unpack what Lenton and Latour mean by "2.0," I will first explain Gaia, using the words of functional medicine interlocutors. Ji described

Gaia as "the theory, put forward by James Lovelock, that living matter on the earth collectively defines and regulates the material conditions necessary for the continuance of life." According to the Gaia hypothesis, Ji elaborates, "the planet, or rather the biosphere, is thus likened to a vast self-regulating organism." When parts of the organism are out of balance (e.g., soil depletion), other parts of the organism suffer (e.g., human health). The Gaia hypothesis adds to my concept of nested ecologies by signaling the intimate "interconnectivity of all life" (Prescott and Logan 2017, 1). Returning to the topic of inter-species communication via microRNAs, Ji notes, "When we drink cow's milk, their microRNA begins to regulate our RNA. Therefore, we are very biologically interconnected with the whole biosphere, and we can begin to take a step back and think about a meta-organism." According to this expanded view of nested ecologies, humans are holobionts, living in the whole biosphere.

When considering the Gaia hypothesis, Timothy Lenton, a geographer, and Bruno Latour, a philosopher, anthropologist, and sociologist, indicate that Earth has entered into the Anthropocene, and humans are becoming aware of how their actions affect the planet's climate and ecosystems. They argue that, as a result, "deliberate self-regulation" is imminently possible. "Making such conscious choices to operate within Gaia constitutes a fundamental new state of Gaia, which we call Gaia 2.0." (Lenton and Latour 2018, 1066). Ultimately, Lenton and Latour position Gaia 2.0 as a potential framework for effectively fostering global sustainability.

Similarly, functional medicine interlocutors emphasize how seemingly inconsequential actions of humans can have enormous effects. In order to illustrate this point, Dr. Prescott and Dr. Logan turn to Darwin's discovery that red clover growth was determined by bee pollination (see Prescott and Logan 2017). In turn, numbers of bees were limited by higher numbers of field mice, enemies of early beehive development. The number of field mice was determined by the number of neighborhood cats. In his lectures, published in 1872, Thomas Henry Huxley, somewhat in jest, added a social sphere to Darwin's discovery. He asserted that the "old maids" who fed the neighborhood cats were, in fact, influencing the status of global affairs. This example illuminates how human social behaviors can effect significant ecological change.

If we are to take Gaia 2.0 seriously, humans must work with nature—and, in turn, microbes—to overcome the many modern challenges facing our planet. According to Dr. Prescott and Dr. Logan, solutions to many pressing planetary dilemmas involve "understanding the complex symbiotic interconnections between all things—from the level of microscopic microbial ecosystems that reside *within us*, to the myriad macroscale environmental ecosystems that *we reside in* and completely *depend on* for our survival" (2017, 2). These words emphasize how the natural laws of interdependence, mutualism, and interconnectivity underpin life in all forms.

Dr. Mayer applies Gaia 2.0 to meat and dairy production when he describes how conventionally raised farm animals are separated from their natural environments and food supplies. These animals are fed foods that are inappropriate for their digestive system, thus leading to chronic inflammation. They may also suffer from acute gastrointestinal infections that require continual antibiotics. Dr. Mayer writes, "We can't escape the suspicions that the products that come from such chronically diseased animals are not good for our gut microbiota and not beneficial for our health" (2016, 243). From a functional medicine perspective, the health of other species is of integral importance to human health.

## REDEFINING "DYSBIOSIS": POLITICAL ECOLOGY AND HUMAN HEALTH

Gaia 2.0 applies to all forms of life, including plant-human interconnections. Functional medicine interlocutors furthermore critique the "absurd amount" of herbicides, fungicides, and pesticides used in conventional farming (see Prescott and Logan 2017). Dr. Lynch indicates, "[In] 2016, 2.2 million pounds of Roundup was sprayed on spring wheat alone." Extending his observations to how systemic use of insecticides has increased over the past decade, Dr. Mayer asserts that these toxins are "ultimately incorporated and expressed in the entire plant and its products" (2016, 244). Then, connecting the health of plants to that of humans, he warns, "The collateral damage on our gut microbiome of the increasing deployment of weed killers (such as the notorious glyphosate, or 'Roundup')—necessary to overcome the weed's resistance to such chemicals—remains largely unknown, at least to the consumer" (2016, 244).[8] Dr. Bush similarly notes that while the public is aware of the dangers of over-prescribing antibiotics, they may be less aware that glyphosate is an antibiotic that is engineered into and sprayed on our food with detrimental effects for the microbiome.

Glyphosate, the active ingredient in Roundup, is used as a broad-spectrum, non-selective, systemic herbicide, pesticide, and crop desiccant. At present, everyone, even those consuming an organic diet, is exposed to glyphosate. Dr. Stephanie Seneff, senior research scientist at the MIT Computer Science and Artificial Intelligence Laboratory and author of

*Toxic Legacy*, emphasizes, "Glyphosate is everywhere in our environment. . . . It's very frustrating that you cannot avoid getting glyphosate exposure in America today." Providing a few examples of glyphosate's ubiquity, Dr. Seneff notes, "It's been found in tampons. It's been found in various cotton products. It's been found in vaccines, which is very disturbing to me, and it's all over the food supply. People tested honey, including organic honey; glyphosate was [a] contaminant in the organic honey." She explains that although organic honey contained significantly less glyphosate than non-organic honey, it makes sense that even organic honey would be contaminated to some degree. Describing a challenge faced by organic farms, she explains, "You can't put fences around [the border of your farm] to say that the air can't blow glyphosate in if your neighbor's spraying it from their airplane." Furthermore, glyphosate-laced water runoff from conventional farms seeps into the soil of organic farms.

Although glyphosate has been registered in the United States as a pesticide since 1974 (US Environmental Protection Agency n.d.), it was not widely used due to its toxicity: it tended to kill everything in its path— including the very crops it is meant to protect from pests and weeds. Hoping to make crops resistant to glyphosate while using glyphosate to indiscriminately kill other life forms, scientists began experimenting with genetically modified seeds. Then, in the late 1990s, scientists successfully produced "Roundup Ready" GMOs by inserting a gene that encodes the glyphosate-tolerant enzyme CP4 EPSP synthase (see Funke et al. 2006). Dr. Seneff explains, "Since about 1998, they have introduced GMO Roundup Ready corn, soy, canola, cotton, alfalfa, [and] sugar beets—a lot of these are really important crops for the processed food industry, and these are all resistant to glyphosate." In addition to GMO crops, farmers spray other crops, especially grains and legumes, with glyphosate just prior to harvest. Since glyphosate acts as a crop desiccant, spraying crops causes them to dry out sooner, thus allowing for earlier harvest.

Glyphosate's prevalence in conventional farming may be traced to industry interests. Dr. Seneff suggests that Monsanto, the company that created Roundup, has known since before the herbicide's approval back in the mid-1970s that their product was toxic for humans. Describing how the company decided to hide this information, Dr. Seneff suggests, "Monsanto managed to get past the regulatory process using what I consider to be unethical methods." Dr. Gentempo adds, "[It] is a disturbance to my conscience when I see what's being perpetrated on humanity and being done through greed and corruption and fraud and lies." Now that glyphosate is approved by the EPA, the government does not monitor how much of the herbicide is in food. According to functional medicine interlocutors like Dr. Seneff, this lack of regulatory control is what makes glyphosate so dangerous.

Glyphosate is effective as a pesticide because it disables the shikimate pathway, which is a seven-step metabolic pathway used by bacteria, archaea, and eukarya for the biosynthesis of folates and aromatic amino acids. Since human cells lack the shikimate pathway, the biotech industry asserts that glyphosate is not dangerous for humans. Nonetheless, after being exposed to glyphosate, the bacteria in the human microbiome are unable to produce essential amino acids that are critical for human life, leaving individual hosts (people) vulnerable to chronic disease—another example of nested ecologies (D'Brant n.d.). Dr. Seneff characterizes glyphosate as "the most important factor in our deterioration of health today in America."

The noxious effects of glyphosate were made public when Bayer, the maker of Roundup, faced ninety-five thousand claims linking their broad-spectrum herbicide and pesticide to non-Hodgkin's lymphoma (Cohen 2020). Bayer bought Monsanto, the original creator of Roundup, in 2016 for $63 billion, thus inheriting the litigation. In June 2020, Bayer agreed to pay $10 billion to settle the claims, making the deal one of the largest settlements in US civil litigation. The settlement included no admission of liability or wrongdoing; therefore, Bayer continues to sell the product without warning labels about its safety. While Bayer has set aside $1.25 billion for potential future claims, it still faces thirty thousand outstanding claims from plaintiffs who have not agreed to join the settlement.

Non-Hodgkin's lymphoma may not be the only disease caused by glyphosate. In fact, many functional medicine practitioners and proponents maintain that glyphosate and GMOs are driving the epidemic of chronic disease. Emphasizing how laypeople are the first to know about environmental health concerns (see Brown 1997), Dr. Gentempo indicates, "Things have changed environmentally, and those environmental changes have literally impacted peoples' lives." The explosion of chronic disease is not due to a sudden change in our genetics, but instead to changes in our environment and especially in our food system.

According to Dr. Seneff's research at MIT, glyphosate may also be a driving factor in the rise of celiac disease, autism, Alzheimer's, and other neurological disorders. Dr. Bush describes work that his lab is doing on how glyphosate interacts with gluten to induce gluten sensitivity. Regarding autism, he notes, "We went from one in five thousand children with autism in 1975, which happens to be the year before we had Roundup. . . . Today we have one in forty [children with autism]. . . . In just [forty-five] years we've developed this epidemic." If the boom in autism persists, this disorder will affect one in three to five children by 2035—a future that Dr. Bush characterizes as "unsustainable."

When paired with the concept of nested ecologies, chemicals like glyphosate point to a need for redefining "dysbiosis," a word used in functional medicine to describe a gut microbiome that is "leaky," out of balance, and overrun with pathogenic bacteria. I reexamine the origins of the word: the Greek prefix "dys-" describes something that is difficult, painful, or troubled, and the Greek root word "bio" means "life." Thus, in the remainder of this chapter, I will be using "dysbiosis" to indicate a state in which life is experiencing difficulty and pain or is otherwise in trouble.

Seen through the lens of nested ecologies, the dysbiosis I describe can be observed everywhere around us, including in the air we breathe. First, environmental pollutants such as particulate matter (airborne chemicals) can cause gut dysbiosis. Second, Dr. Prescott and Dr. Logan (2017) note that birch trees exposed to high ozone levels produce pollen that is more allergenic due to alterations in the microbiome of the pollen itself. In essence, the dysbiosis of birch trees and other living organisms in our environment frame and potentiate dysbiosis in humans.

Examples like these have led functional medicine interlocutors to assert, extending Gaia 2.0, that the health and longevity of humans depend on addressing environmental degradation. Krishnan states, "One of the things we know about autoimmune disease is that you have to have some sort of genetic predisposition, which most of us actually do. Then, the second part is you have to have some sort of intestinal dysbiosis. Then, the third part is an environmental trigger." He then links autoimmune disease to "being exposed to certain things like glyphosate or other weed killers and pesticides that can start causing perturbations in the ecology, which will then amplify itself into this dysbiotic system called a disease." What Krishnan refers to as an "environmental trigger," I call a dysbiotic external ecology. What he labels a "dysbiotic system," I identify as a dysbiotic internal ecology. His etiological description elucidates the nested consequences of a dysbiotic environment.

My approach to the dysbiotic environment supports what Dr. Prescott and Dr. Logan call the "dysbiosphere." They write, "We are in the midst of massive biodiversity losses, global environmental degradation, rapid urbanization, and, of course, the reality of climate change. . . . Current species loss, by some estimates, is one thousand times higher than normal oscillations" (2017, 30, 33). In our present-day dysbiosphere, rapid industrial growth causes environmental degradation and provokes biodiversity loss, with detrimental effects to human health. This situation led Ceballos et al. to assert, "If the currently elevated extinction pace is allowed to continue, humans will soon (in as little as three human lifetimes) be deprived of many biodiversity benefits" (2015, 4). They affirm that on a human time scale, biodiversity loss would be permanent since, in the aftermath of past mass extinction, millions of years passed before the earth was able to rediversify. The question becomes: What has led earth's life forms to the brink of mass extinction?

From a functional medicine perspective, the answer may be humans' apathy to the well-being of non-human life (i.e., a failure to embrace Gaia 2.0). Dr. Prescott and Dr. Logan write, "There are global outcries when Apple moves a headphone jack—[meanwhile,] bees, fireflies, butterflies, and amphibians are all disappearing from our midst" (2017, 95). According to Dr. Prescott and Dr. Logan, these species are "beautiful to look at," but we only tend to notice them when they disappear. All have joined the endangered species list. Dr. Prescott and Dr. Logan take great pains to signal why we *should* care. Turning to the life work of Tari Haahtela, they note an ominous trend: "As butterfly species declined in certain areas, rates of allergies increased" (2017, 107). In contrast, "[a]llergy is rare where butterflies flourish in a biodiverse environment."[9] Functional medicine interlocutors build on Gaia 2.0 to emphasize how and why the health of other species sets the stage for human health.

Furthermore, functional medicine interlocutors often turn to the food system to signal the relationship between political ecology and human health. That is, our food system affects the integrity of the natural environment, determines the quality of our health, and has an enormous economic impact on our globe. Dr. Mayer writes, "Through our food supply, this system connects us closely to the world around us, picking up vital information about how our food is grown, what we put in our soil, and what chemicals were added to it before we buy it in the supermarket" (2016, 73). Furthermore, food is the language by which internal and external microbial ecologies communicate. Speaking to my concept of nested ecologies, Dr. Miller indicates, "The microbiome is a nerdy, scientific way of tracking that connection. It is a way of telling that story." Dr. Lynch adds, "We have a microbiome in our digestive system. Soils also have a microbiome. If we don't have a microbiome, we're sick. If the soils don't have a microbiome, it's sick. If the soil's sick, we're sick." The external microbiome in the natural environment affects the internal microbiome within our human bodies—the very essence of nested ecologies.

Thus, from a functional medicine perspective, "conventional" (read:

non-organic) farming techniques such as monoculture have extremely detrimental effects on human health. Dr. Hyman explains that present-day conventional farming is "hurting the soil that we grow our food in, so our soil is depleted and our food is depleted." Dr. Logan and Dr. Prescott analogize continuous monoculture to a "steady diet of fast food" for the microbiome of soil. "Apple varieties that are less common to North American supermarkets have a hundred times more phytonutrients than the standard fare. Older variants of organic yellow corn had sixty times more beta-carotene" (2017, 158–159). Agricultural practices determine the health of our crops, which, in turn, determines the health of humans.

This perspective reframes regenerative agriculture and conservation strategies for microbial diversity as public health interventions. Current farming practices are destroying our fresh water supply, and runoff from nitrogen-based fertilizers has created swaths of marine dead zones. According to the Food and Agriculture Organization of the United Nations, losses in agrobiodiversity sum to 90 percent of plant varieties and half of livestock varieties (Food and Agriculture Organization of the United Nations n.d.). Dr. Hyman explains why this is important: "No more bees, no more pollination, no more plants, no more animals—no more humans" (Hyman 2020, 18).

Agrobiodiversity losses demonstrate how factory farming of animals is bad for plants, animals, humans, and the planet. Dr. Prescott and Dr. Logan write, "Biodiversity loss leads to reduced interaction between environmental and human microbiotas. This in turn may lead to immune dysfunction and impaired tolerance mechanisms in humans" (2017, 131). Their assertion is supported by the 2015 World Health Organization Biodiversity Report, which reads: "Reduced contact of people with the natural environment and biodiversity, and biodiversity loss in the wide environment, leads to reduced diversity in the human microbiota, which itself can lead to immune dysfunction and disease" (World Health Organization and Secretariat of the Convention on Biological Diversity 2015, 8). Thus, public health interventions may include increasing contact between the natural environment and biodiversity.

Without ongoing contact with nature, individuals' mental health may suffer. Referring to "solastalgia"—a term coined by Australian philosopher Glen Albrecht to describe a loss of place that provokes nostalgia—Dr. Prescott and Dr. Logan write, "Environmental degradation from mining leaves visible scars on the land, and potentially on the less visible minds of those living in the affected areas" (2017, 110). The solution to solastalgia, from the perspective of functional medicine, is embracing nature and dirt (see Hunger, Gillespie, and Chen 2019). Krishnan suggests "getting a little bit dirtier" in order to reduce the incidence of allergies, asthma, and other immune dysfunctions. "We don't have to keep sanitizing our hands; we don't necessarily have to sanitize our environment around us." His assertions, combined with those expressed in the 2015 World Health Organization Biodiversity Report, represent a radical reframing of what public health might look like in the future.

Future public health interventions may embrace findings that a thriving external ecology leads to thriving human health. One example of this would be building more green spaces in urban environments. Dr. Prescott and Dr. Logan indicate, "Green spaces contribute unique and diverse bacterial signatures to the urban environment, and such vegetation makes a significant contribution to the airborne microbial content—up to tenfold higher than nearby non-vegetated built areas" (2017, 132). The creation of more green spaces would represent a nested ecologies approach to public health.

At present, unequal access to green space is a form of ecological injustice that manifests in unequal health outcomes. Dr. Prescott and Dr. Logan indicate that communities with more green space access generally have healthier dietary habits and are more physically active. This results in a lower risk of blood glucose and insulin imbalances. In contrast, communities with less green space access have a "greater density of fast-food outlets (and fewer fresh food stores) to promote noncommunicable diseases, especially in the disadvantaged neighborhoods" (2017, 59).

## EXPOSURE SCIENCE: "UNREASONABLE RISKS" AND HEALTH DISPARITIES

I similarly point to the relationship among poverty, toxic exposure, and the need for environmental justice. Intersectionally vulnerable individuals—for example, minorities, low income, women and children—are more likely to suffer the effects of multiple, overlapping toxic exposure. For example, Sobo and Loustaunau (2010) note that certain genetically linked disease states may in fact be triggered by manmade environmental conditions such as diet and toxic exposure (see also Gillman 2005; Weinhold 2006). This observation lies at the heart of environmental justice arguments. Thus, I critique the limited attempts made by many functional medicine practitioners to advocate for environmental justice, even while arguing for scientific exploration of the "exposome."

Existing toxicology tends to investigate single environmental exposures in isolation; however, this is not representative of the simultaneous exposures humans constantly face (see Stingone et al. 2017). In contrast, the exposome describes the sum total of toxic exposures over the course of an individual's life span. The term "exposome" was first coined in 2005 by Dr. Christopher Wild, a molecular epidemiologist, to highlight the role of cumulative environmental exposures in driving diseases. As Dr. Robert Verkerk, founder, executive, and scientific director at the Alliance for Natural Health International, explains, "The amount of chemicals that we are exposed to has increased exponentially. There are now 100 million substances [and] compounds used in products, and 75 percent of these were added in the last ten years." Individuals may be exposed to 100,000–200,000 fat-soluble toxins at any one phase of their lives. Timothy Frie, an inclusive health care and policy activist, asserts, "Our health is under attack. Profits are valued more than our lives and the well-being of our communities. There are toxicants in our water, pollutants in our air, carcinogens in our food, and rampant systemic social injustice in our communities." In his opinion, our increasingly toxic environment is the reason why Americans are struggling with greater incidences of chronic diseases than ever before, despite spending an exorbitant amount on health care.

The Toxic Substances Control Act (TSCA), signed into law by President Ford in 1976, grandfathered in the vast majority of "existing chemicals" with little to no safety data. Sarah Vogel (2013), a sociomedical scientist and public health scholar, describes how the TSCA furthermore created a catch-22 for the Environmental Protection Agency: "The agency can't make a finding of potential risk or significant exposure without data, but it can't get data without evidence that an 'unreasonable risk' may exist." Due to this high burden of proving that an existing chemical presents a significant risk, almost all chemicals have remained on the market. The US Government Accountability Office has highlighted the TSCA as an area of "high risk" for abuse and mismanagement, while the chemical industry trade associations maintain that the TSCA is a highly effective statute.

Dr. Cindy Fallon worked in industry until she realized that "I was inadvertently destroying my own health by consuming the toxins that came from the very company that had employed me for twenty-five years." Dr. Fallon argues that people working in industry "play by the rules" so they believe what they are doing is right. However, after struggling with fibromyalgia, eczema, allergies, and hypothyroidism, Dr. Fallon has learned to distinguish between what is legal and what is right. "Regulatory agencies like the EPA and FDA, in spite of being filled with really smart people of good intent, are currently designed to fail on their mission to protect public health and environmental health." Health problems stemming from exposures to multiple toxins do not figure into existing research protocols. She asserts, "The EPA comes right out and states that several studies have tested herbicide formulations, including Roundup, for mutagenic and genotoxic potential, and they say, 'Although positive responses have been reported, the testing systems used may not be adequate for regulatory purposes because ... exposures vary from the required testing protocols.'" The EPA must follow an existing protocol, and to get a change of protocol involves an act of Congress—however, an act of Congress requires sufficient evidence, which is not available using existing protocols. This catch-22 is not due to some moral failing of the people on the EPA board. Rather, the problem is systemic.

To clarify the extent of the problem, I offer the following analogy. Our current environmental protection system is like a legal system in which criminal defendants are innocent until proven guilty, and it is also up to the criminal defendant to gather evidence and prove his or her guilt. In contrast, Europe implemented REACH (Registration, Evaluation, Authorisation, and Restriction of Chemicals) in 2007. This "no data, no chemicals" policy emerged in response to European NGOs—Friends of the Earth, Greenpeace, the World Wildlife Fund, the European Environmental Bureau, and Women in Europe for a Common Future, among others—demanding data for all chemicals in production, placing the burden on industry to generate the data, and taking a precautionary approach to chemicals management.

"Unreasonable risk" and "precautionary" approaches differ fundamentally with regard to the burden of proof for action. While the first requires certainty of human causation of disease, the second necessitates only a critical level of concern. Exposure science redefines the terms of the debate since, instead of considering the potential risk of each chemical or toxin in isolation, scientists are evaluating the effects of a lifetime of toxins on human health.

From the perspective of functional medicine, advances in exposure science are beneficial to the whole of society since everyone is exposed to harmful environmental pollutants in our air and waterways. Dr. LePine describes how the exposures of individuals living in society are inextricably linked to one another. Individuals excrete antibiotics, synthetic hormones, and antidepressants into our water system, and this pharmaceutical-laden water is later consumed by others. This perspective is rooted in systems biology and emphasizes the interconnectedness of all life.

At the same time, the exposome represents the height of personalized medicine. Environmental exposures produce a range of different biological effects in different people. Dr. LePine indicates that who gets sick and who stays well, given these ubiquitous environmental exposures, "is a little bit of survival of the fittest." He explains, "The people who can detoxify well will actually survive in modern society better." He jokingly suggests that in order to live a long life in our modern-day environment, individuals need to be like DDT-resistant cockroaches. This focus on an individual's ability to detoxify runs the risk of obscuring environmental (in)justice.[10]

Pushing back against this tendency, I emphasize how disparate toxic exposures result in health disparities. For example, lead-poisoned children serve as visible reminders of how race- and class-based inequalities are inscribed on the bodies of future generations (Lanphear et al. 1998; Shostak 2013). Furthermore, certain populations face greater risks. The research of Hyland et al. (2021), based in California's Salinas Valley, points to how hidden class and racialized inequalities play a determining role in individuals' exposomes. Families living in Salinas Valley, one of the most productive agriculture regions in California, are mostly working class and Hispanic. These families live in close proximity to where agricultural pesticides are sprayed.

Essentially, the concept of nested ecologies adds a relational layer to the holobiont theory.[11] This layer is supported by Dr. Prescott and Dr. Logan, who define health as mutually imbricated with "the health of society and the health of the planet itself" (2017, 4). According to Dr. Kellman, "[v]iewing ourselves in this way—interconnected with loved ones, our community, our planet—is actually very healthy, with significant benefits for your immune system and your resilience, as well as your microbiome" (2018, 8). Thus, nested ecologies is a tool for thinking of each "individual" as multiple and destabilizing how "we" interact with the world around us. That is, nested ecologies provide a vocabulary for viewing ourselves as collaborators with other humans, other organisms, and microbiota—advocates for Gaia 2.0 with literal skin in the game.

## THE SOCIAL MICROBIOME

Seen through the lens of nested ecologies, the "social microbiome" has four layers. The first layer considers microbiota as communicating, "social" life forms. Dr. Prescott and Dr. Logan explain how, according to emerging microbiome research, microbiota possess "vast networks of intracellular machinery, signaling capabilities, and all sorts of regulatory chains within microbes" (2017, 274). These communicative mechanisms allow microbiota to work together in a collaborative and social manner, thus ensuring the survival of the community.

The second layer examines how microbiomes are created and shared through social interaction. This layer builds upon the first layer by illuminating how communities of "social" microbes are shaped and determined by our social behavior. That is, as much as people exist in and through nested ecologies, individuals and their bacteria also have "nested socialities." Dr. Kellman writes, "Family members tend to have similar microbiomes—not through genetics . . . but because they live in the same house" (2018, 9). Similarly, Krishnan notes, "We now know that there's a centralized kind of microbiome cloud, if you will. . . . When you're living in a household with other people, you've got a microbial community." This "microbiome cloud" also applies to other types of social collectives. Dr. Kellman notes, "One study even found that a woman's roller derby team shared common elements of their microbiome!" (2018, 9). Given that the gut microbiomes of individuals are socially constituted and socially maintained by those with whom they interact the most, this second layer gives new meaning to biosociality (see Rabinow 1996).

The perspective afforded by the second layer of the social microbiome tasks individuals with new responsibilities. Not only is a healthy microbiome a personal project, it is also an obligation to one's community. Dr. Prescott and Dr. Logan write, "Just like vaccination, your personal connection to nature and the steps you take to nourish the diversity of your gut microbes is good for the herd. For all of us" (2017, 9). Their words signal how proper microbiome management can eventually edge into the territory of public surveillance and control over individual bodies (think biopower; see Foucault 1998).

The third layer takes an expanded view of how human behavior shapes and determines the types of bacteria existing around, on, and within us. At the individual level, a culture of cleanliness leads people to use a battery of antibacterial personal hygiene and household disinfecting products, thus weakening the human microbiome to the point of disease vulnerability.[12] At the societal level, monocropping has led to an absence of beneficial bacteria (e.g., soil depletion, resulting in less nutritious food). At the same time, antimicrobial warfare in the form of broad-spectrum antibiotics has prompted the emergence of hyper-virulent bacteria (e.g., drug-resistant "germs").

The fourth and, in my view, most provocative and illuminating layer positions microbiomes as lenses for viewing and analyzing social inequality. Dr. Prescott and Dr. Logan explain, "Dysbiosis exists on a sliding scale, and that burden is shouldered by the disadvantaged. Lower levels of microbial diversity are found among socioeconomically deprived groups" (2017, 118). From an anthropological perspective, Amato et al. (2021) note that a wide range of minorities—including those whose minority status is based on race, sexual identity, gender, and socioeconomic status—experience a higher prevalence of many diseases. They note that the gut microbiome is shaped by the host's environment and in turn affects the host's metabolic, immune, and neuroendocrine functions. As such, the gut microbiome is an important pathway by which social, political, and economic forces can contribute to health inequalities. With an eye toward health policy, the authors foreground the role of host-gut microbe interactions in producing health inequalities, thus linking the microbiome to population health. With all this in mind, I argue that dysbiosis is a matter of environmental justice and social equity.

Furthermore, I argue alongside fellow anthropologists and functional medicine interlocutors that the health of humans, the environment, and the economy are interdependent. Anthropologist Katherine R. Amato opines that gut microbiome research will likely provide insight into underlying biological mechanisms that drive human health. At the same time, she emphasizes the importance of broader ecological and evolutionary contexts that frame how microbes and humans affect each other (Amato 2017). Ceballos et al. contribute to the discussion of environmental overexploitation for economic gain, notable habitat loss, and climate change: "All of these are related to human population size and growth, which increases consumption (especially among the rich), and economic inequality" (2015, 4). Dr. Prescott and Dr. Logan apply this socioeconomic perspective to marketing, along with other forces, that promotes dysbiosis in an unjust "societal womb." They connect dysbiosis to income inequality and argue that lack of exposure to diverse microbes is, in and of itself, a form of impoverishment (2017, 87). Overlapping microbial and socioeconomic poverty, in turn, undergirds booming rates of noncommunicable diseases such as type 2 diabetes, cardiovascular disease, asthma, allergies, autism, depression and other mental disorders, autoimmune conditions (e.g., Crohn's disease, ulcerative colitis, celiac disease), and neurodegenerative diseases.

Socioeconomic poverty (and thus microbial poverty) can be observed at the neighborhood level. Simply put, poverty maps onto dysbiosis. The impoverished neighborhoods Dr. Prescott and Dr. Logan have academically defined as "grey space" are characterized by clusters of fast food outlets serving ultra-processed foods, sedentary screen time, lack of access to quality health care, factories, pollution, and billboards promoting an unhealthy lifestyle.[13] In contrast, describing the work of their friend and colleague,

Richard Mitchell, Dr. Prescott and Dr. Logan emphasize how neighborhood greenness is a marker of socioeconomic privilege. They write, "Satellite images can help to identify green and quantify trees, but they have a hard time revealing the lifestyle intersections of green space and grey space" (2017, 99). While I support their cartographic description of socioeconomic privilege and contact with nature, I critique their use of the word "lifestyle."

I furthermore disagree with the proposal by Mitchell et al. (2015) that access to "green space" is an answer to socioeconomic inequality and health inequality. Mitchell found that mental well-being is socioeconomically determined, but that the effects of socioeconomic inequality can be ameliorated by up to 40 percent if individuals have good access to green areas. Mitchell et al. write, "If societies cannot, or will not, narrow socioeconomic inequality, research should explore the so-called equigenic environments—those that can disrupt the usual conversion of socioeconomic inequality to health inequality" (2015, 84). Dr. Prescott and Dr. Logan support this assertion. "In an urban environment, a vegetation-rich shared commons with some water and diverse wildlife is a living, breathing, omnipresent disruptor of inequality" (2017, 100). From this perspective, the simple remediation of vacant urban lots with trees and vegetation can result in less stress and decreased level of violence. Dr. Prescott and Dr. Logan assert, "The financial return to society on violence reduction alone, never mind healthcare in general, is estimated at hundreds of dollars for every single dollar invested in remediation" (2017, 111). While I am by no means against the "greening" of poor neighborhoods, I argue that planting trees is *not* a sufficient response to the pressing concern of socioeconomic inequality.

It is not enough to ameliorate the effects of poverty by dressing up poor neighborhoods with leafy parks. Green areas in poor neighborhoods are required, but this cannot be used as an "easy fix" to let society off the hook for social inequalities that unduly affect disadvantaged citizens. I agree with Dr. Prescott and Dr. Logan that "inequalities stand in the way of access to biodiversity" (2017, 292). However, I furthermore argue that "taking back the microbiome" through equal opportunities requires a multifaceted approach involving multiple social programs.

## DIVERSITY

Lessons learned from nature are useful tools for examining society. According to emerging microbiome research, microbial diversity is crucial to human health. In the same vein, I argue that social diversity is critical for the health of society (Montgomery 2020a and 2020b).[14] Furthermore, social diversity and microbial diversity are intertwined. Interactions between different groups of people quite literally diversify the gut microbiome of diverse actors. Through equitable access to nutritious food and natural environments, a socially just society promotes equitable access to microbial diversity.

Functional medicine interlocutors unequivocally assert that microbial diversity is integral to human health (see Li 2019, 40, 47). Dr. Mayer writes, "One of the generally agreed-upon criteria for a healthy gut microbiome has been its diversity and the abundance of microbial species present in it. As in the natural ecosystems around us, high diversity of the microbiome means resilience and low diversity means vulnerability to perturbations" (2016, 271–272). Dr. Prescott and Dr. Logan add, "There is little doubt that the sustainability of life on Earth is maintained by diversity" (2017, 93). Over the course of my ethnographic research, the importance of microbial diversity for human health emerged as a consistent theme in functional medicine discourse.[15]

Nonetheless, the importance of microbial diversity has only recently been established. According to Dr. Kharrazian, the major microbiome breakthrough of recent years has been the shift away from a binary approach (i.e., "good bacteria" vs. "bad bacteria") to a model that emphasizes diversity. In this new model, Dr. William Li explains, diversity is what separates people who "get sick all the time" from people who "seem to never get sick." Similarly, Krishnan explains, "Low diversity equals high risk for chronic illness, [while] high diversity equals high degree of protection against chronic illness, including longevity." This new model validates functional medicine's focus on nutrition since diet directly shapes the microbiome. Moving forward, functional medicine will continue to focus on nutrition as a "modifiable target" since the "North American diet" is responsible for up to a one-third decrease in microbial diversity (Mayer 2016, 206).

To this end, functional medicine practitioners and proponents have developed analogies to explain why diet is so important to patients. Patel provides the following financial analogy to explain how low microbial diversity places people at risk for disease: "We take this very diverse microbiome . . . and we narrow the strains of the bacteria. It's like taking the diversity out of your stock portfolio—you are more prone to fluctuations in the stock market." In contrast, Dr. Li describes a diverse microbiome to a "dazzling coral reef that thrives with many species living in close proximity" (2019, 241). Viewing the microbiome as an ecosystem not only folds beautifully into the nested ecologies concept, it also signals how, through effective collaborations among bacteria, microbial diversity is protective of health.

Functional medicine interlocutors' view of microbial diversity is supported by emerging research into the impact of the microbiome on longevity. According to Krishnan, scholars such as Jiangchao Zhao are examining how gut microbiota signatures modulate longevity. Krishnan explains, "They were looking at a certain Chinese population of people [who] . . . actually live active and very healthy lives even in their 90s and 100s. And one of the things that they found was the diversity of their gut microbiota was greater than that of even young adults." Dr. Li describes a similar study on "super-healthy super-agers," individuals who lived into their seventies, eighties, and nineties with no health issues. He indicates that when researchers compared the gut microbiomes of these "super-agers" to young, healthy athletes, "their gut microbiomes were remarkably similar—they were almost identical!" Krishnan sums up these findings: "Diversity is paramount to health. We cannot overstate that because study after study has confirmed that." According to recent microbiome research, maintaining higher microbial diversity over the life course supports longevity.

As an ethnographer listening to functional medicine interlocutors' descriptions of microbiome research, I couldn't help but think of the microbiome as a microcosm of society. I apply lessons learned from the microbiome to society as a whole. Thus, I contend that social diversity determines the well-being of a society, while less diversity sets the stage for inequality, conflict, violence, and hate. I embrace the political nature of this argument; however, at the same time, I ask, why is it political? Dr. Prescott and Dr. Logan's biological concept of diverse microorganisms living together and working together "socially" and "altruistically" to create a healthy microbiome is not political. Dr. Li's ecological concept of diverse species living together in harmony to create a thriving coral reef is not political. Patel's financial concept of a diverse stock portfolio to maximize earnings and minimize risk is not political. So why would the social argument that a just society is built through collaborations among diverse communities of people be considered political? More broadly, how does knowledge circulate—temporally, socially, and politically?

To answer this question, I turn to the work of anthropologist Lesley Green. Green (2019) argues that the Anthropocene pushes us to problematize what is considered valid vs. illegitimate knowledge and who is considered expert vs. non-expert. Doing so allows us to embrace multiple sensibilities, to engage in a South-to-North dialogue regarding the scale of conceptual shifts needed to address the Anthropocene, and to address inequality and racism inherited by environmental sciences. Furthermore, Green points to how economics have been hijacked by finance. Pointing to "ekos" as a common root, she argues instead for reclaiming "ecological economics." In essence, Green demonstrates how the questions I have posed may not be political and yet are produced as political economical approaches to life. Building upon Green's argument, I suggest that alleviating social inequality can produce better outcomes in almost every area of life, ranging from economic productivity to health outcomes.

As if responding to Green, Dr. Prescott and Dr. Logan indicate that "socioeconomically advantaged groups are much less likely to consider the economics of the disadvantaged unless empathy is provoked" (2017, 46). From a functional medicine perspective, dysbiotic environments can make people less empathetic to the plight of others (see Prescott and Logan 2017, 250). As a medical anthropologist, I argue that this approach runs the risk of biologizing callousness instead of holding individuals responsible for their lack of concern for others. Furthermore, as someone who teaches sociocultural anthropology, I observe on a daily basis how ethnography stimulates learners to consider the lived realities of those who face distinct socioeconomic conditions. While Dr. Prescott and Dr. Logan lament a "a systemic slide in empathy" and describe how this "represents yet one more barrier in the quest to narrowing social and health inequalities," I argue that anthropology "provokes" empathy and demands action.

# ∾ *Interlude* ∾

## TOXICITY

I read in Amy Myers's book, *The Autoimmune Solution*, that removing toxins hidden in my everyday environment was key to reversing my autoimmunity. From the perspective of functional medicine, autoimmunity is the body's logical response to an environment that has been contaminated beyond recognition. I went into my bathroom and began examining all my personal care and beauty products, using the Environmental Working Group's Skin Deep database to identify any health hazards. Immediately, I discovered that even the products I considered to be "clean" were filled with ingredients that pose risk for cancer, developmental and reproductive toxicity, and allergies and immunotoxicity.

Once you know, you can't unknow. I felt an urgent need to purge my bathroom—and my entire house—of all these harmful chemicals, and I spent several days feverishly searching the database. When a certain product was not listed, I searched for its ingredients one by one. Inevitably, I found a hazardous ingredient. I started this "spring cleaning" project assuming I was going to weed out the bad ones. It soon became clear that I was bathed (literally and figuratively) in carcinogens and toxins.

When I finished purging, there was almost nothing left. I had to start fresh—this time by searching the database for the safest products and filling my home with these. This process was expensive, and I was hyperaware of my privilege. At the same time, I recognized that purchasing all these items might not be sustainable in the long term. I created a table in which I listed all the clean products that I purchased, their unit prices, recipes for DIY alternatives, and their respective unit prices. Over the coming months, I set out to transition to as many DIY alternatives as possible. "Product formulator" became a role I adopted as part of my health journey.

During my next follow-up visit in San Antonio, my doctor was running late. We waited an hour and a half past my appointment time before she came into the exam room, and then we had only a few minutes to consult with her before she rushed off to the next patient. She asked her physician's assistant to print out some handouts for me to take home. We waited for another half hour, feeling hungry, tired, and annoyed. We were eager to get back on the road for our four-hour trek back to McAllen. When the physician's assistant finally came into the exam room, she handed me a few handouts and briskly escorted us to the exit door.

The next day, while sitting at my dining room table, I examined the handouts. Among them was an info sheet about glyphosate and a second sheet comparing the highest glyphosate foods at the grocery store. Glyphosate, a chemical that was initially used as a chelating agent in plumbing, is now commonly used as an herbicide in the US food system. My doctor had hurriedly suggested that I switch to an all-organic diet. Perhaps this handout was her way of explaining to me why eating organic is important and arming me with the information I needed to identify glyphosate hidden in everyday food items? Given what I had learned about my genomic profile—specifically, my lessened ability to conjugate glutathione to toxins for removal from the body—I knew I couldn't afford "normal" amounts of exposure to glyphosate through conventional food. I filed away the handouts in an accordion folder, but I continued to mull over this information for the next few days.

The next time Rikin and I were at our local big box grocery store, I mentioned to him that I wanted to switch to an all-organic diet as the doctor had briefly suggested. He blurted out, "We can't afford that!" In his view, an all-organic diet is for folks much richer than we are, and the doctor demonstrated her personal privilege by making this suggestion. Her doctor's salary gave her easy access to things that are out of reach for most patients, and she was out of touch with her patients' reality.

Rikin's initial reaction hurt my feelings. I felt that, by expressing anxiety about making ends meet, he was not prioritizing my health and well-being. However, after speaking more with him, I realized he had not read the handouts, and he didn't make the connection between conventional food and my chronic health issues. From his perspective, we had both been eating conventional food our whole lives—along with everyone else who is not superrich. If the doctor had prescribed a medication or offered me a medical procedure, he would immediately recognize these as valid costs. However, in his view, conventional food is just a part of normal life, while organic food is a status marker for the wealthy.

We talked more about the relationship between glyphosate and chronic illness, especially within the context of my genome. After reviewing the science, we both made the switch to a plant-based, nutrient-dense, and organic diet. Our grocery bill nearly doubled. We have both seen improvements in our health, and we consider this to be a worthwhile investment. What we spend on groceries now we will hopefully save in medical expenses later. At the same time, I have sought ways to reduce our grocery bills where possible. For example, we now buy most of our groceries through a local community supported agriculture (CSA) program and online wholesalers. We often eat produce that is surplus or "imperfect" (e.g., misshapen, scarred, and oddly sized), but regardless of the aesthetics, we are grateful for the nourishment this food provides.

The experience left me thinking about people who are less privileged than we are. In our case, budgeting for organic food was a matter of changing our priorities, habits, and expectations. For many, paying double upfront to protect their health is not an option. Instead, they pay through pain, suffering, disease, and medical bills after their health has already deteriorated. If they are recipients of Medicare or Medicaid, taxpayer dollars pick up the tab for extraordinary health care costs. Wouldn't it make more sense—from both the perspective of socioeconomics and human dignity (and rights and compassion!)—to make sure everyone has access to clean food and a nontoxic environment?

# CONCLUSION
# FOOD JUSTICE

The physicians are the natural attorneys of the poor, and the social problems should largely be solved by them.

Medicine, as a social science, as the science of human beings, has the obligation to point out problems and to attempt their theoretical solution. If medicine is to fulfill her great task, then she must enter the political and social life.

DR. RUDOLF VIRCHOW (1821–1902), PHYSICIAN, ANTHRO-POLOGIST, PATHOLOGIST, AND POLITICIAN, AS WELL AS THE FOUNDER OF SOCIAL MEDICINE[1]

In this book, I have advanced the concept of nested ecologies as a heuristic tool for understanding how functional medicine uses systems biology to contextualize bodies within ecological environments. At the same time, I have argued for an expanded view of "external" ecologies. That is, the complex inner workings of the human body are framed and shaped by the physical, cultural, and socioeconomic contexts in which they are nested. Individual health relies on the health of society and the health of the planet itself.

The concept of nested ecologies has many potential applications. For example, nested ecologies can be used as a lens for exploring the importance of environmental conservation for human health and for reframing access to green spaces as a matter of social justice. Nested ecologies can be harnessed as a critique of industries that pollute our environment and our bodies, including those that produce everyday consumer items like cosmetics and household cleaning products. The concept can be leveraged to examine the inner workings of government agencies like the Food and Drug Administration and the Environmental Protection Agency and to interrogate the relationships among funding structures, legislation, and human health. Nested ecologies can be politicized to champion for greater regulation of chemicals, beyond what currently exists under the Toxic Substances

Control Act (TSCA). The concept offers key insights into the shortcomings of the existing health care system, including the logics that define what services are accessible through Medicare and Medicaid.[2] In every instance, nested ecologies highlight the unfortunate link between privilege and health in our neoliberal society.

While the concept of nested ecologies can be applied to many areas of life, food is a valuable lens for examining the Anthropocene and how human health is nested in political ecology. I have noted the epigenetic impact of food on the human body; how socioeconomic and racialized structures undergird food access; how existing food policies drive chronic disease among lower-income and minority communities; and how the gut is being positioned as the site of contestation by those who identify genetic modification as a likely cause of chronic disease. In this concluding chapter, I delve deeper into how the food system is described by functional medicine interlocutors in order to further illuminate some of the implications of nested ecologies for our world.

Functional medicine practitioners often say, "food is medicine." From this perspective, ill health can often be attributed to an unwholesome diet. Approaching the problem as a systems thinker, Dr. Hyman asked himself, "What causes the food?" The answer was the food system. However, this led him to another question: "What causes the food system?" The answer to this question was food policies. This led him to a final question: "What causes the food policies?" Then it dawned on Dr. Hyman that, in our current neoliberal system, food policies are shaped by the food industry, and industry interests are wreaking havoc on human health.

Problems with the food system require urgent action. Dr. Hyman indicates, "In ten years, 83 million Americans will have three or more chronic diseases, compared to 30 million in 2015" (Hyman 2020, 13). Increase in chronic disease is correlated to loss of quality-adjusted life years and life in general. Stated differently, "The average child born today will live five fewer years than their parents, and if they are poor or socially disadvantaged, they will live [ten] to [twenty] fewer years than their parents" (Hyman 2020, 46). Being overfed and undernourished is the leading cause of death worldwide, and for the first time in history, life expectancy in the United States is on the decline.

Dr. Hyman argues that by fixing the food system, the United States would not only reduce the incidence of chronic disease and obesity, but could also address the $22 trillion national debt, reverse the destruction of our environment, seek social justice by minimizing poverty, improve children's ability to learn and develop, increase political stability, and fortify communities. He even goes as far as to affirm that "[i]f we were to identify one big lever to pull to improve global health, create economic abundance, reduce social injustice and mental illness, restore environmental health, and reverse climate change, it would be transforming our entire food system" (Hyman 2020, 7). In his view, how our society grows, processes, produces, distributes, consumes, and wastes food is *the* biggest issue today.

Dr. Hyman is on an urgent mission to transform the food system. "When I graduated medical school, there was not a single state with an obesity rate over 20 percent. Now there is not a single state with an obesity rate under 20 percent" (Hyman 2020, 42). In conversation with Dr. Anand Parekh, chief medical advisor at the Bipartisan Policy Center, Dr. Hyman notes that, according to his estimates, 40 to 50 percent of people die from diet-related diseases such as obesity, diabetes, and heart disease. Dr. Parekh adds, "I call obesity the public health challenge of our century." Dr. Hyman's mission to "fix the food system" and Dr. Parekh's vision of bipartisan public health policy that focuses on prevention are informed by their experiences as doctors.

However, Dr. Hyman realized he could not cure obesity and diabetes in his office. "I felt like I was mopping up the floor while the sink is overflowing and never getting anywhere because people were in a toxic food environment." True to his functional medicine training, Dr. Hyman asked why the food system is structured as it is. He concludes, "As a doctor, it is increasingly clear to me that the health of our citizens, the health of our society and our planet, depends on disruptive innovations that decentralize and democratize food production and consumption" (Hyman 2020, 7). The "disruptive innovations" Dr. Hyman envisions include producing real food at scale; restoring the health of soils, water, air, and the biodiversity of our planet; halting climate change; and preventing and reversing disease.

## BIG FOOD AND BIG AG

The expansive reach of the food system cannot be underestimated. It encompasses all companies that are involved in the production of food before it lands on our plates. These include (genetically modified) seed companies; factory farms; companies that produce fertilizer, pesticides, and herbicides; and processed food companies. Operating together, these companies create an unparalleled industrial behemoth. Dr. Hyman explains that the food system is "the biggest industry on the planet because everybody eats." The food and beverage industries hold the largest shares of the gross domestic product in emerging economies such as Brazil, Russia, India, China, and South Africa (see Otero 2018).

The power of the food industry, however, is not merely a feature of its breadth and the fact that everyone must consume the food industry's products every day for sustenance. Since the 1990s, heavy concentration of food processors has led to consolidation and mega-mergers. Dr. Hyman writes, "The consolidation and monopolization of the food industry over the last 40 years from hundreds of different processed-food companies, seed companies, and chemical fertilizer companies into just a few dozen companies make it the largest collective industry in the world, valued at approximately $15 trillion, or about 17 percent of the world's economy" (2020, 5). In 2014, Arlene Spark reported that four pork processors slaughtered 64 percent of the pork in the United States. Three of the same companies, plus National Beef, slaughtered 81 percent of the beef. Similarly, four companies slaughtered more than half of broiler chickens (Spark 2014, 45). In 2009, the top ten food processors accounted for 28 percent of the world market share (Otero 2018, 17). As a result, a few dozen CEOs control an important aspect of human health.

Functional medicine interlocutors advocate for the de-monopolization of food. Dennis Kucinich, a former US representative from Ohio (1997 to 2013), argues that horizontal and vertical monopolies have created an agribusiness monolith that has "destroyed family farmers, and has actually made America a less democratic nation." He continues, "We need to stop the vertical and horizontal integration that has gone on financially, to the detriment of a lot of small producers. We need to help people go back to the farms, and we need to put limits on the amount of farmland that any one company can own." At the same time, Kucinich links agribusiness to allied industries such as the chemical industry, the biotech industry, and the banks that back them up.

## COMMODITY CROPS AND GOVERNMENT SUBSIDIES

Glyphosate is hyper-prevalent in the food system because GMO and glyphosate-laden crops—namely, corn, wheat, and soy, also referred to as "commodity crops"—are subsidized by the US government. Otero writes, "These crops are subsidized because powerful lobby groups get immense profits from them" (Otero 2018, 16, citing Baines 2015; Winders 2009a, 2009b). Due to these subsidies, much of what Otero calls "the neoliberal diet" can be traced to GMO crops.

While consumers may avoid glyphosate-laden GMO crops, they may still be exposed to the harmful effects of these crops through meat consumption. Again, this practice is driven by government subsidies. Dr. Neil Barnard, president of the Physicians Committee for Responsible Medicine, indicates, "Up until this point, the US government gives almost nothing to vegetables and fruits, and it gives huge subsidies to animal agriculture." These subsidies are indirect. While conducting an interview with Kucinich, John Robbins explains, "In the United States, the federal government subsidizes genetically engineered feed grains—mainly corn and soy, which are fed to livestock in factory farms" (Robbins and Robbins 2013, 183). Stated differently, the majority of GMO soybeans and corn are used to feed livestock because government subsidies lead farmers to grow more commodity crops than American citizens can consume.

Functional medicine practitioners and proponents note a stark mismatch between official dietary recommendations and the way government subsidies are structured. John Robbins notes, "In fact, almost two-thirds of federal subsidy funding currently ends up supporting meat and dairy products, and a great deal also ends up lowering the price of things like high-fructose corn syrup. Less than 1 percent goes to fruits and vegetables" (Robbins and Robbins 2013). Dr. Hyman explains, "We tell everybody to eat five to nine servings of fruits and vegetables, yet 1 percent of government support is for that." Dr. Hyman goes on to say that funding influences how farmland is used: only 2 percent of our land grows fruits and vegetables. As a result, there is not enough produce grown in the United States for every American to follow the official dietary recommendations.

Functional medicine interlocutors, food scholars, and politicians alike have used the dinner plate to emphasize this mismatch. Marion Nestle writes, "More than three quarters of your plate would be taken up by a massive corn fritter (80 percent of benefits go to corn, grains, and soy oil). You'd have a Dixie cup of milk (dairy gets 3 percent), a hamburger the size of a half dollar (livestock: 2 percent), two peas (fruits and vegetables: 0.45 percent), and an after-dinner cigarette (tobacco: 2 percent). Oh, and a really big linen napkin (cotton: 13 percent) to dab your lips" (Nestle 2016).

Essentially, government subsidies are a political economic structure buttressing chronic disease. Dr. Hyman emphasizes, "The food we are growing . . . ends up causing all this chronic disease at the other end of the spectrum." Delving into details, Robbins notes, "At a time when we have the highest rates of obesity of any country in the world, and when one in three US children is expected to get diabetes, we subsidize the foods that make us sick" (Robbins and Robbins 2013, 183). However, questions remain: Why has the

state not addressed this obvious mismatch between official recommendations and government subsidies? More broadly, how does the food industry
dominate public policy?

## INFORMATION WARFARE

According to Dr. Hyman, money rules politics—a reality that has resulted
in subsidies that facilitate Big Food and Big Ag's interests to the detriment
of human health and our environment. "Big Ag and Big Food co-opt politicians, public health groups, grassroots advocacy groups, scientists, and
schools and pollute science and public opinion with vast amounts of dollars
and misinformation campaigns" (Hyman 2020, 5). Offering the Farm Bill
as one example, Dr. Hyman notes how "over six hundred companies spent
$500 million to influence the 2014 Farm Bill to get what they wanted. Almost
seventy-three percent of the members of the Senate Committee on Agriculture, Nutrition and Forestry and ninety percent of the House Agricultural
Committee receive donations from Monsanto (Bayer) and Syngenta. If you
add in all the other food and agriculture companies, one hundred percent
of members would have received donations" (Hyman 2020, 32). He furthermore indicates that from 2015 to 2018, the House Agriculture Committee,
consisting of forty-six members of Congress, accepted roughly $1.2 mil-
lion in campaign contributions from the soda and sugar industries (Sessa-
Hawkins 2017).

Dr. Hyman signals the "revolving door" problem in government. Former industry lobbyists are appointed to government positions and return
to their lobbying careers after leaving their government posts. For example,
the USDA hired sugar, corn, and snack food lobbyist Kailee Tkacz to work
as an adviser on its 2020 dietary guidelines. Dr. Hyman addresses this practice: "Thirteen out of the twenty members of the new guideline committee
have worked for industry and the one who is overseeing it for the government used to be the head of the Corn Refiner's Association that makes
high-fructose corn syrup and the Snack Food Association. It's like the fox
guarding the hen house!" Using this analogy, the "hen house" is positively
overrun with "foxes." Dr. Hyman notes, "There just happens to be about 187
lobbyists for every member of Congress." Dr. Hyman argues that grassroots
efforts are needed to impel lobby reform, including restricting government
officials from becoming lobbyists and lobbyists from taking government
jobs, implementing taxes on excessive lobbying, and prohibiting personal
gifts to public officials.

The powerful influence of food industry lobbyists on legislation has not gone unnoticed by food activists, who are interpellated as interlocutors in the functional medicine movement. When Timothy Frie ran for the Florida state senate in 2020, Big Ag corporations began contacting him immediately after he filed for office. He thought, "Where are the advocacy groups for nutrition and regenerative agriculture and functional medicine?" Robbins interviewed Morgan Spurlock, the documentary filmmaker who directed and starred in the 2004 documentary, *Super Size Me.* During his interview, Spurlock asked Robbins, "What do you think is the biggest thing that's keeping these misguided subsidies in place? Is it just the big business lobby? Is it all the money that's basically pumping into our system in D.C. . . . ?" Robbins responded, "It's big agribusiness and big lobbying dollars from institutions like the Sugar Association, the National Livestock and Meat Board, National Beef Council, National Dairy Council, the Milk Board, and the Grocery Manufacturers Association." As if responding to Robbins's comment, Dr. Hyman concludes, "We don't have a government for the people, by the people, of the people. We have a government for the corporations, by the corporations, and of the corporations." Functional medicine interlocutors and food activists agree that the billions of dollars spent by lobbyists corrupt the government and determine subsidies.

In fact, given the dire effects of the food system on clinical outcomes, some functional medicine interlocutors consider food activism to be an integral part of their role as doctors and health educators. (In this chapter, I will refer to these individuals as "functional medicine interlocutors qua food activists.") Dr. Hyman is, perhaps, the most visible among them. He has increasingly used his public platform for discussing the impact of food policy on health. In 2020, Dr. Hyman sat down with Bill Frist, former Republican senator from Tennessee and former US Senate majority leader. The two established a rapport as fellow doctors. Senator Frist, a heart and lung transplant surgeon and the author of more than one hundred peer-reviewed medical articles, was the first physician to serve in the US Senate since 1928. Dr. Hyman took the opportunity to ask Senator Frist about the problem of lobbying, pointing specifically to the $192 million that the food industry spent to block the GMO labeling bill. In response, Senator Frist suggested that lobbying is not an insurmountable obstacle. In his opinion, the GMO labeling bill failed to pass due to a lack of scientific understanding. In response, I argue the role of lobbying should not be minimized or ignored. However, Senator Frist's point about "scientific understanding" also deserves deeper exploration.

Calling out what he terms "information warfare," Dr. Hyman asserts that the food industry co-opts public health and distorts nutrition science. To support his claim, Dr. Hyman notes that, from 2008 to 2016, Coca-Cola funded 389 articles in 169 journals that concluded that physical activity is the primary determinant of health while diet is essentially harmless (see Serôdio, McKee, and Stuckler 2018). The food industry spends more than $12 billion a year funding nutrition studies, while the National Institutes of Health (NIH) spends a mere $1 billion. With this in mind, Dr. Hyman asks whether science is, in fact, propaganda.

Dr. Hyman furthermore reveals the insidious ways Big Food buys partnerships and thus control over medical "science." For example, the American Diabetes Association has signed a number of major agreements with companies like General Mills, Coca-Cola, Kraft Foods, and Campbell's (Low and Hacker 2013). Between 2009 and 2015, Coca-Cola gave the American Academy of Pediatrics approximately $3 million. In 2017, the American Heart Association received $182 million from PepsiCo, Kraft Foods, Monsanto, Unilever, Mars, Kellogg's, Domino's Pizza, Subway, and General Mills, among others. The Academy of Nutrition and Dietetics allows food corporations to teach dietitians: Coca-Cola Beverage Institute for Health and Wellness, Kraft Foods Global, PepsiCo Health & Nutrition, Nestlé Healthcare Nutrition, and General Mills Bell Institute of Health & Nutrition are among accredited continuing education providers. To fix this situation, Dr. Hyman argues for the ethical sponsorship of professional societies and associations.

In addition to these efforts to control medical "science," the food industry also aims to control public opinion. Dr. Hyman argues that Big Food hides behind benevolently named front groups and thus gains control over public opinion. Groups like the Coalition for Safe and Affordable Food (funded by General Mills and Monsanto) and the Center for Food Integrity (funded by Monsanto, National Restaurant Association, and United Soybean Board) disparage organic food production, defend pesticides and antibiotics in animal production, and promote the trans fats, GMO foods, and artificial sweeteners.

Seen from an anthropological perspective, what Dr. Hyman describes is biopolitics in action—the mechanisms through which human life is managed under regimes of authority. According to anthropologists Paul Rabinow and Nikolas Rose, three key elements constitute biopolitics: "Knowledge of vital life processes, power relations that make humans as living beings as their object, and the modes of subjectivation through which subjects work on themselves qua living beings" (Rabinow and Rose 2006, 215). Given this definition, nothing is more biopolitical than control over public policies regarding food and "scientific" knowledge regarding the effects of food on health. The food industry directly influences the "framework of ideas, standards, formal procedures, and unarticulated understandings that specify how concerns about health, medicine, and the body are made the simultaneous focus of biomedicine and state policy" (Epstein 2007, 17). Through control over public policy, medical "science," and public opinion, the food industry has successfully manipulated the biomedical paradigm and relocated the ultimate source of biopower from the state to corporations.

The food industry exercises capitalist biopower par excellence. Corporations place profit before human health when controlling "scientific" knowledge and state policy. As Robbins and Robbins indicate, "Agrichemical companies, factory farms, and junk food manufacturers are profiting from a status quo that makes us sick, pollutes the environment, and leaves workers impoverished" (Robbins and Robbins 2013, 161). From their perspective, this has resulted in massive illness, trillions of dollars in health care expenses, and widespread hunger. As if in response, Dr. Barnard points out that despite the exorbitant cost of food policies to individuals and our society, "[o]ur government has reinforced and supported the industrial food machine: feedlot agriculture, Monsanto, McDonald's, factory farms, and even now, genetically engineered foods" (quoted in Robbins and Robbins 2013, 38). The food system's hold on public policy affects every person living in America; however, capitalist biopower is certainly not new.

I argue that industry has used unethical means to gain a powerful hold on "science" for decades (see, for example, Carson 1962 and Brodeur 1985). Attempts to deny and suppress information, control research, and manipulate science about the toxic nature of their products were rampant in the tobacco, automobile, asbestos, lead, vinyl, and nuclear power industries during the twentieth century (see Markowitz and Rosner 2002). I suggest that in our contemporary era of neoliberal privatization, deregulation, and globalization, the threat from unregulated industry goes even deeper.

The food industry, in particular, has long had success in shaping nutritional "science" and influencing legislation. Similar to the sleight of hand described by Ralph Nader (1965) with regard to the automobile industry, the food industry has blamed individuals for their food "choices" and ill health. That is, the ill health that results from consuming industrial food products is framed as a problem of overconsumption and insufficient physical activity on the part of consumers. Then, other products—lower fat, lower sugar products labeled with buzzwords such as "diet," "lite," "light," "natural," and "healthy"—are marketed as solutions to other processed foods (Gálvez 2018, 12). Given the power of epigenetics to determine our gene expression, the consequences of these predatory marketing strategies on human health can last for generations.

The issue of GMO seeds represents a powerful lens for viewing the food industry's tactical engagements in "information warfare." Jeffrey Smith, founder and executive director of the Institute for Responsible Technology, explains that scientists are often unable to conduct experiments on GMOs because they are denied access to patented seeds by the companies that own them. Furthermore, when scientists do discover problems, they face personal repercussions.

Smith describes the experience of Russian Academy of Sciences senior researcher Irina Ermakova. Ermakova conducted an experiment in which she fed female rats genetically modified soy. Many of their offspring died, while others were sterile. According to Smith, "She told me that her boss, under pressure from his boss, forbade her from doing any further GMO research. There were methods used to try to intimidate her, documents stolen from her laboratory and burnt on her desk, and samples stolen" (quoted in Robbins and Robbins 2013, 74).

Smith then offers Andrés Carrasco as an example of a scientist who had been silenced and physically attacked. "An organized mob of more than a hundred people attacked him and his friends when he tried to give a talk on the birth defect links to Roundup, Monsanto's herbicide that is used in conjunction with crops" (quoted in Robbins and Robbins 2013, 74). From the perspective of functional medicine interlocutors like Smith, the GMO industry threatens the safety of scientists and the integrity of science itself.

## GENETIC COLONIZATION

Functional medicine interlocutors qua food activists furthermore point to the effects of the GMO industry on farmers and on democratic society. Dr. Vandana Shiva, author and founder of Research Foundation for Science, Technology and Ecology, argues that companies like Monsanto unethically patent life forms on the false grounds of having invented seeds. Shiva insists that, in fact, "they poison the seeds, and they should be treated as polluters and fined, not rewarded with a monopoly." Her analogy of poisoning the seeds describes how GM seeds are created by inserting a gene that encodes for glyphosate-tolerant enzymes.

Dr. Shiva equates the patenting of life forms to colonization. Referring to the histories of India, Africa, and Latin America, Dr. Shiva explains that colonization involved the misappropriation of land and the dispossession of people. "Today the colonization is of the seeds themselves" (quoted in Robbins and Robbins 2013, 89). Leah Penniman, a Black creole farmer and food justice activist, expresses similar concerns in describing the "imposition of European control, power, and norms over our food system." According to Penniman, contemporary colonization of the food system is pervasive.

Functional medicine interlocutors qua food activists simultaneously critique the dire consequences of seed patents on human well-being. Dr. Shiva asserts that "Monsanto's superprofits and royalties have trapped our farmers in debt, and a quarter-million Indian farmers, mostly in the cotton areas, have committed suicide. Patents on seed mean genocide" (quoted in Robbins and Robbins 2013, 89). Meanwhile, people in the United States also face dispossession. Although sustainable farming practices can be traced to African and Indigenous roots, Black people make up only 2 percent of farmers and 1 percent of rural land owners in the United States. Kaya Purohit, chief content officer for Hyman Digital LLC explains, "This is largely the result of discriminatory government laws and funding as well as a lack of legal and financial resources due to systemic racism." From a functional medicine perspective, this decline in Black and Brown farmers leads to disconnection from cultural practices that connect people to the land. Furthermore, it produces unequal access to health-sustaining foods and ultimately causes health disparities.

According to Dr. Hyman and Penniman, food has been weaponized against people of color for decades. Penniman describes how the Greenwood Food Blockade punished civil rights activists by cutting off food supplies to Black communities in the 1960s. Referring to our contemporary moment, Dr. Hyman indicates that the racialization of chronic disease is "not an accident" and calls processed foods "biological weapons of mass destruction." Similarly, Dr. Logan and Dr. Prescott argue that "junk food adherence" is a vicious cycle that ensures suppressed diversity. Penniman agrees and adds that urban schools and prisons are intentionally filled with highly processed foods because "a population that is not well is not going to resist." She explains, "If I'm not feeling well, and I'm dealing with diabetes [and] kidney issues, I'm not going to show up for town hall and tell my senator what they should be doing." Harking back to how Black farmers provided the "material sustenance" for the civil rights movement, Penniman asserts that land ownership is vital not only to health, but also to "our capacity to resist and to make ourselves free."

I find functional medicine interlocutors qua food activists' descriptions of "colonizing the seeds" as a contemporary form of colonization that harms both land and people to be very compelling. However, in order to distinguish sociohistorical forms of colonization from those discussed in this book, I offer the term "genetic colonization." In so doing, I am providing new meaning to a technical term, which as defined by *Oxford Reference* is the "introduction of genetic material from a parasite into a host, thereby inducing the host to synthesize products that only the parasite can use." This technical term applies to GMO seeds since genetic material engineered by Monsanto is inserted into the seeds, thereby inducing the seeds to synthesize glyphosate-tolerant enzymes. However, my use of the term "genetic colonization" layers on a second meaning. I am signaling how companies lay claim to genetic sequences and life forms through patents. I am furthermore critiquing how life becomes a commercial object that can be manipulated for financial profit. Thus, my use of the term "genetic colonization" emphasizes the role of corporate greed in threatening humanity, with people of color—whether dispossessed farmers, underpaid workers, or low-income consumers—suffering the worst effects.

The concept of genetic colonization also serves as a lens for how companies use patents on genetic sequences and life forms to manipulate public policy. As I have argued, food corporations use financial power to infiltrate government processes. In this vein, Dr. Shiva asserts that Monsanto "has taken over the USDA, and it has even taken over our Indian Prime Minister's office." She describes how the Global Food Security Act of 2009 provided a $7.7 billion subsidy to Monsanto. "Our entire seed and agriculture policy is being drafted by these companies." Her critique is not merely of neoliberalism since she argues that economics is no longer about competition. Instead, Dr. Shiva says, "[Economics] has come to be about stealing of governments, stealing democracy, stealing our seeds, and stealing our freedom" (quoted in Robbins and Robbins 2013, 91). From this perspective, the neoliberal promise of a free market (i.e., competition without stealing) would be the lesser of two evils.

Given this backdrop, readers may feel pessimistic about the future of genetic colonization. However, functional medicine interlocutors are hopeful. Smith describes the experiences of Dr. Árpád Pusztai, a researcher tasked with creating protocols that would inform EU law regarding how to test for the safety of GMOs. While conducting research under a UK government grant, Dr. Pusztai inadvertently discovered that GMOs were unsafe and he made his concerns public. He was "fired from his job, gagged with threats, and maligned and attacked for seven months." However, the lifting of his gag order by an order of Parliament in 1999 unleashed a tremendous shift in public opinion. Smith noted more than seven hundred articles about GMOs were published within a month in England alone. He concludes, "The resulting consumer awareness about GMOs and their possible health impacts was sufficient to create a tipping point of consumer rejection. Within ten weeks after the gag order was lifted, virtually every major food company in England committed to stop using GM ingredients" (quoted in Robbins and Robbins 2013, 84). Is a similar shift in public awareness possible in the United States?

## CONSUMPTION-BASED ACTIVISM?

Currently, market-based consumption is the primary way bioconsumers obtain functional medicine services and the resources needed to restore health in the functional medicine modality (lab testing, supplements, and healthy food).[3] This neoliberal model also manifests through the functional medicine emphasis on the role of individuals as stewards of their own health. With respect to food, functional medicine practitioners and proponents have emphasized bioconsumers' role in purchasing the right foods. Dr. Seneff says, for example, "My husband and I practice a 100 percent certified organic diet. When we shop at the grocery store, we buy everything certified organic." According to this logic, it is up to the bioconsumer to "choose" a health-protecting diet.[4]

The underlying argument is that consumption is, in and of itself, a form of activism. Dr. Accurso explains, "A lot of times these companies are producing things because people want them. If we just change our needs, change our wants, then it changes the demand." Dr. Seneff concurs, saying that change in the food system will occur through consumer-driven efforts since "we have a lot of power with our pocketbooks." While their approach is well-intentioned, I argue that it is embedded in structural myopia. Certain individuals have more power with their pocketbooks than others. Consumption-based power is unequal power.

However, functional medicine interlocutors who adhere to consumption-based activism—also referred to as "market-as-movement" (see Pollan 2006)—argue that the power of consumers (those who can afford to buy organic) will have a trickle-down effect. Dr. Seneff instructs others to "buy organic for yourself, for your family, but buy it also because you will be a forcing function to get the farmers to grow more organic food, and that will also lower the price." She argues that if individuals flex their purchasing power, "organic will become affordable for more and more people over time." Her comments reveal a hidden truth: People attracted to functional medicine are more likely to be middle- and upper-class bio-consumers—individuals who are "empowered" by their privilege. Given the demographics of this audience, consumerism seems like a powerful form of activism. I acknowledge their good intentions; however, I argue that universal access to health-protecting foods depends on the dismantlement of social inequalities.

Unfortunately, the majority of functional medicine discourse on food access promotes consumption-based activism. For example, Dr. Hyman urges readers to stop drinking sugary beverages and try his "sugar detox challenge" as a way to sway fiscal policies while addressing individual health. When calling out the "dirty politics" of Big Food, Dr. Hyman suggests that consumers buy non-GMO and USDA organic foods, use refillable containers, buy locally sourced meats, and donate to campaigns with integrity. Regarding the problem of antibiotic overuse in the food system and the looming threat of superbugs, Dr. Hyman suggests that consumers buy meat from a trusted local farm, find certified grass-fed products online, and verify foods are labeled hormone- and antibiotic-free. He asks consumers to support farmworkers by buying fair trade products and supporting advocacy groups that ensure safe and fair working conditions. In order to protect the environment, Dr. Hyman suggests individual citizen-consumers shop at farmers markets, eat at farm-to-table restaurants, start home and community gardens, educate themselves about regenerative agriculture, reduce food waste, start a compost pile, and change their banking and investment strategy to support regenerative and sustainable businesses.[5]

Other functional medicine interlocutors are celebrating the early success of this consumption-based strategy. For example, John and Ocean Robbins write, "But thanks to a passionate resurgence of interest in local foods and food systems, and a shifting economic context, things are beginning to change. Farmers markets, Community Supported Agriculture, organic farms, community gardens, food-justice organizations, and small-scale family farms are on the rise" (Robbins and Robbins 2013, 161–162). Their observations are echoed by Carolyn Dimitri and Lydia Oberholtzer (2009), food studies and agricultural economics scholars, who note that retail sales of organic products in the United States increased from $3.6 billion in 1997 to $21.1 billion in 2009. In the same vein, Alkon and Guthman indicate that while big box stores like Walmart and Safeway were once considered inherently contrary to organic philosophies, they are now major retailers of organic products (2017, 4). Along with these scholars, I argue that while organic foods are becoming more commonplace in restaurants, health food stores, and supermarkets, these positive changes have primarily taken place in affluent areas.[6]

The issue of neighborhood access to organic foods is often missing from functional medicine discourse. Instead, functional medicine interlocutors argue that the continued success of consumer-driven change depends on consumer education. John and Ocean Robbins indicate, "Consumers are taking an interest in knowing where their food comes from, and who grew it. If you want a world where food policy lines up with the health of our bodies, our communities, and our earth, then it's time to get informed, and get activated" (Robbins and Robbins 2013, 162). Smith agrees: "We saw what happened as we and others educated US consumers about the health risks of genetically engineered Bovine Growth Hormone and how it is linked to cancer. It has now been kicked out of Walmart, Starbucks, Yoplait, Dannon, and most American dairies" (quoted in Robbins and Robbins 2013, 84). These functional medicine interlocutors argue that consumers who are armed with knowledge regarding the harmful effects of the conventional food system are more likely to engage in consumer-based activism, thus resulting in change to the food system.

According to other functional medicine interlocutors, the knowledge consumers need goes even deeper. Dr. Hyman indicates that consumers must be hyper-aware of "information warfare" and suggests individuals find the funding sources for specific studies on PubMed. This suggestion makes sense for functional medicine patients who are highly educated and who possess the legal-scientific acumen to suss out conflicts of interest underlying peer-reviewed literature via PubMed. However, this suggestion may be more difficult for less-educated individuals. Given how educational achievement often overlaps with class standing, I argue these types of approaches are primarily available to privileged individuals.[7] By focusing on (self-)education regarding the harmful effects of conventional food, functional medicine interlocutors are neglecting how class inequality structures access to educational resources.

Similarly, functional medicine interlocutors homogenize class-stratified consumers when they suggest that consumer rejection of harmful ingredients can determine how corporations produce foods. Noting how major US food companies have already removed GMOs from their European brands in response to consumer rejection, Smith argues, "I think that any drop in market share whatsoever that a Kraft Food manager can attribute to the growing anti-GMO sentiment in the United States would be sufficient to cause them to quickly abandon GM ingredients" (quoted in Robbins and Robbins 2013, 84–85). Smith estimates that only 5 percent of US shoppers would need to avoid brands containing GM ingredients before food corporations begin removing such ingredients from their US brands as well. According to this argument, consumer knowledge leads to a shift in consumption patterns, which determines the actions of food corporations.

I am hopeful due to the success of consumer rejection in prompting the European Union to place comprehensive legal restrictions on GMOs. However, while consumer rejection produced beneficial effects for all Europeans, the same might not be true for Americans. Instead, consumer rejection in the United States may result in access to organic and non-GMO foods in communities where consumers have the luxury of using the "power of their pocketbooks" (i.e., wealthier neighborhoods) and conventional foods elsewhere (i.e., low-income and minority communities). Income inequality is much worse in the United States (Horsley 2019); thus, while many Europeans may be able to exercise their power as consumers, the same is not true for many Americans.

I am wary of how education is often framed as the answer to many public health problems. For example, health education programs often assume that if individuals only knew about the importance of condom use, this would result in fewer STDs and unwanted pregnancies. These programs do not examine underlying issues of social inequality that drive STDs and unwanted pregnancies. Socioeconomic precariousness and gender inequality can both result in unequal power between sexual partners during moments of negotiation around condom use. Likewise, health education programs may assume that if only individuals were educated about nutrition, they would choose a healthy diet. This approach ignores how socioeconomic and racial inequality undergirds neighborhood food access and food access in general. I argue that a focus on health education too often results in inattention to social structures that predetermine "choice."

More broadly, when food activists focus on a politics of consumption, they are limiting activism to relatively apolitical strategies (Alkon 2012; Guthman 2011). I agree with Alkon and Guthman when they characterize these strategies as primarily accessible to those with wealth and white skin. They argue that the politics of consumption is a "pay to play" approach because "the imaginaries put forward by advocates of the sustainable agriculture movement tend to romanticize the histories of whites, while eliding the contributions of people of color who have labored in past and present agricultural systems" (Alkon and Guthman 2017, 1, citing Alkon 2012;

Allen 2004; Guthman 2008a, 2008b; Slocum 2007). Consumption-based activism based on consumer "choice" and "voting with our forks" is insufficient for addressing structural inequalities.

## HOW THE FOOD SYSTEM TARGETS THE MOST VULNERABLE: THE NEED FOR FOOD JUSTICE

Functional medicine interlocutors qua food activists—a small but raucous subset of functional medicine interlocutors—point to a high prevalence of food insecurity in the United States. According to the USDA Economic Research Service report, "Household Food Security in the United States in 2020," 10.5 percent of US households (13.8 million households) were food insecure and 3.9 percent of US households (5.1 million households) had very low food security. However, from the perspective of functional medicine interlocutors qua food activists, food insecurity is underreported since official statistics focus on caloric sufficiency instead of nutritional sufficiency. They argue that while food insecurity in the past meant that the "insecure" did not have access to sufficient calories, food insecurity today is better described as insufficient access to quality food. Nutritional insufficiency plagues low-income and minority communities, thus acting as a likely driver of chronic disease among these communities (Seligman et al. 2010).

Divergent class diets and, as a result, divergent class health outcomes, are inadvertently buttressed by state policies. Government policy favors industrial agribusiness to the detriment of small-scale farmers, leaving workers impoverished. In this context, the sustainable agriculture movement aims to ensure stable livelihoods for farmers and, as a result, argues for higher prices on organic produce (Allen 2004; Guthman et al. 2006). Meanwhile, cheap foods accessible to the poor—usually packaged and processed—tend to be energy-dense and nutritionally compromised. Ultimately, the upper classes can afford "luxury foods" such as hormone- and antibiotic-free meats and non-GMO, glyphosate-free fruits and vegetables, while lower- and middle-class people are "priced out" and forced into energy-dense diets based on refined sugars, processed foods, and trans fats (see Otero 2018, 23). To make matters worse, the poor are even less able to afford healthy food when they face increasing health care costs due to obesity, diabetes, heart disease, and other chronic diseases.

While poor individuals are the least nourished and the most likely to suffer from chronic disease, subgroups among the poor are vulnerable in unique ways (think: intersectionality; Crenshaw 2014). For example, functional medicine practitioners and proponents argue that the food industry deliberately preys on children. Robbins emphasizes, "The industrial food machine is spewing out and advertising to our kids some of the most unhealthy food-like substances imaginable" (Robbins and Robbins 2013, 38). Dr. Hyman unpacks Robbins's assertion by explaining how junk food companies use effective digital marketing tactics like "advergames" (augmented reality games: e.g., Pokémon GO) to lure players to sponsors' chain restaurants (e.g., McDonald's). Dr. Hyman notes the consequence of unrestricted food marketing: overconsumption of junk food among children.

While processed and fast food companies target children as consumers through increasingly diverse advertising techniques, they also make their way into children's diets through school lunches. Dr. Hyman indicates that half of the budget for the School Nutrition Association (SNA) comes from big food companies such as Kraft, Cook's, Conagra Brands, and Domino's Pizza. Thus, it is no mystery why 50 percent of schools serve brand-name fast foods in their cafeterias and 80 percent have contracts with soda companies. Dr. Hyman notes, "Domino's gave the Houston school district $8 million in exchange for the right to sell these branded pizzas—served in Domino's-emblazoned cardboard boxes and sleeves—in school cafeterias" (Hyman 2020, 144). Due to lobbying efforts, toaster waffles with syrup, tater tots, Uno pepperoni pizza, chicken nuggets, funnel cakes, chocolate muffins, and Slush Puppie beverages are among the food items offered in schools. According to Dr. Hyman, the economic influence of Big Food corporations has detrimental long-term effects on children's intellectual development, mood, and behavior. More specifically, the diet of processed foods and sugar served in schools restrains children's ability to learn and, thus, leads to an achievement gap that reproduces inequality based on "race" and socioeconomic class.

For example, neighborhood access to healthy food (or lack thereof) is an important determining factor when it comes to diet. Dr. Hyman recounts, "There are 23 million Americans that live in food deserts that can't even get a fresh vegetable. I met a girl in Cleveland whose mother wanted to feed her healthy food. She had to take four buses, two hours round trip, to get a vegetable!" In response, Mia Lux, host of *The Conscious-ish Show* and Dr. Hyman's wife, indicates that in some neighborhoods, residents are literally surrounded by fast food. "Is food truly a free choice if we are living in a country swimming with junk?" My answer to this question is a resounding "No!"

Class and "race" map on to neighborhood access to food and furthermore structure "choices." Otero writes, "People live in obesogenic places because their class status does not allow them to do otherwise. Class and "race" are key factors in determining where one can live" (Otero 2018, 4). Given the lack of fresh produce in low-income areas, the high price of fresh compared to processed foods, and the disproportionate health consequences for intersectionally vulnerable people based on class and "race," food activists argue the industrial food system is both unethical and dangerous (see Alkon and Guthman 2017). At the same time, merely supplying fresh food without addressing the underlying problem of poverty can lead to unintended consequences, such as the gentrification of low-income neighborhoods (see Guthman 2011, 87–90).

Instead, it is important to understand how neoliberalism is embodied through diet by socioeconomically vulnerable people. Julie Guthman, a geographer and social scientist, writes, "It is critical to think about the body as a site where the biological and the social constantly remake each other. . . . This is true even for class, the most indisputably social of all categories of difference" (2011, 97). People from different classes have differentiated access to nutrients and health care. At the same time, they are subjected to different labor regimes, exposed to different levels of toxins,[8] and at risk for developing different diseases. For these reasons, food "choices" are structurally conditioned by income and wealth inequality (see Otero 2018).

Turning to Paul Farmer's concept of structural violence (see Farmer 2009), Dr. Hyman characterizes our food system as an invisible form of oppression since it breeds social injustice, exacerbates poverty, and reproduces racism. In so doing, Dr. Hyman rejects how desert imagery naturalizes underlying political and economic processes leading to "food deserts" (see Beaulac, Kristjansson, and Cummins 2009). He writes, "Food deserts imply a natural phenomenon, like an unfortunate desert somehow just occurred. Nothing is less true" (Hyman 2020, 225). In contrast, the term "food swamps" has been used to describe places with high concentrations of fast food, which are predictive of obesity and illness. These "swamps" result from long-standing disinvestment by the state in communities of color (McClintock 2011).

Building on these concepts, Dr. Hyman goes on to introduce "food apartheid." He writes, "We talk of food deserts and food swamps, but perhaps a better term is 'food apartheid,' an embedded social and political form of discrimination that recognizes that these areas of food disparity are not a natural phenomenon like deserts" (Hyman 2020, 226). He explains "food apartheid" is increasingly used to describe how, through lack of real food and overabundance of processed foods, food oppression makes people of color sick, fat, and disabled (see Freeman 2007). Paulette Jordan, former

Idaho state representative and member of the Coeur d'Alene tribe, remarks, "This deeply impacts our rural communities. Especially those like mine because we have more people who are dying of cancer or diabetes. They are just plagued with chronic illness." Both Dr. Hyman and Jordan contribute to food justice critiques regarding the whiteness of community food security and argue for food access in low-income communities of color (Alkon and Guthman 2017, 7–8). Dr. Hyman suggests that Black church leaders link the struggles of minority communities to racial targeting by the food industry. "Black lives matter. But black health matters, too" (Hyman 2020, 236). In his view, food apartheid disables and kills more people of color than anything else.

The injurious and even fatal effects of food apartheid are well documented. Dr. Hyman notes, "If you are African American, you are 80 percent more likely to be diagnosed with type 2 diabetes. You are four times as likely to have kidney failure. You are three and a half times more likely to have amputations from diabetes as whites." From a functional medicine perspective, lack of access to nutritious food is a form of oppression that predisposes communities to generations of illness and suffering. Food apartheid is the ultimate cause of health disparities among people of color.

Furthermore, the existing food system is predicated on the reproduction of poverty and "race" inequality since conventional agribusiness relies on the exploitation of minority farm workers. These workers—often undocumented Mexicans—are among the lowest-paid workers in the United States. Tom Colicchio, a restauranteur, explains, "Our food system was originally built on slavery. . . . It hasn't changed that much. It's using low-pay workers to produce food." Commenting on how the COVID-19 pandemic has changed public perception of farm workers and food preparers, Colicchio says, "All of a sudden, they are in the position where they are essential. Well, why weren't they essential all along? And why weren't they being paid more all along?" The answers to these questions do not rest in farmers' malevolence.

Instead, processed food corporations and food distributors set prices that farmers must accept in order to sell their products. In general, these prices are set so low that they force farmers into debt and, sometimes, out of business. Alkon and Guthman write, "In the case of fruit and vegetable farmers, those who remain often operate on narrow margins, surviving off what agricultural economists call the 'immigrant subsidy'—that is, the ability to pay undocumented migrant workers far less than citizens receive (and far less than the value of their work), let alone a living wage" (2017, 3, referring to Martin and Taylor 1997). Thus, the problem is systemic: minority farm workers are paid dismal wages due to a system that profits from farmers' economic precariousness.

Exploitation extends not only to pay below minimum wage, but also to verbal abuse, sexual abuse, physical violence, and toxic exposure. Turning to "the neglected victims of our food system," Dr. Hyman explains that being a farmworker is one of the most dangerous jobs in the United States since farm workers die at seven times the rate of other workers. These farmers use herbicides and pesticides that are neurotoxins, carcinogens, and hormone disruptors, leading Dr. Shiva to refer to Big Ag as the "poison cartel." The chemical exposure farm workers experience results in acute pesticide poisoning and long-term health effects such as cancer, type 2 diabetes, neurodegenerative diseases, and developmental disorders. According to the CHAMACOS study[9] in Salinas, California, Hispanic farm workers were 59 percent more likely to get leukemia, 70 percent more likely to get stomach cancer, and 63 percent more likely to get cervical cancer when compared to the average population. At the same time, farm workers ironically suffer from hunger and develop diet-related diseases (Brown and Getz 2011; Gray 2014; Holmes 2013).

In essence, these functional medicine interlocutors qua food activists are arguing for food justice. Agricultural development scholar Rasheed Hislop describes it as "the struggle against racism, exploitation, and oppression taking place within the food system that addresses inequality's root causes both within and beyond the food chain" (2014, 19). Food justice activism is an outgrowth of the environmental justice movement. Penniman explains, "Environmental justice is a huge issue because we are talking about who is getting environmental benefits and who is suffering from environmental harms—pesticide exposure, extreme heat . . . ." Low-income communities and minority populations, acting as "popular epidemiologists" (Brown and Mikkelsen 1997), document their disproportionate exposure to environmental toxins and argue for a safe, healthy, and clean environment.[10] At the same time, activists point to how marginalized communities are less likely to have access to neighborhood green spaces and healthy food (Agyeman 2005; Park and Pellow 2011; Pellow and Brulle 2005).[11] Thus, food justice goes beyond food provisioning to address the underlying causes of injustice in the food system: environmental unsustainability and social inequality.

Human rights are at stake. During his *Doctor's Farmacy* interview with Dr. Miller, Dr. Hyman refers to the CHAMACOS statistics. "You are seeing the harm that our current agricultural production system does to the workers because of toxic use of chemicals, because of poor working conditions, because of being almost indentured servants." Dr. Hyman first learned about the intimate connection between environmental challenges and social injustices when he attended the Institute for Social Ecology in college. This experience has shaped his thinking, including how he approaches his work as a doctor. In response to Dr. Hyman's assertion, Dr. Miller links the exploitation of workers to the exploitation of the soil and the exploitation of consumers' bodies. She argues, "We can't heal communities unless we actually take care of farm workers and take care of soil. . . . We cannot bring the world along to start to change our practices and protect the planet unless we all have a minimum level of health and welfare." I agree that seeking food justice begins with an unwavering commitment to the health and welfare of all humans.

Multiple actors can play a role in ensuring workers' human rights. Colicchio insists that the problem of low wages can be fixed by breaking up monopolies and placing food processors back in communities. Meanwhile, Dr. Hyman argues that restaurant and food retailers must pressure growers to adhere to the Fair Food Program. This includes no forced labor, child labor, or violence; minimum wage payments; no sexual harassment or verbal abuse; access to shade, clean drinking water, and bathrooms; time to rest; and permission to leave the fields during pesticide spraying and other dangerous conditions. Responding to Dr. Hyman, Penniman indicates that while farmers are not solely responsible for the solution, they do have a unique role to play. "We have the opportunity to make sure that our farm workers are treated fairly . . . and we have a unique voice where we can really get bipartisan ears [to tell] policy makers about the shifts that need to happen on a systemic level." Her words reiterate that food justice can only be achieved through systemic change.

Ultimately, everyone is responsible for bringing about systemic change. For this reason, functional medicine interlocutors qua food activists encourage others to engage in a politicized, community-based struggle for food justice. Dr. Hyman recommends individuals play a community-level role in changing food habits by becoming agents of change in their workplaces, unions, private associations, faith communities, and the family. Harking back to his comment that diabetes and obesity are not cured in the doctor's office, he writes, "[They are] cured on the farm, in the grocery store, in the restaurant, in our kitchens, schools, workplaces, and faith-based communities" (Hyman 2020, 7). In addition, Dr. Hyman suggests individuals engage representatives to enforce lobbying restrictions, support ballot initiatives, promote regenerative agriculture, and "vote with their vote."

## FOOD POLICY RECOMMENDATIONS AND THE "NANNY STATE"

Functional medicine interlocutors qua food activists and food scholars agree that food activism must be politicized. Dr. Hyman asserts, "It's clear that our food policies and our ag[ricultural] policies are promoting the production, the marketing, and distribution of all the wrong foods." He unpacks this statement when he critiques the expenditure of billions of dollars in subsidies on commodity crops, $75 billion a year in food stamp payments that are mostly spent on processed food and soda, unregulated marketing of the worst foods, and industry-influenced dietary guidelines. Dr. Hyman writes, "Changes to our own diet are necessary but not sufficient to truly create the shifts needed to create a healthy, sustainable, just world. The policies and businesses that drive our current system must change to support a reimagined food system from field to fork and beyond" (Hyman 2020, 7). Thus, Dr. Hyman proposes extensive reforms to modernize outdated policies.

Nonetheless, Dr. Hyman contends that these harmful food policies were originally created with the best of intentions. In the case of crop insurance subsidies, he explains that these policies historically protected farmers from weather and price fluctuations while supporting increased crop production. According to Dr. Hyman, over time these same policies inadvertently became the number one cause of climate change. Meanwhile, they "deplete global water resources, and drive environmental destruction and the production of cheap ingredients that are mostly turned into processed disease-promoting food-like substances" (Hyman 2020, 35). In his view, subsidies for commodity crops have long since served their purpose and are overdue for much-needed transformation. He proposes that the USDA be reinvented as the US Department of Food, Health, and Well-Being and that this new agency support regenerative agriculture—especially of "specialty crops" such as fruits and vegetables, whole grains, beans, nuts, and seeds.

Functional medicine practitioners and proponents also recommend updating policies regarding food labels. Smith contends that if companies were required to label GM ingredients in food, this would prove a "watershed moment in the struggle." He cites a poll in which 90 percent of Americans said they want GMOs to be labeled and 53 percent said they would not eat GM foods if they were labeled. Indicating how public policy is upstream to consumer behavior and, thus, corporate decision making, Smith suggests, "If they see that Americans are going to remove their brands from their shopping carts over GMOs, then these companies would rather eliminate GMOs than admit that they use them" (quoted in Robbins and Robbins 2013, 85). In a similar vein, Dr. Hyman discusses current efforts to require labeling added sugars on all food labels. Dr. Anand Parekh agrees with Dr. Hyman that this policy change would change consumer behavior, which may then motivate food manufacturers to reformulate their recipes to reduce added sugars. Fewer added sugars in processed food could, in turn, save millions of lives that are currently being lost to diabetes, heart disease, cancer, and other chronic diseases. While I maintain that behavior is shaped by structural factors—not purely knowledge—I fully agree that foods should be properly labeled regarding their ingredients.

According to functional medicine proponents, nutritional education and stricter requirements for food labeling are merely two facets of a multi-pronged strategy for revamping the food system. Dr. Aseem Malhotra, Dr. Robert Lustig, and Dr. Grant Schofield suggest that in addition to public education regarding the harmful effects of sugar and food labels that list sugar in teaspoons, the diabetes crisis can be reversed through banning companies that make sugary products from sponsoring sporting events, extending soda taxes to sugary foods, banning ads on sugary drinks, discontinuing government food subsidies for commodity crops, and preventing all professional dietetic organizations from accepting money or endorsing companies that market processed foods (see Hyman 2020).

When arguing for clearer food labels and restrictions on junk food ads, Dr. Hyman turns to examples from the United States and beyond and argues that, although multinational food companies will not change voluntarily, they can be forced into change by stricter regulations and taxation. He writes, "In the United Kingdom, for example, food companies complied with new regulations forcing them to reduce the amount of sodium in their products. But they did not make those same changes with their products in the United States until New York City Health Department under Michael Bloomberg required similar changes" (Hyman 2020, 75). This pattern held true for trans fats. Dr. Hyman continues, "Even though they had the technology to replace these deadly fats with healthier ingredients, many food companies refused to make the change until laws in various countries required them to do so" (Hyman 2020, 75). Turning specifically to how the food industry preys on children, Dr. Hyman suggests that the US government limit food advertisements aimed at children younger than fourteen. In so doing, the United States would follow in the footsteps of countries that have already taken aggressive regulatory steps (including Quebec, Sweden, and the United Kingdom). He furthermore suggests schools introduce salad bars, eliminate junk foods, support farm-to-school programs, and reintroduce cooking skills into the school curriculum.

Dr. Hyman argues that since chronic disease is the single biggest threat to global economic development, fixing the food system is an economic imperative. His argument highlights the need for linkages between food policy and health care policy. Specifically, he frames needed fixes to the food system as a bipartisan issue and argues for politicians on both sides to "stop the flow of sick people into the system and the harm to our environment and climate by fixing the cause: our food system" (Hyman 2020, 14). In so doing, he intervenes in an ongoing debate that pits creating Medicare for All against reducing national debt through limited entitlements. He suggests that both Democrats and Republicans fail to consider the underlying cause of high health care costs.

He proposes changes to our food policy based on "true cost accounting." Specifically, he indicates, "Instead of just treating rampant chronic diseases with medication and surgery, we have to start preventing and treating with food." Dr. Hyman explains, "If we can get food reimbursed by health care, it's a game changer. Actually, I am working on that at the Cleveland Clinic with the Food Farmacy, which is the idea of paying for food for people instead of drugs to help reverse disease—and that actually help saves lives and money." He proposes health care innovations such as medical reimbursements for food as medicine through all federal and state health insurance programs; creating Food Savings Accounts where tax-free money can be stored for whole, real, health-promoting foods; research funding and reimbursements for functional medicine; and integrating nutrition education in medical schools.

Furthermore, functional medicine practitioners and proponents have honed in on the Supplemental Nutrition Assistance Program (SNAP), commonly referred to as "food stamps," as a misguided program that inadvertently contributes to nutritional deficiency. SNAP accounts for the largest portion of the Farm Bill. While the program emerged to address hunger and malnutrition, functional medicine interlocutors qua food activists argue that it now drives obesity and disease for 46 million Americans. Speaking in different digital spaces, Dr. Barnard, Dr. Parekh, and Dr. Hyman express that, despite its name, SNAP has jettisoned nutrition as a priority. Dr. Barnard explains, "The program has become largely a service for the junk food industry." Dr. Hyman offers evidence to support Dr. Barnard's assertion, noting how Big Cola earns 30 percent of its revenue from food stamps, resulting in more health consequences for SNAP recipients.

Due to limited resources, SNAP recipients face economic pressure to buy the worst foods.[12] At the same time, SNAP recipients are targets of food industry marketing. Given these external forces, Dr. Hyman is careful not to insinuate that SNAP recipients are culpable for their poor food "choices." In so doing, he turns to a 2018 study in the *American Journal of Preventative Medicine* to document how shoppers in poor New York City neighborhoods were two to four times more likely to encounter grocery store displays and advertisements for sugary drinks during the first week of every month—the same week they receive their food stamps (see Moran et al. 2018). Dr. Hyman writes, "Big Food aims its junk food ads at low-income Americans with laser focus. The retailers target SNAP recipients with the worst and most profitable foods" (Hyman 2020, 95). As a result, SNAP recipients, who account for 65 percent of the adults on Medicaid, have twice the rate of heart disease and are three times more likely to die of diabetes compared to other Americans (Dobbs et al. 2014). Dr. Hyman asserts, "The math is simple: Providing healthy and nutritious foods to SNAP recipients would reduce chronic disease rates . . . benefit the millions of people who depend on SNAP, and ultimately save taxpayers billions or potentially even trillions of dollars" (Hyman 2020, 96). When making these points, Dr. Hyman argues that food is a social justice issue and advocates for a shift from "blame the victim" to "change the system" approach.

Functional medicine interlocutors qua food activists credit SNAP for substantially reducing traditional food insecurity (i.e., caloric deficiency) in the United States. However, Dr. Parekh notes, "With our obesogenic environment in the last several decades, the program has not evolved to make sure that nutrition and diet quality are paramount as well." Functional medicine interlocutors qua food activists agree with Dr. Parekh that by putting the "N" back in SNAP, the program can be updated to support the health of the 40 million Americans who depend on it. They furthermore suggest that emphasis on quality can potentially be accomplished by offering incentives for purchasing nutritious foods.

Such incentives have already proven successful in some places and have produced better health outcomes and health cost savings. For example, Dr. Hyman describes programs in twenty-eight states that offer extra money for every dollar spent on fruits and vegetables. Experts at the Tufts University Friedman School of Nutrition Science and Policy found a 20 percent incentive for fruit and vegetable purchases to Medicaid and Medicare beneficiaries would produce a net savings of $39.7 billion in health care costs and prevent at least 1.93 million cardiovascular disease events. Broadening the 20 percent incentive to include nuts, fish, whole grains, and olive oil would prevent 3.28 million cardiovascular events and save $100.2 billion in health care costs after deducting the cost of the healthy food incentives (Lee et al. 2019).

In addition, many functional medicine proponents agree that SNAP should limit foods that are harmful. Dr. Barnard indicates, "We would like to limit the SNAP program to those foods that are healthy: grains, beans, vegetables, and fruits, whether they are fresh, frozen, or perhaps in a can." Meanwhile, Dr. Hyman asserts, "In a taxpayer program, sugar-sweetened beverages should not be included." Dr. Barnard explains that if retailers were only compensated with government money for healthy foods, "[i]t would spell the end to food deserts. The result would be that needy folks who are now paying a terrible price for the junk food avalanche that is all around them could instead become the healthiest people in America" (quoted in Robbins and Robbins 2013, 39–40). While functional medicine interlocutors qua food activists support Dr. Barnard's conclusion, critics may argue that limiting harmful foods impinges on individuals' free choice.

These policy recommendations beg the following questions: When is it appropriate for the state to place restrictions on consumer choice? To what degree should government regulate private companies to ensure that they act in accordance with broader public interests? How do regulations figure into public health? How can government and industry create incentives for responsible corporate behavior?

At the very core of the debate about food and the "nanny state" is the dilemma of whether to govern or not to govern (Vallgårda 2015; see also Calman 2008; Sparks 2011; Wiley, Berman, and Blanke 2013). A neoliberal approach emphasizes the importance of individual choice with respect to foods. In contrast, I, along with functional medicine interlocutors, argue that government policies should steer the population toward healthy foods and away from those that lead to chronic disease. In Dr. Hyman's view, taxation of unhealthy products coincides with the state's responsibility to protect the health of its citizens. He refutes the notion that these types of taxes force people to live in a "nanny state" by pointing to mandatory seat belt laws, vaccinations, and car seats for children. Initially, mandatory car seats, air bags, and fuel emission standards were all opposed by the car industry, but they are now viewed as policies that are good for society, save lives, and protect the environment.

At present, not only are there no restrictions on unhealthy foods, but the state also pays for sugary and ultra-processed foods that cause chronic disease. Each year, $7 billion in food stamps are spent on sugary beverages (O'Connor 2017). SNAP households devote a greater percentage of their expenditures to sweetened beverages, snacks, deserts, prepared foods, cereals, and sugars than non-SNAP households. Meanwhile, SNAP households spend less on fruits, vegetables, nuts, and seeds than non-SNAP households (US Department of Agriculture 2016). Dr. Hyman writes, "While Uncle Sam can't force anyone to eat fruits and veggies, the government can at least make sure that taxpayer dollars aren't used to subsidize the Frankenfoods that are driving the belt-popping rates of obesity and chronic disease" (Hyman 2020, 93). While critics argue such restrictions would stigmatize people using SNAP by limiting their consumer choice, Dr. Hyman notes that SNAP already excludes harmful substances such as cigarettes.

Proponents of greater regulation point to tobacco as an example of how public policies and regulations can work in the favor of public health. The comparison between tobacco and processed food is fitting since, in both cases, existing statistics do not even begin to take into account the true burden of disease: the disability, suffering, and immeasurable psychological, social, and economic toll on families and communities. For every tobacco-related death, there are twenty people suffering with chronic disease, and most of the total burden is concentrated among the poor, less educated, and racial minorities (Gostin 2014). This pattern of social inequality holds true for processed foods. In 2018, the former treasury secretary Lawrence Summers and others launched the Task Force on Fiscal Policy for Health. The task force advocates for taxing unhealthy foods, such as soda, as a solution to rising health care costs and the obesity crisis. To support their efforts, they point to how taxing tobacco not only discourages tobacco sales, but also raises awareness about the threat tobacco poses to health.

In contrast, critics (often Big Food corporations and their beneficiaries) argue that soda taxes are regressive since they disproportionately affect low- and middle-income families. In response to this critique, Dr. Hyman insists that the money from taxes on sugary foods should be spent on social programs for poor communities. In addition, these taxes must be combined with price reductions on healthy foods, business incentives for research and development, and marketing and distribution of protective healing foods. He turns to the Philadelphia soda tax, where tax revenue has provided more than $500 million to fund universal pre-K, public schools, and recreation centers, as an example of how soda taxes can produce benefits for the most affected. Furthermore, in San Francisco, the $10 million in annual revenue from the penny-per-ounce soda tax has helped to pay for nutritious school meals made with locally grown produce, water hydration stations in schools and public buildings, and healthy eating vouchers for low-income San Franciscans. Dr. Hyman asserts that every government should institute a junk food tax of some kind, use tax income to subsidize nutritious foods, and create soda-free zones.

Big Food companies resist state regulation and, instead, argue for consumer "choice" (see Pollan 2006, 2008; Nestle 2006, 2013). These companies deride state intervention under the banner of the "nanny state," which they argue threatens individual freedom and liberal democracy. At the same time, these companies spend hundreds of millions on lobbying to influence (non) regulation and ensure their interests are represented through subsidies. This situation leads Otero to note how, by most accounts, "state regulation (if any) and intervention such as subsidies are meant primarily to enhance the profitability of corporations and rarely to protect citizens" (2018, 14). At the same time, I, along with Otero, argue that despite the dominance of oligopolies in the food industry, the state can intervene to protect the health of its citizens. The food system is changeable through policy reform. However, I argue that policy reform will be motivated from below, by grassroots movements.

## GRASSROOTS MOVEMENTS

Food activist Vani Hari is one prominent example of how a single person can do a great deal to address problems in the food industry.[13] Hari exposed the harmful chemicals in fast foods such as Chick-fil-A. In response to Hari, the company removed artificial dyes, high-fructose corn syrup, chicken treated with antibiotics, and TBHQ from their food. She then outed Chipotle for using trans fats and GMO ingredients. Thousands signed Hari's petition, leading Chipotle to remove GMO ingredients from their foods. She also revealed how Kraft Foods uses artificial dyes and preservatives in their macaroni and cheese in the United States but not in the United Kingdom, where these chemicals are prohibited. She collected hundreds of thousands of signatures and forced Kraft to remove the chemicals from the US version. Due to Hari's efforts, Subway, McDonald's Wendy's, Jack in the Box, Chick-fil-A, and White Castle have removed azodicarbonamide—sometimes referred to as the "yoga mat" chemical because of its use in plastic and rubber products—from their food. In addition, Starbucks has stopped using a carcinogenic caramel color in their pumpkin spice latte, and General Mills and Kellogg's no longer use the toxic preservative BHT.

Extrapolating from Hari's experience, functional medicine practitioners and proponents assert that government will not act unless it is impelled from below. With regard to her concern about glyphosate, Dr. Seneff indicates that "the power of the money in the chemical industry seems to have paralyzed the government, so I do not believe it's going to happen top-down." Similarly, Dr. David Brady, a naturopathic medical physician, suggests that rapid increases in chronic disease will not be reversed by a "magic drug," but instead through changes to our diet, food supply, and environment. He asserts, "That is not going to happen because the powers that control the food supply . . . are going to make those changes for us. It is going to be driven grassroots by people who are chronically ill and are fed up and need the system to change." These assertions from the functional medicine realm coincide with social science and food scholars' perspectives.

While it is the state's responsibility to protect the well-being of its citizens, those citizens must spur the state to action. According to Otero (2018), policies have primarily promoted the interests of Big Food; thus, the challenge of society is to push state intervention toward promoting public health. Otero writes, "The progressive sectors of civil society must mobilize to exert pressure on the state for it to become a societal actor in the wider public interest" (2018, 8). Echoing these sentiments, Senator Frist states, "You don't have to be a politician to participate in the public sector." Harking back to the example of tobacco, he contends that if politicians are faced with data about the harmful effects of conventional food, they will act in the best interests of citizens. However, it is up to concerned citizens to bring this knowledge to their representatives.

Reiterating these sentiments, I signal the vital importance of grassroots efforts for galvanizing state action. Furthermore, I argue that the state will face bottom-up pressure to change the food system only when food activists transcend individualistic and consumption-oriented approaches (see Otero 2018). When this is not the case, food activists unwittingly emphasize self-responsibility, thus perpetuating neoliberal notions of good citizenship (Alkon and Guthman 2017, 14, citing Bondi and Laurie 2005; Dean 1999; Larner and Craig 2005; Rose 1999). I will provide examples to clarify this point.

Food justice organizations, attempting to do the abandoned work of the neoliberal state, take responsibility for the provisioning of food in low-income and minority communities. In so doing, they inadvertently allow the dismantling of food assistance programs. These groups effectively serve their communities. At the same time, however, they implicitly argue that it is their role, not the state's, to ensure access to healthy food (see Alkon and Guthman 2017, 13). Harking back to Robbins and Robbins's celebratory remarks about how farmers markets, community supported agriculture, organic farms, community gardens, food justice organizations, and small-scale family farms are on the rise, these creative alternatives do not contest state and corporate power and may thus reproduce neoliberal forms of governance (Guthman 2008c). While these examples of community action are beneficial, they can also reinforce the idea that community groups are responsible for addressing problems that are systemic in nature (Alkon and Guthman 2017, 15).

At the same time, these strategies can neglect socioeconomic and racialized inequality. Food scholars have described how farmers markets and other sustainable agriculture venues are primarily frequented by whites and, through discourse circulated in these spaces, become culturally coded as white (Alkon and Guthman 2017, 9, citing Alkon and McCullen 2010; Guthman 2008a; Slocum 2006, 2007). Alkon and Guthman write, "Phrases common to the sustainable agriculture movement, such as 'getting your hands dirty in the soil' and 'looking the farmer in the eye,' all point to 'an agrarian past that is far more easily romanticized by whites than others'" (2017, 9, citing Guthman 2008b, 394). As an intersectional scholar, I point to the socioeconomic privilege of patrons at farmers markets and of health-protecting foods in general.

Furthermore, I argue for the role of the state in mainstreaming regenerative agriculture. Since food policies shape both the natural environment and human health, food policy reform must address human-environment linkages. In making this argument, I agree with the Union of Concerned Scientists, who affirm that national food policy should ensure that all Americans have access to healthy food; that our food supply is free of pathogenic bacteria, chemicals, and drugs; that food production and marketing are transparent; that the food industry pays a fair wage to its employees; that the food system's carbon footprint is reduced; that carbon sequestration is increased; and that farm policies are designed to support public health and environmental objectives.

The concept of nested ecologies frames regenerative farming as integral to both environmental stewardship and human health. Dr. Hyman comments, "Remarkably, food that is good for you is also good for the environment, our depleted soil, our scarce water resources, and the biodiversity of plants, animals, and pollinators, and it helps reverse climate change" (Hyman 2020, 55). In so doing, he argues that regenerative farming can restore ecosystems. Dr. Miller similarly connects human health to how food is produced. From a functional medicine perspective, the very principles used for protecting soil can be applied to treating patients.

The future of regenerative farming is hopeful. Dr. Hyman describes how large companies are beginning to understand the need for regenerative agriculture. He explains, "Dannon and General Mills are funding farmers to turn their conventional farms into regenerative farms because they understand that if we keep farming the way we are, we won't actually be able to grow food anymore—we will deplete the soil." While the transition to regenerative farming can be costly, Dr. Hyman affirms that once the two-to four-year transition is complete, regenerative farms "make more money, they produce better food, more nutritious food, and everybody wins!" He adds, "It revitalizes rural communities, it revitalizes farmers, and it is just such an obvious solution—and the side effect is less environmental degradation." From this perspective, regenerative farming is an investment in both human and environmental capital.

Unfortunately, the movement currently unfolds through neoliberally oriented negotiations among corporations, farmers, and bioconsumers. In this context, supporters of regenerative agriculture call out the state's failure to protect the public from environmental toxins. Dr. Hyman asserts that the Food and Drug Administration and the Environmental Protection Agency "are not doing their job" when it comes to regulating herbicides and pesticides (Hyman 2020, 17). In particular, he points to how the FDA allows harmful ingredients, including more than ninety-five hundred additives that have never been tested for safety, in our food. Like other food activists, he indicates that consumers can protect themselves and their families by purchasing organic food from trusted local farmers (see also Szasz 2007). Fortunately, Dr. Hyman does not stop there. Instead, he argues FDA reforms should prevent antibiotic overuse, stop companies from making false claims on food labels, and strengthen regulation of chemical food additives.

I argue that the state should invest in regenerative agriculture. This can be accomplished by redirecting the $20 billion per year in subsidies from GMO and glyphosate-laden crops (corn, soy, wheat) to regenerative agriculture, with a focus on fruits, vegetables, nuts, seeds, whole grains, and legumes. Such a change would reframe the regenerative food movement and would demonstrate the state's commitment to the health and well-being of its citizens.

I furthermore argue that the state has a responsibility to ensure the integrity of nutritional science. This can be accomplished by redirecting some of the NIH funds currently spent on research and development for pharmaceuticals to increasing rigor (and removing corporate interests) in nutrition science. Dr. William Li notes, "The great thing is that we are now able to benefit from all the research that has been done over the years directed at developing new jobs by pharmaceutical companies, and we can use those same tools in a toolbox to study food. When you do that, you start developing the answer to why something works." In essence, this switch from research and development for "blockbuster drugs" to improving nutritional science would facilitate a transition from treating disease to preventing illness. It would take seriously the adage that "food is medicine" by identifying the specific compounds within food that produce well-being.

In essence, state intervention is needed to transform the food system and the socio-environmental inequalities that it both depends upon and (re)produces. The policy changes I envision would clarify the state's responsibility for ensuring equitable access to healthy food. In order to open up the possibility of individuals changing their eating habits, food policies must be informed by the social structures that shape food choices (see Johnston and Baumann 2014). Food policy reform should equitably incorporate the thoughts, opinions, and needs of those who have historically faced the greatest burden. That is, food policies should not be designed by white, class-privileged actors and should target low-income communities and communities of color (see Alkon 2012, Guthman 2008a). Finally, to create a society in which everyone has access to healthy food, food policies must dismantle the neoliberal structures that constrict true freedom of choice. This involves placing new restrictions on the harmful practices of food processers and producers, such as the use of toxic chemicals and poor labor conditions (Guthman 2011).[14] Social justice can only be achieved through holding the state accountable for the regulation of industrial food. At issue are not only the harmful practices of food corporations, but also how these practices, through a lack of regulation, prey upon individuals who are vulnerable due to age, class, and "race" inequality.

By arguing for a multiracial, class-inflected movement that (re)politicizes food activism and demands state action, I am pushing for an expanded "politics of the possible" (Guthman 2008a). When food activists celebrate the merits of sustainable food alternatives without considering how they inadvertently reproduce socioeconomic and racialized inequality, they unwittingly adopt a neoliberal mindset in which confronting the state and food corporations in the interest of human and environmental health is not a possibility. I wholeheartedly agree with Alkon and Guthman, who write, "We believe that collective campaigns rooted in the realities of those most harmed by the industrial food system and alternatives that push back against neoliberal strategies and subjectivities can nourish new political possibilities within the world of food activism" (2017, 20). That is, a socially just food system, achieved through state intervention, is only rendered possible through our collective imagination of it *as a possibility*.

Anti-racist, anti-classist organizing is needed to protect the common good. Although Big Food targets the most vulnerable in society, the noxious effects of the food industry affect us all. Dr. Hyman writes, "Whether you are the CEO of Bayer or Coca-Cola or the head of the Sustainable Food Trust or the Environmental Working Group, or Republican, Democrat, Muslim, Christian, Jewish, any "race" or any ethnicity. . . . Our collective actions and behaviors will move things in the right direction, and our children and their children might enjoy a sustainable future of good food and a safe climate" (2020, 336). Referring to how conventional food causes disease, reduces productivity, and harms the environment, Dr. Barnard asserts, "We need to work for societal change, because the price . . . is simply too high" (quoted in Robbins and Robbins 2013, 37). Given what is at stake, people separated by politics, culture, "race," and class must come together to challenge corporations and demand state action.

I conclude this book with a few thoughts for future research. How does access to epigenetic testing expand or constrain agency and notions of what it means to be an individual? In our capitalist system, who is able to "control their own fate?" Furthermore, as disruptive technologies allow patient-consumers to more readily access information about their bioindividuality, how are patient-provider relationships affected? With nested ecologies in mind, I suggest that the direct-to-consumer structure of companies like 23andMe subjects individuals to a bioconsumptive regime that produces multiple layers of exclusion. The relationship between privilege and agency in functional medicine merits further inquiry.

At the same time, I ask how the emerging technologies used in functional medicine can be reconfigured to deliver a broader, more equitable impact. Genetic therapies and public health interventions have been characterized as at odds, so how might we use the concept of nested ecologies to disrupt the "me" vs. "we" medicine binary (see Dickenson 2014). Instead of characterizing precision medicine as "a distraction from the goal of producing a healthier population" (Bayer and Galea 2018, 243), I ask how epi(genomic) medicine might be placed at the service of public health. For example, how might public health officials embrace "precision public health" as a way to identify and address individual risk factors, and prevent deaths, amid a pandemic? My hope is for improved population-wide health outcomes through more equitable access to functional medicine.[15]

> Never doubt that a small group of thoughtful, committed citizens
> can change the world. Indeed, it is the only thing that ever has.[16]
> MARGARET MEAD

*Postlude*

# HEALTH IS A PROCESS

A t the time of this writing, I have come through to the other end of a health crisis. I am stronger than I have ever been and healthier than I was even as a small child. Over the course of this journey, my month-long Medical Symptom/Toxicity score has fallen from 103 to eight. Less than ten is considered optimal. Looking back, I am in awe of how extraordinary my recovery has been. During the healing process, however, my improvement was not always linear—I often felt like, for every few steps forward, I took one step back.

I didn't fully realize how much more resilient my health is until about six months ago after a family trip. Up until that point, coming down sick immediately after returning home from a trip was a regular occurrence. On this occasion, it was my mother who was sick with a nasty cold on our flight home. Within a few days, my husband caught it as well. Although I was living with both of them at the time, I was the only person in the household who was well. A week later, my husband told me that, although he was still symptomatic, he was likely no longer contagious. I kissed him, and within a couple hours, I felt the virus slinking down my throat. However, even though I caught the cold, my symptoms were very mild in comparison to my mother and husband. In the past, viruses have knocked me off my feet for weeks, months, and sometimes even years. This time, the virus was a passing annoyance, and I was able to continue with life as usual.

Additionally, chronic viruses I have struggled with have settled into a latent state. A recent polymerase chain reaction test found that Epstein-Barr viral DNA is not replicating in my body. At the same time, my EBV titers have fallen across the board—my immune system still remembers, but it is not in high alarm.

These results were accompanied by other welcome news. My last two laboratory tests have been negative for autoimmunity. My blood levels for heavy metals were in the normal range. My most recent pap smear did not detect any HPV or cervical dysplasia. Beyond merely addressing nutritional deficiencies, changes to my diet have optimized my methylation. Concurrently, my symptoms of estrogen dominance are melting away.

I occasionally have some neck and shoulder pain, which is easily resolved with a massage. Although my arthritis and disc disease are degenerative, I have not noticed any progression in my symptoms. In fact, my symptoms have improved, and I no longer have migraines, blurred vision, nausea, or faintness.

While I am no longer taking thyroid medication, my thyroid symptoms have also improved. I do not feel fatigued and my hair is long and strong. By ceasing the medication, my irregular heart arrhythmia has stabilized.

I no longer have histamine intolerance, seasonal allergies, disordered activation of my mast cells, or cholinergic urticaria—allergies to the sun. In the past, sun exposure would have caused me to break out into hives in a matter of minutes—sometimes seconds. Over the last seventeen months, I have enjoyed a broad range of outdoor activities, spending hours in the sun with no symptoms. I have not experienced anaphylaxis since those terrible nights when I was experiencing withdrawal from antihistamine medications. When my EpiPen expired, I removed it from my purse. I have not refilled my prescription because I am confident I no longer need it.

My test results were also negative for leaky gut and small intestinal bacterial overgrowth (SIBO). I have not experienced any IBS symptoms in more than a year and a half, and I consider that I no longer have IBS. I told my conventional internal medicine physician that I am cured of both IBS and cholinergic urticaria, but he did not remove either from my "active conditions" list. Perhaps he, along with Harvard Health, believes chronic conditions like IBS cannot be cured, and I have simply learned to manage my symptoms so they do not interfere with my overall health and quality of life (Harvard Health 2021). Unfortunately, the possibility of recovery from chronic disease has been stamped out in many conventional clinical contexts. In response, I reject the tyranny of permanent diagnoses and the biomedical authority upon which they rest. Instead, I save space for the possibility of full recovery and, in so doing, I create the conditions that make this a possibility.

I began this research project when I needed to apply ethnographic research methods to my own health problems. I needed to use my skills as an anthropologist to recover my own health. Now that the health crisis has passed, I am determined to continue growing my good health. This will be a lifelong project, which will require further adaptations on my part. Health, I have learned, is a process, not a destination.[1]

By far the most joyful outcome of this process so far has been a natural, unassisted pregnancy. Rikin and I were recently blessed with a beautiful and bright-eyed baby girl, Madelena. She fills our home with giggles and smiles. I am still in complete awe. My body made this incredible little person and she is ours to love forever.

# ACKNOWLEDGMENTS

In spring 2019, I applied for a Faculty Development Leave from the University of Texas Rio Grande Valley (UTRGV). My plan for the proposed leave was to write a book on medical migration across the US-Mexico border. My application was approved for spring 2020. However, as the semester came to a close, I began toying with another book idea—something much more personal. I confided in my two "writing buddies"— Andrés Amado and Marisa Palacios Knox—both of whom emboldened me to seek permission to change the book project for my upcoming leave.

My first step was to reach out to Casey Kittrell, senior editor at the University of Texas Press. Casey nurtured and guided my first book, *No Alternative*, beginning when I was doctoral candidate. In many ways he helped me become the author I am today. I was incredibly inspired by this new idea, but what I was proposing felt so far off the beaten path that I was unsure if others would recognize its value as a scholarly monograph. It felt like a risk. We spoke on the phone and he wholeheartedly supported my idea. If not for his support in this moment, I would not have had the confidence to pursue my "passion project."

I wrote the first draft of this book at my dining room table, while in lockdown during the COVID-19 pandemic. When my husband, Rikin, came into the kitchen to heat his meals, I carried my laptop into the bathroom, where I would continue writing. I am sure he found my behavior somewhat strange, but he has always respected how important my writing is to me. (And if there was ever any doubt, certainly none remains after being each other's sole companion for more than a year in lockdown!) I am grateful to Rikin for his support and encouragement after my daily visits to my at-home "writing café." Also, more than anything else in our marriage so far, I am thankful for his role in facilitating my recovery from chronic disease. Without his partnership during my healing journey, this book would not exist, and I would not be well today.

Although I was by myself, I was not alone. I was accompanied by Andrés and Marisa in the at-home "writing café." Before the pandemic, we met in person, taking turns for picking the café of the day or visiting each other's homes. During the pandemic, we met every weekday afternoon via Zoom. We took breaks every forty-five minutes or so to catch up, exchange ideas, and insert a few moments of levity into our otherwise focused sessions. We used technology to adapt to the circumstances, and it was almost as if they were at my kitchen table with me—like "old times" when I occasionally hosted our writing meetups and invited them to explore my fairly extensive tea collection. (However, they might say it was if they were hosting me in their homes!) Although we are in different fields, these two colleagues provided me with ongoing feedback throughout the writing process. I deeply value their insights and I cherish their friendship.

When I was putting together the first draft, I wrote about one chapter per week. My close friend from graduate school, James Battle, invited me to join his virtual writing group on Friday mornings. At the beginning of each week, two writing group members submitted a chapter or article draft to the entire group via email, allowing the others to read the submitted work and provide comments and suggestions at the Friday meeting. Over the course of several months, I submitted most of the chapters in this book to the group and I benefited greatly from their generative comments. In addition to James, I am indebted to Sandra Harvey, Victoria Massie, and Dennis Browe for their close reading of my work. Sandra encouraged me to write in an experimental style, Victoria asked thought-provoking questions, Dennis pushed me to hone my critique of the phenomena I was observing, and James shared his honest opinions about when a chapter was still lacking versus when I had "found my stride."

One of the questions James asked me was whether or not the 241 practitioners included in my ethnography indeed formed a social network. Is there a functional medicine community? Or are the practitioners included in my ethnography random individuals that I happen to have come across? Having conducted the ethnography, I knew I was observing a cohesive functional medicine community; however, James's question pointed to the need for graphic visualizations of the cohesion I observed. I enlisted the help of my favorite computer wiz—my younger brother, Jason Vega. He was completing his bachelor's degree in Computer Science at UC San Diego. I sent Jason the data table in the appendix and he was able to produce the people- and source-centric social networks. The job was more than he bargained for and I am very appreciative of his hard work.

As I continued writing the first draft, it quickly became clear that the book was too long for publication. I wrote much more than three hundred thousand words. Part of the problem was that I was, in fact, writing two books. Even after untangling the two manuscripts, my writing still needed serious tightening. Each week, I emailed a new chapter draft to my mother, Tuen Wong. My mom is a former English major. While I was producing words, she was eliminating them. We did not see each other for sixteen months during the pandemic and, in some way, her involvement in my writing process helped me to feel her presence. Moreover, my mom was supportive of every decision I made during my healing journey. She never questioned my judgment or doubted the "alternative" methods I was pursuing. She repeatedly told me that I knew what was best for my body. Her faith gave me faith.

After this pruning process, I shared drafts of my work with a trusted colleague at UTRGV, Bill Yaworsky. Since I joined the anthropology department, Bill and I developed a habit of exchanging manuscripts and offering each other feedback. Bill is a social and cultural anthropologist with research interests in Latin America, politics, and social psychology. He is humble to a fault. Every time he reads my work, he reminds me that he is not a medical anthropologist, so his opinion is simply that of an educated lay reader—then he delivers feedback that is invariably useful and constructive. I often needed the perspective of an anthropologist who is not positioned squarely within my own subdiscipline, and Bill's comments helped me to gauge how my work would be perceived by the wider audience I was hoping to write for.

This manuscript greatly benefited from the generous and insightful comments of two supportive reviewers. The first, Jennifer Rogerson, urged me to deepen my analysis of privilege. The second, an anonymous reviewer, suggested I make the book even more accessible to a broad audience—for example, by providing definitions for biological and medical terms with which the average reader may be unfamiliar. Both reviewers helped me to engage more deeply with the existing literature in medical anthropology. I am incredibly indebted to them both.

I am indebted to the staff at University of Texas Press, including the acquisitions; editorial, design, and production; marketing and sales; and rights and permissions teams. I am grateful to Sally Furgeson for her incredibly thorough copyediting of this manuscript.

I revised this book while caring for my newborn daughter, Madelena. Either my mom or my husband gave Madelena one bottle of pumped breastmilk per day, thus allowing me precious time for focused work. I am so grateful for how they have contributed to my finishing this book. Madelena and I are blessed with their love.

# APPENDIX

# PERSONS DESCRIBED

# IN THIS BOOK

This list consists of individuals included in the book because of their positionality vis-à-vis functional medicine, food justice, and public discourse. It does not include the social scientists I reference, nor does it list my family members or friends.

| Person | Source | Role |
|---|---|---|
| Matthew Accurso | *The Human Longevity Project* docuseries | Entrepreneur, health consultant |
| Ted Achacoso | *The Human Longevity Project* docuseries | MD |
| Michael Ash | *The Human Longevity Project* docuseries | DO; ND |
| Josh Axe | *Dr. Josh Axe* YouTube channel | DC; DNM; CNS |
| Neil Barnard | *Voices of the Food Revolution* | MD |
| Paul Beaver | Interpreting Your Genetics Summit | PhD, materials engineering; co-founder and chief scientific officer, Fitgenes Ltd.; founder and director, 3P Healthcare Pty Ltd. |

| | | |
|---|---|---|
| Jeffrey Bland | *FxMed* podcast; *The Human Longevity Project* docuseries; September 2017 *Functional Forum*; Interpreting Your Genetics Summit; Simplexity Medicine: Health Care Reimagined Conference | PhD; FACN; CNS |
| Michael Bloomberg | His role is described by Hyman in *Food Fix* | Former mayor, New York City; participant, Task Force on Fiscal Policy for Health |
| Tom Blue | *The Human Longevity Project* docuseries | Strategic advisor, Institute for Functional Medicine |
| David Brady | *Betrayal: The Autoimmune Disease Solution They're Not Telling You About* docuseries | ND |
| Kelly Brogan | *The Human Longevity Project* docuseries; *Betrayal: The Autoimmune Disease Solution They're Not Telling You About* docuseries; "Tantalizing Evidence of a Brain Microbiome" blog post | MD |
| Zach Bush | Food Revolution Network interview; EMF Summit; *Autoimmune Secrets* docuseries; "Intrinsic Health Coaching Program" webpage; "The Virome: A Template for A Regenerative Future" webinar; Eat4Earth online event | MD |
| Nessa Carey | *The Epigenetics Revolution: How Modern Biology Is Rewriting Our Understanding of Genetics, Disease, and Inheritance* | PhD, virology; international director, PraxisAuril; lecturer, Molecular Biology, Imperial College London |

| | | |
|---|---|---|
| Andrés Carrasco (1946–2014) | His role is described by Smith in *Voices of the Food Revolution* | MD; head of the Molecular Embryology Lab, University of Buenos Aires; chief scientist, National Council for Science and Technology, Argentina |
| Benjamin Chan | *FxMed* podcast | PhD, biology; associate research scientist, Paul Turner Lab |
| Rangan Chatterjee | *The Human Longevity Project* docuseries | MD |
| Nalini Chilkov | *The Human Longevity Project* docuseries | Doctor of Oriental medicine |
| Gail Cresci | *The Human Longevity Project* docuseries | PhD, nutrition; RD |
| Pete Cummings | "Nutrition: The Gut Brain Axis and Human Performance" webinar | MD; MSc; forensic pathologist |
| Jay Davidson | Mitochondrial Summit; Viral and Retroviral Summit; Microbe Formulas, Facebook ad; *Autoimmune Secrets* docuseries | DC; PScD; co-founder, Microbe Formulas |
| William Davis | *Autoimmune Secrets* docuseries | MD |
| Jeanne D'Brant | "The Shikimate Pathway, the Microbiome, and Disease: Health Effects of GMOs on Humans" PowerPoint | DACBN; DC; CTN; RH (AHG); associate professor, Biology and Allied Health, State University of New York. |
| John Dempster | *The Gut Solution* docuseries | ND; FAARFM; ABAAHP |
| Lorenzo Drago | *The Human Longevity Project* docuseries | PhD, clinical microbiology; professor, clinical microbiology, University of Milan |
| Marvin Edeas | *The Human Longevity Project* docuseries | MD; PhD; microbiome researcher |
| Yousef Elyaman | Interpreting Your Genetics Summit | MD |

| | | |
|---|---|---|
| Irina Ermakova | Her role is described by Smith in *Voices of the Food Revolution* | PhD; Dr. Sc.; leading scientist, Institute of Higher Nervous Activity and Neurophysiology, Russian Academy of Sciences |
| Cindy Fallon | "The Innate Immune System" webinar | PhD, organic chemistry |
| Paul Farmer (1959–2022) | Described by Hyman in "Application of Functional Medicine in a Large Medical System (Cleveland Clinic)"; *Food Fix* | MD; PhD, medical anthropology; Kolokotrones University; professor and chair, Department of Global Health and Social Medicine, Harvard Medical School |
| Kara Fitzgerald | *FxMed* podcast and email newsletter | ND |
| Leigh Frame | *George Washington School of Medicine and Health Sciences Integrative Medicine* podcast | PhD, human nutrition; MHS; director, Integrative Medicine Program, George Washington University School of Medicine and Health Sciences |
| Timothy Frie | November 2020 Functional Forum | Membership Chair of the American Public Health Association (APHA) Human Rights Forum; Member of the Association for Public Policy Analysis and Management (APPAM) |
| Bill Frist | *The Doctor's Farmacy* podcast | MD; former senator and US Senate majority leader |
| Joel Fuhrman | *Autoimmune Secrets* docuseries | MD; president, Nutritional Research Foundation; faculty, Northern Arizona University, Health Sciences Division |
| Jason Fung | *The Human Longevity Project* docuseries | MD |
| Leo Galland | His contribution is described by Dr. Bland | MD |
| Donna Gates | BodyEcology.com; *Body Ecology* email; Interpreting Your Genetics Summit | EdM; ABAAH; nutritional consultant |

| | | |
|---|---|---|
| Tracy Gaudet | Institute for Functional Medicine's Annual International Conference 2020 | MD |
| Patrick Gentempo | *The Human Longevity Project* docuseries | DO; founder, Creating Wellness |
| Bryan Glick | Interpreting Your Genetics Summit | DO |
| Niki Gratrix | *Autoimmune Secrets* docuseries | Co-founder, Optimum Health Clinic; nutritionist and health coach |
| John Gray | *The Gut Solution* docuseries | PhD, psychology |
| David Haase | Interpreting Your Genetics Summit | MD |
| Vani Hari | You Can Heal Your Life 2020 Summit; her role is described by Hyman in *Food Fix* | Food activist who, by exposing harmful chemicals, has changed dozens of multi-billion dollar food corporations |
| Stanley Hazen | *The Doctor's Farmacy* podcast | MD; chair, Department of Cellular and Molecular Medicine, Lerner Research Institute; section head, Preventive Cardiology and Rehabilitation, Heart and Vascular Institute, Cleveland Clinic |
| Martha Herbert | Healthy Gut Summit | MD; PhD; assistant professor, neurology, Harvard Medical School |
| Andrew Heyman | *George Washington School of Medicine and Health Sciences Integrative Medicine* podcast; Advances in Mitochondrial Medicine Symposium | MD; MHSA |
| Leroy Hood | His contribution is described by Dr. Bland and Maskell | PhD; biologist, California Institute of Technology and University of Washington |

| Mark Hyman | *The Doctor's Farmacy* podcast; *The Human Longevity Project* docuseries; "Application of Functional Medicine in a Large Medical System (Cleveland Clinic)" presentation; *Food Fix*; *The Conscious-ish Show;* Institute for Functional Medicine Annual International Conference 2020 | MD |
|---|---|---|
| Felice Jacka | Her role is described by Dr. Prescott and Dr. Logan | PhD; professor, nutritional and epidemiological psychiatry, Deakin University; director, Food and Mood Centre; founder and president, International Society for Nutritional Psychiatry Research |
| Sayer Ji | GreenMedInfo email; Interpreting Your Genetics Summit; "How Raw Honey Could Save Your Microbiome (and Travel Back In Time)" article; *The Human Longevity Project* docuseries | Founder, GreenMedInfo |
| Randy Jirtle | *FxMed* podcast | PhD, radiation biology; professor, epigenetics, Department of Biological Sciences, North Carolina State University; senior scientist, McArdle Laboratory for Cancer Research, University of Wisconsin, Madison |
| Yael Joffe | Interpreting Your Genetics Summit | PhD, nutrigenomics; director, Centre for Translational Genomics |

| | | |
|---|---|---|
| Janice Joneja | *The Health Professional's Guide to Food Allergies and Intolerances* | PhD, medical microbiology and immunology; prior to retiring: faculty, School of Biomedical and Molecular Sciences, University of Surrey, England; head of the Allergy Nutrition Program, Vancouver Hospital and Health Sciences Center |
| David Scott Jones | *Betrayal: The Autoimmune Disease Solution They're Not Telling You About* docuseries | MD; president emeritus, Medical Education, Institute for Functional Medicine |
| Paulette Jordan | November 2020 Functional Forum | Idaho state representative (2014–2018) |
| David Katz | Functional Forum conference | MD; MPH; FACPM; FACP; FACLM |
| Raphael Kellman | *The Microbiome Breakthrough* | MD |
| Datis Kharrazian | *The Human Longevity Project* docuseries; *FxMed* email newsletter | PhD; DHSc; DC; MS; MMSc; FACN |
| Peter Konturek | *The Human Longevity Project* docuseries | MD; professor, gastroenterology, University Erlangen; director, Department of Medicine, Thuringia Clinic |
| Chris Kresser | *FxMed* podcast; *The Human Longevity Project* docuseries; *Unconventional Medicine* | LAc; functional health coach |
| Kiran Krishnan | *The Human Longevity Project* docuseries; Genius of Your Genes Summit | BS, microbiology |
| Dennis Kucinich | *Voices of the Food Revolution* | Former US representative (1997–2013) |
| Vishen Lakhiani | *The Doctor's Farmacy* podcast | Entrepreneur |
| Beth Lambert | *The Human Longevity Project* docuseries | Executive director, Parents Ending America's Childhood Epidemic (PEACE) |

| | | |
|---|---|---|
| Todd LePine | *The Doctor's Farmacy* podcast; "The Gut and Skin Microbes," HealthMeans interview | MD |
| Cynthia Li | *The Doctor's Farmacy* podcast | MD |
| William Li | TED Talks; *The Doctor's Farmacy* podcast; *Eat to Beat Disease* | MD |
| Grace Liu | *The Human Longevity Project* docuseries | PharmD; founder, Gut Institute |
| Alan Logan | *The Secret Life of Your Microbiome* | ND |
| Ritamarie Loscalzo | Interpreting Your Genetics Summit | MS; DC; CCN; DACBN |
| Robert Luby | *FxMed* email newsletter | MD; director, Medical Education Initiatives, Institute for Functional Medicine |
| Max Lugavere | *The Human Longevity Project* docuseries | Health science journalist |
| Robert Lustig | His role is described by Hyman in *Food Fix* | MD; pediatric endocrinologist, UC San Francisco |
| Mia Lux | *The Conscious-ish Show* | Host, *The Conscious-ish Show* |
| Ben Lynch | *The Human Longevity Project* docuseries | ND |
| Aseem Malhotra | His role is described by Hyman in *Food Fix* | MD; cardiologist |
| Molly Maloof | Functional Forum conference | MD; lecturer, Stanford University |

| | | |
|---|---|---|
| James Maskell | Fatigue Super Conference; *The Energy Blueprint* podcast; 2017 Functional Forum; email newsletter; "Enhancing Patient Care with Virtual Group Visits" webinar; *The Human Longevity Project*; *The Community Cure*; *Rogue Health Economist* daily live-cast; TEDMED; JP Morgan Healthcare Conference; Advances in Mitochondrial Medicine Symposium | Entrepreneur; functional medicine advocate |
| Emeran Mayer | *The Mind-Gut Connection* | MD; director, G. Oppen-heimer Center for Neurobiol-ogy of Stress and Resilience; co-director, Digestive Diseases Research Center; professor, Medicine, Physiol-ogy, and Psychiatry, UCLA |
| Sarkis Mazmanian | TEDMED: "Why Science Says to Listen to Your Gut" | PhD, microbiology; Luis B. and Nelly Soux Professor of Microbiology, Caltech |
| Rollin McCraty | *The Human Longevity Project* docuseries | PhD; psychophysiologist and director of research, Heart-Math Institute; professor, Florida Atlantic University |
| Michael McEvoy | *The Human Longevity Project* docuseries | Founder, CEO, and head clinician, Metabolic Healing, Inc. |
| Helen Messier | Interpreting Your Genetics Summit | MD; PhD, molecular immunology |
| Daphne Miller | *FxMed* podcast | MD; associate clinical profes-sor, University of California San Francisco |
| Deanna Minich | *The Human Longevity Project* docuseries | PhD, nutrition; certified nutritionist, trained by the Institute for Functional Medicine |

| | | |
|---|---|---|
| Richard Mitchell | His role is described by Dr. Prescott and Dr. Logan | PhD, geography; professor, Social and Public Health Sciences Unit, University of Glasgow; honorary professor, College of Medicine and Veterinary Medicine, University of Edinburgh |
| Josh Mitteldorf | *FxMed* email newsletter | PhD, astrophysics; member, Life Extension Board |
| Rodger Murphree | *The Gut Solution* docuseries; *Autoimmune Secrets* docuseries | DC |
| Andrea Nakayama | *The Human Longevity Project* docuseries; *FxNutrition* email newsletter; Fatigue Super Conference; Interpreting Your Genetics Summit; *Betrayal: The Autoimmune Disease Solution They're Not Telling You About* docuseries | Functional medicine nutritionist |
| Robert Naviaux | Advances in Mitochondrial Medicine Symposium | MD |
| Neil Nedley | *Autoimmune Secrets* docuseries | MD |
| Marion Nestle | Cited by Hyman in *Food Fix* | PhD, molecular biology; MPH, public health nutrition; Paulette Goddard Professor, Nutrition, Food Studies, and Public Health, New York University |
| Tom O'Bryan | *Autoimmune Secrets* docuseries; *The Human Longevity Project* docuseries; *Betrayal: The Autoimmune Disease Solution They're Not Telling You About* docuseries | DC, CCN, DACBN |

| | | |
|---|---|---|
| Peter Osborne | *Betrayal: The Autoimmune Disease Solution They're Not Telling You About* docuseries | PScD; board-certified clinical nutritionist |
| Jonathan Otto | *Autoimmune Secrets* docuseries | Filmmaker |
| George Papanicolaou | *The Doctor's Farmacy* podcast | DO |
| Anand Parekh | *The Doctor's Farmacy* podcast | MD; chief medical advisor, Bipartisan Policy Center (BPC); former deputy assistant secretary for health, US Department of Health and Human Services |
| Kirk Robert Parsley | *The Human Longevity Project* docuseries | MD |
| Sachin Patel | *The Human Longevity Project* docuseries | Functional health coach; founder, Living Proof Institute |
| Linus Pauling (1901–1995) | His contribution is described by Dr. Bland | PhD; quantum chemist and molecular biologist, California Institute of Technology |
| Vincent Pedre | *FxMed* podcast, email; *The Gut Solution* docuseries | MD |
| Leah Penniman | *The Doctor's Farmacy* podcast | Farmer, educator, author, and food justice activist, Soul Fire Farm |
| David Perlmutter | His contribution to *Betrayal: The Autoimmune Disease Solution They're Not Telling You About* docuseries is described by Dr. Nandi; *The Doctor's Farmacy* podcast | MD; FACN; ABIHM |
| Martin Picard | *The Energy Blueprint* podcast | PhD; neurology researcher, Columbia University |
| Susan Prescott | *The Secret Life of Your Microbiome*; Institute for Functional Medicine Annual International Conference 2020 | MD |

| | | |
|---|---|---|
| Árpád Pusztai | His role is described by Smith in *Voices of the Food Revolution* | PhD, biochemistry; biochemist and nutritionist, Rowett Research Institute, Aberdeen, Scotland (1963–1999) |
| David Quig | *FxMed* podcast | PhD, nutritional biochemistry |
| Matt Riemann | *The Human Longevity Project* docuseries | Founder and CEO, Ultimate Human Foundation |
| John Robbins | *Voices of the Food Revolution* | Co-founder and president, Food Revolution Network |
| Ocean Robbins | Food Revolution Network email | CEO and co-founder, Food Revolution Network |
| Rosalinda Roberts | Her role is described by Dr. Brogan's team | PhD, biology; professor, Behavioral Psychology, University of Alabama School of Medicine |
| Marwan Sabbagh | *The Doctor's Farmacy* podcast | MD |
| Grant Schofield | His role is described by Hyman in *Food Fix* | PhD; professor, public health; director, Human Potential Centre (HPC), Auckland University of Technology |
| Stephanie Seneff | *The Human Longevity Project* docuseries | PhD, electrical engineering; PhD, computer science; senior research scientist, MIT |
| David Servan-Schreiber (1961–2011) | *Anti-Cancer: A New Way of Life* | MD |
| Jason Shepherd | TEDMED | PhD, neurobiology; neurobiology researcher, University of Utah School of Medicine |
| Maya Shetreat | *The Gut Solution* docuseries | MD |
| Vandana Shiva | *Voices of the Food Revolution* | PhD, philosophy; founder, Researcher Foundation for Science, Technology, and Ecology; founder, Navdanya |

| | | |
|---|---|---|
| David Sinclair | *The Doctor's Farmacy* pod-cast; *Impact Theory* YouTube channel; *Dr. Josh Axe* You-Tube channel | PhD; professor, genetics, Harvard Medical School |
| George Slavich | Interpreting Your Genetics Summit | PhD, clinical psychology; director, UCLA Laboratory for Stress Assessment and Research; associate professor, Psychiatry and Behavioral Sciences, UCLA |
| Jeffrey Smith | *Voices of the Food Revolution* | Vice president, GMO testing company, Genetic ID; founder and executive director, Institute for Responsible Technology |
| Morgan Spurlock | *Voices of the Food Revolution* | Documentary filmmaker; director and star, *Super Size Me* |
| Lawrence Summers | His role is described by Hyman in *Food Fix* | Former US treasury secretary; president, Harvard University; participant, Task Force on Fiscal Policy for Health |
| Moshe Szyf | *FxMed* podcast | PhD; geneticist, McGill University |
| Dimitris Tsoukalas | *The Human Longevity Project* docuseries | MD |
| Paul Turner | *FxMed* podcast | PhD; virology researcher at Yale University |
| Robert Verkerk | "What Happened to 'Do No Harm'?" article; Interpreting Your Genetics Summit | PhD; founder, executive and scientific director, Alliance for Natural Health International |
| Alison Vickery | online blog | Functional health coach |
| Rudolf Virchow (1821–1902) | Cited by Dr. Prescott and Dr. Logan in *The Secret Life of Your Microbiome* | MD; anthropologist, patholo-gist, politician, and founder of social medicine |

| | | |
|---|---|---|
| Terry Wahls | *Betrayal: The Autoimmune Disease Solution They're Not Telling You About* docuseries; Toxic Mold Summit; Mitochondrial Summit; *FxMed* podcast; TerryWahls .com; email newsletter; The Wahls Protocol Facebook group; *The Community Cure*; *Health Theory* YouTube channel | MD |
| Courtney Walker | Her role is described by Dr. Brogan's team | Undergraduate researcher, University of Alabama |
| Volkmar Weissig | *The Human Longevity Project* docuseries | PhD; professor, Pharmaceutical Sciences, Midwestern University |
| Ari Whitten | *The Energy Blueprint* podcast | PhD candidate; health coach and fatigue specialist |
| Christopher Wild | His role is described by Kresser | PhD; director, International Agency for Research on Cancer |
| Yasmina Ykelenstam | online blog | Health coach and histamine specialist |

# NOTES

PRELUDE: ANTHOPOLOGY OF AND FOR HEALING

1. This was before the COVID-19 pandemic, when remote instruction via video platforms was still very unusual.

INTRODUCTION

1. Vickery is the mentee of Dietrich Klinghardt. As a physician and scientific advisor, Dr. Klinghardt develops and employs diagnostic and treatment modalities for autism, chronic infections, metal toxicity, and more.

2. Discussed further in chapter 1.

3. In chapter 1, I demonstrate how conducting in-depth interviews, listening, and observing are considered valued diagnostic tools among functional medicine practitioners.

4. In *Accessing Recovery*, a manuscript in progress, I explore the illness narrative of wounded healers as another important discursive form in functional medicine.

5. See chapter 1.

6. A similar concept, implicit bias, has emerged from behavioral psychology to describe how a lifetime of experiences with social groups results in hidden biases about race, ethnicity, age, gender, religion, socioeconomic class, sexuality, disability status, and nationality (see Banaji and Greenwald 2013).

7. While this amount represented a significant burden for my family, it pales in comparison to the $42,000 to $100,000 annual cost for autoimmune medications, which are taken for life, as Dr. Terry Wahls pointed out in an August 6, 2019, email.

CHAPTER 1. PARADIGM SHIFTS

1. In *Accessing Recovery*, I provide an in-depth discussion of functional medicine as personalized medicine. Although personalized medicine offers clear benefits, it is inaccessible to many due to high costs.

2. I would not be surprised if the United States has already surpassed the 20 percent figure. While we do not yet have nationwide statistics, I expect that health costs have increased precipitously due to the COVID pandemic.

3. I offer a critique of how "lifestyle" is portrayed in functional medicine discourse later in this chapter. I further critique the use of "lifestyle" in functional medicine in chapters 3 and 5, as well as in *Accessing Recovery*.

4. I discuss the Cleveland Clinic's application of functional medicine in detail in *Accessing Recovery*.

5. Functional medicine embraces much of the philosophy of integrative medicine (emphasizing the therapeutic relationship between practitioner and patient, prioritizing evidence, and integrating all appropriate therapies) while also incorporating a systems biology approach (see chapter 2).

6. See chapter 2 regarding systems biology.

7. In *Accessing Recovery*, I use ethnographic evidence to demonstrate how functional

medicine interlocutors position patients as "the doctors of the future." That is, functional medicine proponents legitimate the embodied knowledge of patients *as* expert knowledge. In this model, patient-clients are responsible for their recovery. Meanwhile, physicians are portrayed as coaches or guides.

8. See chapter 2.

9. See my comments in the introduction regarding hyper-self-reflexivity. I acknowledge how troubling it is that my privilege is what allowed me to purchase my recovery.

10. For a detailed description of systems biology, see chapter 2.

11. The reconfigured role of bioconsumers in functional medicine is a theme of *Accessing Recovery*. Stated simply, bioconsumers leverage their financial capital in private markets in order to obtain goods and services and to gain self-knowledge. As a result, they effect change on their biology, seek belonging, and accrue greater social capital.

12. For a more in-depth description, see the section in this chapter titled "Listening and Observing: Adopting Anthropological Methods."

13. Using the concept of nested ecologies, I will be expanding on the interface of internal and external factors throughout the book.

14. See *Accessing Recovery* for an in-depth description of how the illness narratives provide functional medicine practitioners with clues for clinical care and how providers' narratives as "wounded healers" constitute a powerful discursive form within functional medicine.

15. These comments about what counts as legitimate scientific knowledge foreground topics presented in the next chapter.

16. Dr. Ingelfinger was the editor of the *New England Journal of Medicine* at the time of publication. Dr. Li also comments on Ingelfinger's essay in her book, *A Brave New Medicine*.

17. In *Accessing Recovery*, I turn to the personal stories of illness and recovery among functional medicine practitioners. Many became functional medicine practitioners precisely because they were unable to heal themselves using the tools they were taught in conventional medicine.

18. Matthiessen (2013) examines two dimensions of medical consultations—stratification and instantiation—thus demonstrating how relationship-centered health care can be interpreted using systemic functional linguistics. Hasty et al. (2012) signal how certain forms of communication are used to negotiate power imbalances in doctor-patient relationships.

19. My Spanish-to-English translation. This is what Menéndez refers to as *proceso salud/enfermedad/atención*.

20. He calls this "*autoatención*," which translates to "self-care." Menéndez developed this term in 2003, long before self-care practices as we currently understand them came into being.

21. See chapter 3.

22. In *Accessing Recovery*, I describe how functional medicine proponents like Maskell position "group medicine" as a cost-effective delivery method for functional medicine care. Ultimately, however, I argue that group medicine and one-on-one care are not equivalent.

23. In May 2020, Maskell offered a similar critique. As host of the webinar, "Enhancing Patient Care with Virtual Group Visits," he stated, "What we call 'lifestyle' is really

an environment that people can't afford to get out of." I discuss how this relates to the (limited) accessibility of functional medicine in *Accessing Recovery*.

24. I explore how social inequalities unduly affect disadvantaged citizens in chapter 5.

INTERLUDE: STUCK IN A WEB OF CHRONIC DISEASE

1. I critically analyze the cost of functional medicine, along with issues of accessibility, in *Accessing Recovery*.

2. In *Accessing* Recovery, I document how my experience is similar to many other individuals seeking functional medicine care.

3. In *Accessing Recovery*, I describe how functional medicine recasts "embodied knowledge" as "authoritative knowledge" (see Jordan 1992).

4. This was before the COVID-19 outbreak; thus, this type of telemedicine was entirely novel to me.

5. I have lightly edited these excerpts for clarity and correctness.

6. In May 1986, the International Committee on the Taxonomy of Viruses decided that the virus that causes AIDS would officially be called HIV (human immunodeficiency virus) instead of HTLV-III/LAV (human T-lymphotropic virus type III/lymphadenopathy-associated virus). In March 1987, the FDA approved the first antiretroviral drug, zidovudine (AZT), as treatment for HIV. I was born in August 1987. See K. Case (1986) and Molotsky (1987).

7. Here, I am using quotes to signal how "natural" *and* synthetic hormones are used at *unnatural* levels in cattle farming.

8. See the conclusion.

9. See chapter 4.

10. See the conclusion.

11. Experiences like mine, unfolding in the absence of HPV, point to new potential therapeutic targets for cervical cancers.

12. Mastocytosis is a rare disease characterized by the accumulation of mast cells in the skin or organs. The immunologist tested me for this disease based on my itching, hives, rapid heartbeat, headaches, and sensitivity to temperature changes.

13. D-ribose is a supplement used to reduce fatigue and improve athletic performance. It is a key component of adenosine triphosphate (ATP) and thus aids in storing and releasing energy.

CHAPTER 2: SYSTEMS BIOLOGY

1. See chapter 5.

2. By using the word "complementary," I am at once pointing to how functional medicine therapies are complementary to existing medical therapies.

3. See chapter 1.

4. See chapter 3 where I discuss epigenetics.

5. See my critique of the functional medicine approach to lifestyle in chapter 1 and later in this chapter.

6. In the comments section for Maurizio Meloni's *Somatosphere* piece, Lock acknowledges that while Atwood Gaines used the term "local biologies" months before she first used the same words, the meaning she attributes to the term is distinct from the meaning attributed to Gaines (Meloni 2014).

7. I develop these arguments in detail in *Accessing Recovery*.

8. I will discuss the food environment further in the conclusion to this book.

9. See my discussion of how functional medicine rejects the Cartesian mind/body split in chapter 1.

10. See Dr. Chilkov's suggestions for incorporating conventional oncology with functional medicine for the treatment of cancer in chapter 1. Dr. Servan-Schreiber made similar remarks in his book, *Anticancer: A New Way of Life* (2009).

INTERLUDE: GENETIC FATE?

1. Both HSV-1 and EBV are viruses in the herpes family.

2. In *Accessing Recovery*, I examine the relationships among bioconsumption, bioentrepreneurship, biocapital, and digital capitalism.

3. I acknowledge that empowerment, including my own, is facilitated by socioeconomic privilege.

4. In an interview posted to YouTube on October 7, 2020, Dr. Jennifer Ashton said, "We've seen other similar syndromes after infection, sometimes after viruses [like] Epstein-Barr and chronic Lyme. We've seen it with chronic fatigue syndrome, and we've even seen it after SARS." Long-hauler symptoms include fatigue, body aches, shortness of breath, difficulty breathing, and inability to be active (*Good Morning America* 2020).

CHAPTER 3: (EPI)GENETICS AND ITS MULTIPLE IMPLICATIONS

1. In *Accessing Recovery*, I explore how functional medicine's use of advanced diagnostics to create personalized treatment protocols often results in recovery from chronic disease for patients who are privileged enough to afford this type of care.

2. See chapter 1.

3. See chapter 1.

4. I argue that privilege and disadvantage are not binary and mutually exclusive (see Atewologun and Sealy 2014). As in chapter 1, I turn to the hyphenated term "privilege-disadvantage" to depict privilege and disadvantage as unfolding along an intersectional continuum, constituted by multiple privileges and advantages (see Crenshaw 2014).

5. Here, McEvoy distinguishes between "genetic mutations" and "genetic variants" (SNPs) in public discourse. While these terms are often used interchangeably, the differences between mutations and variants are vast. I explain SNPs below in chapter 3.

6. See chapter 2.

7. See Jablonka and Lamb 2014, 246–247, for more detail on cell differentiation.

8. See Jablonka and Lamb 2014, 111–151, for more detail on epigenetic inheritance systems.

9. Skinner et al. 2013 define transgenerational epigenetic effects as "the germline transmission of epigenetic information between generations in the absence of direct environmental exposures."

10. As Mattingly writes, "The moral is always historical, always shaped by social context." (Mattingly 2012, 164). Furthermore, the moral is a communal enterprise. "The moral in any society is dependent upon the cultivation of virtues that are developed in and through social practices" (Mattingly 2012, 164).

11. A feminist critique might signal a patriarchal undertone in Dr. Lynch's comments.

12. Niewöhner (2011) observed Dr. Szyf's epigenetic research team. His team is also referenced in the footnotes of Meloni (2014).

13. However, building upon Waggoner's 2017 argument regarding the "zero trimester," I can imagine interventions that aim to address trauma in future parents—especially mothers—prior to pregnancy. Unfortunately, these interventions would likely be focused on individual traumas and not structural violence, thus eclipsing the opportunity to argue for social justice.

14. Here, I am placing the word "choices" within quotation marks because, as an anthropologist, I am constantly attentive to how "free choice" is never truly free. Individuals' "choices" are always already structured by capital (see Bourdieu 1984; Althusser 1970), along with racializing and gendering logics.

15. Later in this chapter, I query who can afford to be "empowered" by genomic profiling. Empowerment is directly tied to capital.

16. Foreshadowing topics discussed in the next chapter, Dr. Perlmutter's research explores the role of the microbiome in shaping neuroplasticity.

17. Hore also indicates excessive supplementation can lead to genetic instability.

18. See chapter 5.

19. See chapter 2.

20. Quote from a sample DNAge® report.

21. See Jablonka and Lamb 2014, 254–256, for more detail on epigenetic variations (e.g., stress) and the selection of genes.

22. Discussed at length in the conclusion.

23. Relying on *The Global Burden of Diseases, Injuries, and Risk Factors Study 2010* (GBD 2010) and 2008 World Health Organization estimates, the 2013 review article published by David Hunter and K. Srinath Reddy in the *New England Journal of Medicine* states that noncommunicable diseases contributed to 63–65 percent of deaths worldwide. However, the article also concludes, "Noncommunicable diseases will be the predominant global public health challenge of the 21st century."

24. Over the course of my ethnographic research, I observed how functional medicine practitioners' admiration of Blue Zones often leads to simultaneous romanticizing and inadvertent othering of non-Western cultures. I explore this tendency further in *Accessing Recovery*.

25. See chapter 5.

26. In chapter 1, I presented an anthropological critique of the Cartesian mind/body split. Here, I continue to insist on the falseness of Cartesian dualism—the mind is in the body and the body is in the mind.

27. See my critique in chapter 5 about providing more "green spaces" as an answer to socioeconomic and racialized inequality.

28. Regarding emotional well-being, I am wary of how this focus can inadvertently "blame the victim." Instead of dismissing patients' complaints as "all in their head," this well-meaning framework could be misused to suggest that patients' illnesses are largely due to their mismanagement of negative emotions. (See chapter 1, where I describe how functional medicine rejects the Cartesian mind/body split.) I have not observed this during my ethnographic fieldwork. Therefore, I am not critiquing functional medicine discourse—I am simply flagging a danger.

29. See discussion on the epigenetics of cancer above.

30. Again, I flag how access to "empowerment" is mediated by socioeconomic privilege.

31. One of my primary critiques in *Accessing Recovery* is that while recovery can often be achieved using functional medicine, our existing health care system renders these tools and techniques largely inaccessible to lower-income and minority communities.

32. See my comments on medical nomenclature in chapter 2.

## CHAPTER 4: THE POLITICAL ECOLOGY OF "HUMAN" MICROBIOLOGY

1. Here, I placed the words "disadvantage" and "unfavorable" in quotes because I am acknowledging the functional medicine argument that individual SNPs also conferred competitive advantage from a historical perspective. See chapter 3.

2. See chapter 3.

3. See chapter 3 regarding how epigenetics can produce intergenerational effects. See chapter 5 for a discussion of "ancestral diets" and *Accessing Recovery* for further problematization of "ancestral knowledge."

4. I am placing "our" within quotes to continue problematizing the binary that separates "us" [humans] from "them" [bacteria].

5. See, for example, Fitzpatrick et al. 2020 on how gut-trained bacteria protect the brain from infection.

6. According to Dr. Li, the microbiome "weigh[s] about three pounds, the equivalent heft of your brain" (2019, 35). Dr. Mayer writes, "If you put all your microbes together and shaped them into an organ, it would weigh between 2 and 6 pounds—on par with the brain, which weighs in at 2.6 pounds" (2016, 17).

7. Again, I am placing "our" within quotes to problematize the us/them binary that separates humans from the bacteria living on and inside them.

8. See the conclusion for an in-depth discussion of food access. In *Accessing Recovery*, I trace how unequal health care access further aggravates disparate health outcomes.

9. Here, I am using quotation marks to reiterate that the "gut" and the "brain" do not operate as distinct entities and may, in fact, be mutually constituted.

10. See chapter 1.

11. See chapter 1.

12. See chapter 5.

13. See Lorimer (2019) for more of an anthropological perspective on the emerging figure of the human as a holobiont.

14. See chapter 5 and the conclusion.

15. In *Accessing Recovery*, I examine how bioentrepreneurship runs the risk of reinscribing racial inequality and venturing into the territory of biopiracy. I also observe how corporate sponsors market to functional medicine providers who, in turn, market to bioconsumers.

## CHAPTER 5: THE SOCIAL MICROBIOME

1. Here, I am using the plural form of "knowledge" to emphasize that there are multiple ways of knowing and to argue for the legitimacy of non-hegemonic forms of knowledge.

2. Later in this chapter, I describe *Clostridium difficile* in the context of Dr. Peter Konturek's work with fecal microbiota transplantation.

3. See discussion of phage therapy in chapter 4.

4. See discussion in chapter 2 regarding root cause(s) and systems biology.

5. See chapter 4 on the gut-brain connection.

6. See the conclusion.

7. I explore these dynamics in depth in *Accessing Recovery*.

8. His assessment of the food system foreshadows some of the arguments in the conclusion.

9. This quote is, in fact, the title of Dr. Haahtela's 2009 article in *Allergy*.

10. Furthermore, functional medicine interlocutors describe how the exposome encompasses all of an individual's exposures, including their stressors, anxious thoughts, and negative internal dialogue. I argue that this framing of the exposome-as-perception inadvertently blames victims by casting their "negative internal dialogue" as a matter of personal responsibility. I agree with the underlying thrust of this argument: mind and body are truly one, and biological and psychological exposures are entangled in one's exposome. However, I extend the notion of the exposome-as-perception by arguing that the exposome also serves as a record of discrimination and social inequalities.

11. I discuss holobiont theory in chapter 4.

12. See chapter 4.

13. See my critiques of "lifestyle" in chapters 1–4.

14. Beronda Montgomery similarly underscores the importance of equity in science, technology, engineering, and medicine using analogies from plant biology and microbiology.

15. Likewise, Krishnan concludes on *The Human Longevity Project*, that "the theme that more diversity improves health in general is a very solid theme."

CONCLUSION: FOOD JUSTICE

1. This quote appeared as part of a much longer quote in Dr. Prescott and Dr. Logan's *The Secret Life of Your Microbiome*.

2. I explore the shortcomings of the health care system in great depth in *Accessing Recovery*.

3. I critique how functional medicine's neoliberal approach—including its emphasis on individual responsibility and market-based consumption—inadvertently excludes low-income individuals in *Accessing Recovery*.

4. See chapters 2–4 for my critiques of diet as a "choice."

5. Alluding to class differences, Dr. Hyman recognizes that not everyone is able to change their banking and investment strategy. In his book, *Food Fix*, Dr. Hyman pairs his consumption-based suggestions with policy recommendations. I will describe these in the "Food Policy Recommendations and the 'Nanny State'" section.

6. See my discussion in the section "How the Food System Targets the Most Vulnerable: The Need for Food Justice" regarding "food deserts," "food swamps," and "food apartheid."

7. In *Accessing Recovery*, I describe how economic capital sometimes facilitates social capital in functional medicine circles. Self-knowledge costs money (through, for example, expensive lab tests, functional medicine care) and (self-)knowledge (knowledge learned on one's own path toward healing that is later shared with others) becomes social capital.

8. See chapter 5 for a description of the exposome and health disparities.

9. CHAMACOS is an acronym for the Center for the Health Assessment of Mothers

and Children of Salinas. It is also a play on words since "chamacos" is a colloquial term meaning "little children" in Mexico. The study analyzes children's development and environmental exposures in the Latino farmworker community of Salinas and includes twenty years of data and nearly three hundred thousand biological samples.

10. See chapter 5.

11. See my comments in chapter 5 about green spaces.

12. While SNAP does cover fruits and vegetables, it also covers cheaper foods like candy, potato chips, and sugary drinks.

13. I encountered Hari's story in Dr. Hyman's *Food Fix* (2020). I also heard Vani Hari describe her activism as an expert at the You Can Heal Your Life 2020 Summit.

14. See chapter 5.

15. This hope is the driving force behind my exploration of access to functional medicine in *Accessing Recovery*.

16. Both James Maskell and Chris Kresser include this quote in their respective books to emphasize how the actions of individuals can bring about meaningful change. See Maskell's *The Community Cure* and Kresser's *Unconventional Medicine*.

**POSTLUDE**

1. See Kellman (2018) on the paradigm shift from "disease as invader" to "health as process."

# WORKS CITED

Aberg, Karolina A., Andrey A. Shabalin, Robin F. Chan, Min Zhao, Gaurav Kumar, Gerard van Grootheest, Shaunna L. Clark, Lin Y. Xie, Yuri Milaneschi, Brenda W. J. H. Penninx, and Edwin J. C. G. van den Oord. 2018. "Convergence of Evidence from Methylome-Wide CpG-SNP Association Study and GWAS of Major Depressive Disorder." *Translational Psychiatry* 8, no. 162, 1–10.

Ablon, Joan. 1981. "Stigmatized Health Conditions." *Social Science & Medicine. Part B: Medical Anthropology* 15, no. 1, 5–9.

Agyeman, Julian. 2005. *Sustainable Communities and the Challenge of Environmental Justice.* New York: NYU Press.

Alkon, Alison Hope. 2012. *Black, White, and Green: Farmer's Markets, Race, and the Green Economy.* Athens: University of Georgia Press.

Alkon, Alison Hope, and Julie Guthman. 2107. *The New Food Activism: Opposition, Cooperation, and Collective Action.* Berkeley: University of California Press.

Alkon, Alison Hope, and Christie Grace McCullen. 2010. "Whiteness and Farmers Markets: Performances, Perpetuations . . . Contestations?" *Antipode* 43, no. 4, 937–959.

Allen, Patricia. 2004. *Together at the Table: Sustainability and Sustenance in the American Agrifood System.* University Park: Penn State University Press.

Althusser, Louis. 1970. "Ideology and Ideological State Apparatuses (Notes Towards an Investigation)." In *Literary Theory: An Anthology,* 2nd ed., edited by Julie Rivkin and Michael Ryan. Malden, MA: Blackwell Publishing.

Amato, K. R. 2017. "An Introduction to Microbiome Analysis for Human Biology Applications." *American Journal of Human Biology* 29, no. 1, e22931, doi: 10.1002/ajhb.22931.

Amato, K. R., M. C. Arrieta, M. B. Azad, M. T. Bailey, J. L. Broussard, C. E. Bruggeling, E. C. Claud, E. K. Costello, E. R. Davenport, B. E. Dutilh, H. A. Swain Ewald, P. Ewald, E. C. Hanlon, W. Julion, A. Keshavarzian, C. F. Maurice, G. E. Miller, G. A. Preidis, L. Segurel, B. Singer, S. Subramanian, L. Zhao, and C. W. Kuzawa. 2021. "The Human Gut Microbiome and Health Inequities." *Proceedings of the National Academies of Science* 118, no. 25.

American Autoimmune Related Diseases Association and National Coalition of Autoimmune Patient Groups. 2011. "The Cost Burden of Autoimmune Disease: The Latest Front in the War on Healthcare Spending." http://www.diabetesed.net /page/_files/autoimmune-diseases.pdf.

*Are You What Your Mother Ate? The Agouti Mouse Study.* 2017. Films Media Group. https://www.youtube.com/watch?v=Ybulqzn6R40.

Arzani, Mahsa, Soodeh Razeghi Johromi, Zeinab Ghorbani, Fahimeh Vahabizad, Paolo Martelletti, Amir Ghaemi, Simona Sacco, and Mansoureh Togha. 2020. "Gut-Brain Axis and Migraine Headache: A Comprehensive Review." *Journal of Headache and Pain* 21, no. 15.

Atewologun, Doyin, and Ruth Sealy. 2014. "Experiencing Privilege at Ethnic, Gender, and Senior Intersections." *Journal of Managerial Psychology* 29, no. 4, 423–439.

Autoimmune Association. n.d. "Autoimmune Disease List." https://autoimmune.org /disease-information/.

Baer, Hans. 1996. "Toward a Political Ecology of Health in Medical Anthropology." *Medical Anthropology Quarterly* 10, no. 4, 451–454.

Baines, Joseph. 2015. "Fuel, Feed, and the Corporate Restructuring of the Food Regime." *Journal of Peasant Studies* 42, no. 2, 295–321.

Banaji, Mahzarin, and Anthony Greenwald. 2013. *Blind Spot: Hidden Biases of Good People*. London: Bantam Press.

Bateson, Gregory. (1972) 2000. *Steps to an Ecology of Mind: Collected Essays in Anthropology, Psychiatry, Evolution, and Epistemology*. Chicago: University of Chicago Press.

Bayer, Ronald, and Sandro Galea. 2018. "Public Health in the Precision-Medicine Era." In *Beyond Bioethics: Toward a New Biopolitics*, edited by Osagie K. Obasogie and Marcy Darnovsky. Berkeley: University of California Press.

Beaulac, Julie, Elizabeth Kristjansson, and Steven Cummins. 2009. "A Systematic Review of Food Deserts, 1966–2007." *Preventing Chronic Disease: Public Health Research, Practice, and Policy* 6, no. 3, A105.

Beidelschies, Michelle, Marilyn Alejandro-Rodriguez, Xinge Ji, Brittany Lapin, Patrick Hanaway, and Michael Rothberg. 2019. "Association of the Functional Medicine Model of Care with Patient-Reported Health-Related Quality-of-Life Outcomes." *Journal of the American Medical Association* 2, no. 10, e1914017.

Bell, Susan E., and Anne E. Figert. 2012. "Medicalization and Pharmaceuticalization at the Intersections: Looking Backward, Sideways, and Forward." *Social Science and Medicine* 75, no. 5, 775–783.

Benbrook, Charles M. 2016. "Trends in Glyphosate Herbicide Use in the United States and Globally." *Environmental Sciences Europe* 28, no. 1, 3.

Benezra, Amber. 2017. "Writing the Microbiome." *Medical Anthropology Quarterly Book Forum Blog Series*. https://medanthroquarterly.org/forums/forumreview /writing-the-microbiome/.

———. 2020. "Race in the Microbiome." *Science, Technology, and Human Values* 45, no. 5, 877–902.

Bestard, Joan. 2004. "Kinship and the New Genetics: The Changing Meaning of Bio-genetic Substance." *Social Anthropology* 12, no. 3, 253–263.

Boas, Franz. 1982. *Race, Language, and Culture*. Chicago: University of Chicago Press.

Boersma, Peter, Lindsey I. Black, and Brian W. Ward. 2020. "Prevalence of Multiple Chronic Conditions Among US Adults, 2018." *Preventing Chronic Disease* 20, 200130.

Bondi, Liz, and Nina Laurie. 2005. *Working the Spaces of Neoliberalism: Activism, Professionalisation, and Incorporation*. Hoboken, NJ: Wiley.

Boon, Sarah. 2017. "21st Century Science Overload." *Canadian Science Publishing*. http://blog.cdnsciencepub.com/21st-century-science-overload/.

Borghol, Nada, Matthew Suderman, Wendy McArdle, Ariane Racine, Michael

Hallett, Marcus Pembrey, Clyde Hertzman, Chris Power, and Moshe Szyf. 2012. "Associations with Early-Life Socio-Economic Position in Adult DNA Methylation." *International Journal of Epidemiology* 41, no. 1, 62–74.

Bourdieu, Pierre. 1984. *Distinction: A Social Critique of the Judgement of Taste*. Cambridge, MA: Harvard University Press.

Briggs, Charles, and Clara Mantini-Briggs. 2003. *Stories in the Time of Cholera: Racial Profiling during a Medical Nightmare*. Berkeley: University of California Press.

Brodeur, Paul. 1985. *Outrageous Misconduct: The Asbestos Industry on Trial*. New York: Pantheon Books.

Brons, Lajos. 2015. "Othering, An Analysis." *Transcience, A Journal of Global Studies* 6, no. 1, 69–90.

Brown, Sandy, and Christy Getz. 2011. "Farmworker Food Insecurity and the Production of Hunger in California." In *Cultivating Food Justice: Race, Class, and Sustainability*, edited by Alison Hope Alkon and Julian Agyeman. Cambridge, MA: MIT Press.

Brown, Hannah, and Alex M. Nading. 2019. "Introduction: Human Animal Health in Medical Anthropology." *Medical Anthropology Quarterly* 33, no. 1, 5–23.

Brown, Phil, and Edwin J. Mikkelsen. 1997. *No Safe Place: Toxic Waste, Leukemia, and Community Action*. Berkeley: University of California Press.

Browner, Carol H. 1999. "On the Medicalization of Medical Anthropology." *Medical Anthropology Quarterly* 13, no. 2, 135–140.

Bygren, Lars Olov, Petter Tinghög, John Carstensen, Sören Edvinsson, Gunnar Kaati, Marcus E. Pembrey, and Michael Sjöström. 2014. "Change in Paternal Grandmothers' Early Food Supply Influenced Cardiovascular Mortality of the Female Grandchildren." *BMC Genetics* 20, no. 15, 12.

Calman, Kenneth. 2008. "Beyond the 'Nanny State': Stewardship and Public Health." *Public Health* 123, no. 1, e6–e10.

Cancer Genome Atlas Research Network. 2017. "Integrated Genomic and Molecular Characterization of Cervical Cancer." *Nature* 543, 378–400.

Cao-Lei, L., K. N. Dancause, G. Elgbeili, R. Massart, M. Szyf, A. Liu, D. P. Laplante, S. King. 2015. "DNA Methylation Mediates the Impact of Exposure to Prenatal Maternal Stress on BMI and Central Adiposity in Children at Age 13\F1/2 Years: Project Ice Storm." *Epigenetics* 10, no. 8, 749–761.

Carey, Nessa. 2012. *The Epigenetics Revolution: How Modern Biology Is Rewriting Our Understanding of Genetics, Disease, and Inheritance*. New York: Columbia University Press.

Carson, Rachel. 1962. *Silent Spring*. Boston: Houghton Mifflin.

Case, K. 1986. "Nomenclature: Human Immunodeficiency Virus." *Annals of Internal Medicine* 105, no. 1, 133. https://www.avert.org/printpdf/node/351.

Ceballos, Gerardo, Paul R. Ehrlich, Anthony D. Barnosky, Andrés García, Robert M. Pringle, and Todd M. Palmer. 2015. "Accelerated Modern Human-Induced Species Losses: Entering the Sixth Mass Extinction." *Science Advances* 1, no. 5.

Centers for Disease Control and Prevention. n.d. "About Epstein-Barr Virus (EBV)." https://www.cdc.gov/epstein-barr/about-ebv.html.

Centers for Disease Control and Prevention. 2021. "Weekly Updates by Select Demographic and Geographic Characteristics: Provisional Death Counts for Coronavirus Disease 2019 (COVID-19)." https://www.cdc.gov/nchs/nvss/vsrr/covid_weekly

/index.htm?fbclid=IwAR3-wrg3tTKK5-9tOHPGAHWFVO3DfslkJ0KsDEPQpW mPbKtp6EsoVV2Qs1Q.

Cleveland Clinic. n.d. "HPV." https://my.clevelandclinic.org/health/diseases/11901 -hpv-human-papilloma-virus.

———. n.d. "Normal Menstruation." https://my.clevelandclinic.org/health/articles /10132-normal-menstruation.

Cohen, Patricia. 2020. "Roundup Maker to Pay \$20 Billion to Settle Cancer Suits." *New York Times*. https://www.nytimes.com/2020/06/24/business/roundup -settlement-lawsuits.html?searchResultPosition=3.

Cole, Steve. 2009. "Social Regulation of Human Gene Expression." *Current Directions in Psychological Science* 18, no. 3, 132–137.

Conching, A., and Z. Thayer. 2019. "Biological Pathways for Historical Trauma to Affect Health: A Conceptual Model Focusing on Epigenetic Modifications." *Social Science & Medicine* 230, 74–82. doi:https://doi.org/10.1016/j.socscimed.2019.04 .001.

Crenshaw, Kimberlé. 2014. "The Structural and Political Dimensions of Intersectional Oppression." In *Intersectionality: A Foundations and Frontiers Reader*, edited by Patrick R. Granzka. Boulder, CO: Westview Press.

Danner, Bridgit. 2018. "How Birth Control Affects Your Gut." https://www .bridgitdanner.com/womens-wellness-blog/how-birth-control-affects-your-gut.

D'Brant, Jeanne. n.d. "The Shikimate Pathway, the Microbiome, and Disease: Health Effects of GMOs on Humans." Powerpoint presentation. https://d3n8a8pro7vhmx .cloudfront.net/yesmaam/pages/680/attachments/original/1466869052/GMO _Shikimate_pathway_gut_flora_and_health.pdf?1466869052.

Dean, Mitchell. 1999. *Governmentality: Power and Rule in Modern Society*. London: Sage.

DelVecchio Good, Mary-Jo. 2010. "The Medical Imaginary and the Biotechnical Embrace: Subjective Experiences of Clinical Scientists and Patients." In *A Reader in Medical Anthropology: Theoretical Trajectories, Emergent Realities*, edited by Byron J. Good, Michael M. J. Fischer, Sarah S. Willen, and Mary-Jo DelVecchio Good. Malden, MA: Wiley-Blackwell.

Demura, Masashi, and Kiyofumi Saijoh. 2017. "The Role of DNA Methylation in Hypertension." *Advances in Experimental Medicine and Biology* 956, 583–598.

Dickenson, Donna. 2014. "In Me We Trust: Public Health, Personalized Medicine, and the Common Good." *Hedgehog Review* 16, no. 1, 64–83.

Dimitri, Carolyn, and Lydia Oberholtzer. 2009. "Marketing U.S. Organic Foods: Recent Trends From Farms to Consumers." *Economic Information Bulletin*, no. EIB-58.

Dobbs, David. 2018. "What Is Your DNA Worth?" In *Beyond Bioethics: Toward a New Biopolitics*, edited by Osagie K. Obasogie and Marcy Darnovsky. Berkeley: University of California Press.

Dobbs R., C. Sawers, F. Thompson, J. Manyika, J. Woetzel, P. Child, S. McKenna, A. Spatharou. 2014. "Overcoming Obesity: An Initial Economic Analysis," McKinsey Global Institute. https://www.mckinsey.com/~/media/McKinsey/Business %20Functions/Economic%20Studies%20TEMP/Our%20Insights/How%20the %20world%20could%20better%20fight%20obesity/MGI_Overcoming_obesity _Full_report.ashx.

Douglas, Michael P., and Stacy W. Gray. 2020. "Private Payer and Medical Coverage for Circulating Tumor DNA Testing: A Historical Analysis of Coverage Policies from 2015 to 2019." *Journal of the National Comprehensive Cancer Network* 18, no. 7, 866–872.

Dressler, W. 1990. "Culture, Stress and Disease." In *Medical Anthropology: Contemporary Theory and Method*, edited by T. Johnson and C. Sargent. New York: Praeger.

Duke University Medical Center. 2010. "Epstein-Barr: Scientists Decode Secrets of a Very Common Virus That Can Cause Cancer." *Science Daily*. https://www.sciencedaily.com/releases/2010/12/101215121905.htm.

Dunn, Jessilyn, Haiwei Qui, Soyeon Kim, Daudi Jjingo, Ryan Hoffman, Chan Woo Kim, Inhwan Jang, Dong Ju Son, Daniel Kim, Chenyi Pan, Yuhon Fan, I. King Jordan, and Hanjoong Jo. 2014. "Flow-Dependent Epigenetic DNA Methylation Regulates Endothelial Gene Expression and Atteroschlerosis." *Journal of Clinical Intervention* 124, no. 7, 3187–3199.

Edwards, Jeanette, Sarah Franklin, Eric Hirsch, Frances Price, and Marilyn Strathern. (1993) 1999. *Technologies of Procreation: Kinship in the Age of Assisted Conception.* New York: Routledge.

Epstein, Steven. 2007. *Inclusion: The Politics of Difference in Medical Research.* Chicago: University of Chicago Press.

Ettore, Elizabeth. 2005. "Gender, Older Female Bodies, and Autoethnography: Finding My Feminist Voice by Telling My Illness Story." *Women's Studies International Forum* 28, no. 6, 535–546.

Fadiman, Anne. 1997. *The Spirit Catches You and You Fall Down: A Hmong Child, Her American Doctors, and the Collision of Two Cultures.* New York: Farrar, Straus and Giroux.

Fahy, Gregory, Robert Brooke, James Watson, Zinaida Good, Shreyas S. Vasanawala, Holden Maecker, Michael D. Leipold, David T. S. Lin, Michael S. Kobor, Steve Horvath. 2019. "Reversal of Epigenetic Aging and Immunosenecent Trends in Humans." *Aging Cell.* https://onlinelibrary.wiley.com/doi/10.1111/acel.13028.

Faircloth, Charlotte. 2017. "'Natural' Breastfeeding in Comparative Perspective: Feminism: Morality, and Adaptive Accountability." *Ethos* 82, no. 1, 19–43.

Farmer, Paul. 2001. *Infections and Inequalities: The Modern Plagues.* Berkeley: University of California Press.

———. 2006. *Aids and Accusation: Haiti and the Geography of Blame.* Berkeley: University of California Press.

———. 2009. "On Suffering and Structural Violence: A View from Below." *Race/Ethnicity: Multidisciplinary Global Contexts* 3, no. 1, 11–28.

Farmer, Paul, Bruce Nizeye, Sara Stulac, and Salmaan Keshavjee. 2006. "Structural Violence and Clinical Medicine." *PLOS Medicine* 3, no. 10, 1686–1691.e449.

Farquhar, Judith. 1994. "Eating Chinese Medicine." *Cultural Anthropology* 9, no. 4, 471–497.

Fitzpatrick, Zachary, Gordon Frazer, Ashley Ferro, Simon Clare, Nicolas Bouladoux, John Ferdinand, Zewen Kelvin Tuong, Maria Luciana Negro-Demontel, Nitin Kumar, Ondrej Suchanek, Tamara Tajsic, Katherine Harcourt, Kirsten Scott, Rachel Bashford-Rogers, Adel Helmy, Daniel S. Reich, Yasmine Belkaid, Trevor D.

Lawley, Dorian B. McGavern, and Menna R. Clatworthy. 2020. "Gut-Educated IgA Plasma Cells Defend the Meningeal Venous Sinuses." *Nature* 587, 472–476.

Food and Agriculture Organization of the United Nations. n.d. "What Is Happening to Agrobiodiversity?" https://www.fao.org/3/y5609e/y5609e02.htm.

Foster, George. 1976. "Disease Etiologies in Non-Western Medical Systems." *American Anthropologist* 78, no. 4, 772–782.

Foucault, Michel. 1998. *The History of Sexuality,* Volume 1: *The Will to Knowledge.* London: Penguin.

———. 2003. In *Society Must Be Defended: Lectures at the College de France.* Lecture 11, March 17, 1976. New York: Picador Press.

Franklin, Sarah. 2013. "From Blood to Genes? Rethinking Consanguinity in the Context of Geneticization." In *Blood and Kinship: Matter for Metaphor from Ancient Rome to the Present,* edited by Christopher H. Johnson, Bernhard Jussen, David Warren Sabean, and Simon Teuscher. New York: Berghahn.

Freeman, A. 2007. "Fast Food: Oppression through Poor Nutrition." *California Legal Review* 95, 2221.

Fuentes, Agustín. 2012. *Race, Monogamy, and Other Lies They Told You: Busting Myths about Human Nature.* Berkeley: University of California Press.

———. 2019. "Holobionts, Multispecies Ecologies, and the Biopolitics of Care: Emerging Landscapes of Praxis in a Medical Anthropology of the Anthropocene." *Medical Anthropology Quarterly* 33, no. 1, 156–162.

Funke, Todd, Huijong Han, Martha L. Healy-Fried, Markus Fischer, and Ernst Schönbrunn. 2006. "Molecular Basis for the Herbicide Resistance of Roundup Ready Crops." *Proceedings of the National Academy of Sciences* 103, no. 35, 13010–13015.

Gálvez, Alyshia. 2018. *Eating NAFTA: Trade, Food Policies, and the Destruction of Mexico.* Berkeley: University of California Press.

Gao, Shijuan, Jiandong Li, Liping Song, Jiaoxiang Wu, and Wenlin Huang. 2017. "Influenza A Virus-induced downregulation of miR-26a contributes to reduced IFNα/β production." *Virologica Sinica* 32, no. 4, 261–270.

Gawande, Atul. 2009. "The Cost Conundrum." *New Yorker, Annals of Medicine.* June 1, 2009.

Geertz, Clifford. 1973. *The Interpretation of Cultures.* New York: Basic Books.

Gil, Sharon, Nikki Jamie Cruz, Dae-Wook Kang, Daniel H. Geschwind, Rosa Krajmalnik-Brown, and Sarkis Mazmanian. 2019. "Human Gut Microbiota from Autism Spectrum Disorder Promote Behavioral Symptoms in Mice." *Cell* 177, no. 6, P1600–1618.e17.

Gillman, M. 2005. "Developmental Origins of Health and Disease." *New England Journal of Medicine* 353, no. 17, 1848–1850.

Gluckman, Peter, and Mark Hanson. 2008. *Mismatch: The Lifestyle Diseases Timebomb.* Oxford, UK: Oxford University Press.

Goldstein, Donna. 2003. *Laughter Out of Place: Race, Class, Violence, and Sexuality in a Rio Shantytown.* Berkeley: University of California Press.

Good, Byron J., and Mary-Jo DelVecchio Good. 1981. "The Semantics of Medical Discourse." In *Sciences and Cultures: Anthropological and Historical Studies of the*

*Sciences*. Edited by Everett Mendelsohn and Yehuda Elkana. Dordrecht, Netherlands: D. Reidel Publishing Company.

Good, Mary-Jo DelVecchio, Byron J. Good, Cynthia Schaffer, and Stuart E. Lind. 1990. "American oncology and the discourse on hope." *Culture, Medicine, and Psychiatry* 14, 59–79.

*Good Morning America*. 2020. "Coronavirus Victims Who Now Suffer Long-Term Symptoms." https://www.youtube.com/watch?v=iu_Gs7N4lGk.

Gostin, Lawrence. 2014. *Global Health Law*. Cambridge, MA: Harvard University Press.

Gray, Margaret. 2014. *Labor and Locavore: The Making of a Comprehensive Food Ethic*. Berkeley: University of California Press.

Green, Lesley. 2019. "A Comment on the Anthropocene Manifesto." *Environmental Humanities* 11, no. 2, 493–497.

Guthman, Julie. 2008a. "Bringing Good Food to Others: Investigating the Subjects of Alternative Food Practice." *Cultural Geographies* 15, 431–447.

———. 2008b. "'If They Only Knew': Color Blindness and Universalism in California Alternative Food Institutions." *Professional Geographer* 60, 387–397.

———. 2008c. "Neoliberalism and the Making of Food Politics in California." *Geoforum* 39, 1171–1183.

———. 2011 *Weighing In: Obesity, Food Justice, and the Limits of Capitalism*. Berkeley: University of California Press.

Guthman, Julie, Amy W. Morris, and Patricia Allen. 2006. "Squaring Farm Security and Food Security in Two Types of Alternative Food Institutions." *Rural Sociology* 7, no. 4, 662–684.

Haraway, Donna. 1988. "Situated Knowledges: The Science Question in Feminism and the Privilege of Partial Perspective." *Feminist Studies* 14, no. 3, 575–599.

Harman, Vicki, and Benedetta Cappellini. 2015. "Mothers on Display: Lunchboxes, Social Class, and Moral Accountability." *Sociology* 49, no. 4, 764–781.

Harrington, Kevin, Daniel J. Freeman, Beth Kelly, James Harper, and Jean-Charles Soria. 2019. "Optimizing Oncolytic Virotherapy in Cancer Treatment." *Nature Reviews Drug Discovery* 18, 689–706.

Harvard Health. 2021. "Soothing Solutions for Irritable Bowel Syndrome." Harvard Health Publishing. https://www.health.harvard.edu/diseases-and-conditions/soothing-solutions-for-irritable-bowel-syndrome.

Hasty, Daniel J., Ashley Hesson, Suzanne Evans Wagner, and Robert Lannon. 2012. "Finding Needles in the Right Haystack: Double Modals in Medical Consultations." *University of Pennsylvania Working Papers in Linguistics* 18, no. 2, article 6.

Helmreich, Stefan. 2009. *Alien Ocean: Anthropological Voyages in Microbial Seas*. Berkeley: University of California Press.

Hislop, Rasheed Salaam. 2014. "Reaping Equity: A Survey of Food Justice Organizations in the U.S.A." Master's thesis, University of California, Davis.

Hobsbawm, Eric J., and Terence O. Ranger. 1992. *The Invention of Tradition*. Cambridge, UK: Cambridge University Press.

Holmes, Seth. 2013. *Fresh Fruit, Broken Bodies: Migrant Farmworkers in the United States*. Berkeley: University of California Press.

Hopper, Susan. 1981. "Diabetes as a Stigmatized Condition: The Case of Low-Income

Clinic Patients in the United States." *Social Science & Medicine. Part B: Medical Anthropology* 15, no. 1, 11–19.

Hore, Timothy. 2017. "Modulating Epigenetic Memory through Vitamins and TET: Implications for Regenerative Medicine and Cancer Treatment." *Epigenomics* 9, no. 6, 863–871.

Horsley, Scott. 2019. "Why America's 1-Percenters Are Richer than Europe's." National Public Radio. https://www.npr.org/2019/12/05/783001561/why-americas -1-percenters-are-richer-than-europe-s.

Horvath, Steven. 2013. "DNA Methylation Age of Human Tissues and Cell Types." *Genome Biology* 14, no. 10, R115.

Hunger, MaryCarol R., Brenda W. Gillespie, and Sophie Yu-Pu Chen. 2019. "Urban Nature Experiences Reduce Stress in the Context of Daily Life Based on Salivary Biomarkers." *Frontiers in Psychology* 10, 722. https://www.frontiersin.org/articles /10.3389/fpsyg.2019.00722/full.

Hunter, David J., and K. Srinath Reddy. 2013. "Noncommunicable Diseases." *New England Journal of Medicine* 369, 1336–1343.

Hyland, Carly, Patrick Bradshaw, Julianna Deardorff, Robert Gunier, Ana-María Mora, Katherine Kogut, Sharon Sagiv, Asa Bradman, Brenda Eskenazi. 2021. "Interactions of Agricultural Pesticide Use Near Home during Pregnancy and Adverse Childhood Experiences on Adolescent Neurobehavioral Development in the CHAMACOS Study." *Environmental Research* 204, no. 3, 111908.

Hyman, Mark. 2020. *Food Fix: How to Save Our Health, Our Economy, Our Communities, and Our Planet—One Bite at a Time*. New York: Little, Brown Spark.

Ingelfinger, Franz J. 1980. "Arrogance." *New England Journal of Medicine* 303, 1507–1511.

Inhorn, Marcia. 1993. "Medical Anthropology and Epidemiology: Divergences or Convergences?" *Social Science & Medicine* 40, no. 3, 285–290.

Jablonka, Eva, and Marion Lamb. 2014. *Evolution in Four Dimensions: Genetic, Epigenetic, Behavioral, and Symbolic Variation in the History of Life*. Cambridge, MA: MIT Press.

Janowitz Koch, I., M. M. Clark, M. J. Thompson, K. A. Deere-Machemer, J. Wang, L. Duarte, G. E. Gnanadesikan, E. L. McCoy, L. Rubbi, D. R. Stahler, M. Pellegrini, E. A. Ostrander, R. K. Wayne, J. S. Sinsheimer, B. M. von Holdt. 2016. "The Concerted Impact of Domestication and Transposon Insertions in Methylation Patterns between Dogs and Grey Wolves." *Molecular Ecology* 25, no. 8, 1838–1855.

Johns Hopkins Medicine. n.d. "Oral Herpes." https://www.hopkinsmedicine.org /health/conditions-and-diseases/herpes-hsv1-and-hsv2/oral-herpes.

Johnston, Josée, and Shyon Baumann. 2014. *Foodies: Democracy and Distinction in the Gourmet Foodscape*. Milton Park, UK: Routledge.

Jordan, Brigitte. 1992. *Birth in Four Cultures*. Long Grove, IL: Waveland Press.

Kaati, Gunnar, Lars Olov Bygren, and Sören Edvinsson. 2002. "Cardiovascular and Diabetes Mortality Determined by Nutrition during Parents' and Grandparents' Slow Growth Period." *European Journal of Human Genetics* 10, 682-688.

Kampourakis, Kostas, and Kevin McCain. 2019. *Uncertainty: How It Makes Science Advance*. New York: Oxford University Press.

Kandil, Caitlin Yoshiko. 2020. "Asian Americans Report Over 650 Racist Attacks

Over Last Week, New Data Says." *NBC News*. https://www.nbcnews.com/news/asian-america/asian-americans-report-nearly-500-racist-acts-over-last-week-n1169821.

Kapoor, Ilan. 2004. "Hyper-Self-Reflexive Development? Spivak on Representing the Third World 'Other.'" *Third World Quarterly* 4, 627–647.

Karachaliou, Niki, Clara Mayo de las Casas, Miguel Angel Molina-Vila, and Rafael Rosell. 2015. "Real-Time Liquid Biopsies Become a Reality in Cancer Treatment." *Annals of Translational Medicine* 3, no. 3, 36.

Kaufman, Joan, Bao-Zhu Yang, Heather Douglas-Palumberi, Shadi Houshyar, Deborah Lipschitz, John H. Krystal, and Joel Gelernter. 2004. "Social Supports and Serotonin Transporter Gene Moderate Depression in Maltreated Children." *Proceedings of the National Academies of Sciences* 101, no. 49, 17317–17321.

Kay, Lily E. 1993. *The Molecular Vision of Life: Caltech, the Rockefeller Foundation, and the New Biology*. Oxford: Oxford University Press.

Kellman, Rafael. 2018. *Microbiome Breakthrough: Harness the Power of Your Gut Bacteria to Boost Your Mood and Heal Your Body*. Boston: Da Capo Lifelong Books.

Kirmayer, Laurence J., and Ana Gómez-Carrillo. 2019. "Agency, Embodiment and Enactment in Psychosomatic Theory and Practice." *Medical Humanities* 45, no. 2, 169–182.

Kleinman, Arthur. 1978. "Concepts and a Model for Comparison of Medical Systems as Cultural Systems." *Social Science & Medicine. Part B: Medical Anthropology* 12, 85–93.

———. 1982. "Neurasthenia and Depression: A Study of Somatization and Culture in China." *Culture, Medicine and Psychiatry* 6, 117–190.

———. 1988. *The Illness Narratives: Suffering, Healing, and the Human Condition*. New York: Basic Books.

———. 2004. "Culture and Depression." *New England Journal of Medicine* 351, 951–953.

Kleinman, Arthur, and Anne Becker. 1998. "'Sociocomatics': The Contributions of Anthropology to Psychosomatic Medicine." *Psychosomatic Medicine: Journal of Biobehavioral Medicine* 60, no. 4, 389–393.

Kresser, Chris. 2017. *Unconventional Medicine: Join the Revolution to Reinvent Healthcare, Reverse Chronic Disease, and Create a Practice You Love*. Austin, TX: Lioncrest Publishing.

Kuhn, Thomas. 1962. *The Structure of Scientific Revolutions*. Chicago: University of Chicago Press.

Kulinski, Joseph M., Dean D. Metcalfe, Michael L. Young, Yun Bai, Yuzhi Yin, Robin Eisch, Linda M. Scott, and Hirsh D. Komarow. 2019. "Elevation in Histamine and Tryptase Following Exercise in Patients with Mastocytosis." *Journal of Allergy and Clinical Immunology* 7, no. 4, 1310–1313.

Kuwaza, Christopher W., and Elizabeth Sweet. 2009. "Epigenetics and the Embodiment of Race: Developmental Origins of US Racial Disparities in Cardiovascular Health." *American Journal of Human Biology* 21, 2–15.

Lakoff, Andrew. 2012. "The Generic Biothreat, Or, How We Became Unprepared." *Cultural Anthropology* 23, no. 3, 399–428.

Lanphear, Bruce P., Thomas D. Matte, John Rogers, Robert P. Clickner, Brian Dietz, Robert L. Bornschein, Paul Succop, Kathryn R. Mahaffey, Sherry Dixon, Warren

Galke, Michael Rabinowitz, Mark Farfel, Charles Rohde, Joel Schwartz, Peter Ashley, David E. Jacobs. 1998. "Dust and Residential Soil to Children's Blood Lead Levels: A Pooled Analysis of 12 Epidemiologic Studies." *Environmental Research* 79, no. 1, 51–68.

Larner, Wendy, and David Craig. 2005. "After Neoliberalism? Community Activism and Local Partnerships in Aotearoa New Zealand." *Antipode* 37, no. 3, 402–424.

Latour, Bruno. 1987. *Science in Action: How to Follow Scientists and Engineers Through Society*. Cambridge, MA: Harvard University Press.

———. 1999. *Pandora's Hope: Essays on the Reality of Science Studies*. Cambridge, MA: Harvard University Press.

Lavin, Chad. 2009. "Pollanated Politics, or, the Neoliberal's Dilemma." *Politics and Culture* 2, 57–67.

Leach, Melissa, and Ian Scoones. 2013. "The Social and Political Lives of Zoonotic Disease Models: Narratives, Science and Policy." *Social Science and Medicine* 88, 10–17.

Lebrun, Lydie A. 2012. "Effects of Length of Stay and Language Proficiency on Health Care Experiences among Immigrants in Canada and the United States." *Social Science & Medicine* 74, no. 7, 1062–1072.

Lee, Sandra Soo-Jin. 2013. "American DNA: The Politics of Potentiality in a Genomic Age." *Current Anthropology* 54, (S7), 77–86.

Lee, Yujin, Dariush Mozaffarian, Stephen Sy, Yue Huang, Junxiu Liu, Park E. Wilde, Shafika Abrahams-Gessel, Thiago de Souza Veiga Jardim, Thomas A. Gaziano, and Renata Micha. 2019. "Cost-Effectiveness of Financial Incentives for Improving Diet and Health through Medicare and Medicaid: A Microsimulation Study." *PLoS Med* 16, no. 3, e1002761.

Lenton, Timothy M., and Bruno Latour. 2018. "Gaia 2.0." *Science* 361, no. 6407, 1066–1068.

Lester, Rebecca. 2019. *Famished: Eating Disorders and Failed Care in America*. Berkeley: University of California Press.

Lévi-Strauss, Claude. (1958) 1963. *Structural Anthropology*, translated by Claire Jacobson and Brooke Grundfest Schoepf. New York: Basic Book Publishers.

Li, William. 2019. *Eat to Beat Disease*. New York: Balance.

Lichtenstein, P., N. V. Holm, P. K. Verkasalo, A. Iliadou, J. Kaprio, M. Koskenvuo, E. Pukkala, A. Skytthe, and K. Hemminki. 2000. "Environmental and Heritable Factors in the Causation of Cancer—Analyses of Cohorts of Twins from Sweden, Denmark, and Finland." *New England Journal of Medicine* 343, no. 2, 78–85.

Lock, Margaret. 1984. *East Asian Medicine in Urban Japan: Varieties of Medical Experience*. Berkeley: University of California Press.

———. 1990. "Rationalization of Japanese Herbal Medication: The Hegemony of Orchestrated Pluralism." *Human Organization: Journal of the Society for Applied Anthropology* 49, no. 1, 41–47.

———. 1993. *Encounters with Aging: Mythologies of Menopause in Japan and North America*. Berkeley: University of California Press.

———. 2001. "The Tempering of Medical Anthropology: Troubling Natural Categories." *Medical Anthropology Quarterly* 15, no. 4, 378–492.

———. 2005. "Eclipse of the Gene and the Return of Divination." *Current Anthropology* 46 (S5), 47–70.

———. 2012. "From Genetics to Postgenomics and the Discovery of the New Social Body." In *Medical Anthropology at the Intersections: Histories, Activisms, and Futures*, edited by Marcia C. Inhorn and Emily A. Wentzell. Durham, NC: Duke University Press.

———. 2013. "The Epigenome and Nature/Nurture Reunification: A Challenge for Anthropology." *Medical Anthropology* 32, no. 4, 291–308.

———. 2015. "Comprehending the Body in the Era of the Epigenome." *Current Anthropology* 56, no. 2, 151–177.

———. 2017. "Recovering the Body." *Annual Review of Anthropology* 46, 1–14.

Lock, Margaret, and Patricia Kaufert. 2001. "Menopause, Local Biologies, and Cultures of Aging." *American Journal of Human Biology* 13, 494–504.

Lonardi, Cristina. 2007. "The Passing Dilemma in Socially Invisible Diseases: Narratives on Chronic Headache." *Social Science and Medicine* 65, no. 8, 1619–1629.

Lorimer, Jamie. 2017. "Why Liberals Love the Microbiome." *Medical Anthropology Quarterly Book Forum Blog Series*. https://medanthroquarterly.org/?p=411.

———. 2019. "Hookworms Make Us Human: The Microbiome, Eco-immunology, and a Probiotic Turn in Western Health Care." *Medical Anthropology Quarterly* 33, no. 1, 60–79.

Low, Ashley P., and George Hacker. 2013. "Selfish Giving: How the Soda Industry Uses Philanthropy to Sweeten Its Profits." https://www.cspinet.org/sites/default /files/attachment/cspi_soda_philanthropy_online.pdf.

Luhrmann, T. M. and Jocelyn Marrow. 2016. *Our Most Troubling Madness: Case Studies in Schizophrenia Across Cultures*. Berkeley: University of California Press.

Lynch, Ben. 2020. *Dirty Genes: A Breakthrough Program to Treat the Root Cause of Illness and Optimize Your Health*. New York: HarperOne.

Lyrenäs, Ebbe. 1985. "Beta-Adrenergic Influence on Esophageal and Colonic Motility in Man." *Scandinavian Journal of Gastroenterology* 20, no. 20, supplement 116.

Mann, Michael. 2013. "Globalizations." In *The Sources of Social Power, vol. 4: Globalizations, 1945–2011*. Cambridge, UK: Cambridge University Press.

Marcus, George E. 1995. "Ethnography in/of the World System: The Emergence of Multi-Sited Ethnography." *Annual Review of Anthropology* 24, no. 1, 95–117.

Markowitz, Gerald, and David Rosner. 2002. *Deceit and Denial: The Deadly Politics of Industrial Pollution*. Berkeley: University of California Press.

Marks, Jonathan. 2013. "The Nature/Culture of Genetic Facts." *Annual Review of Anthropology* 42, 247–267.

Marmot, Michael. 2005. *The Status Syndrome: How Your Social Standing Directly Affects Your Health*. London: Bloomsbury Publishing.

———. 2015. *The Health Gap: The Challenge of an Unequal World*. London: Bloomsbury Publishing.

Martin, Emily. 1994. *Flexible Bodies: Tracking Immunity in American Culture from the Days of Polio to the Age of AIDS*. Boston: Beacon Press.

Martin, Kay. 2018. *Social DNA: Rethinking Our Evolutionary Past*. New York: Berghahn.

Martin, Philip L., and J. Edward Taylor. 1998. "Poverty amid Prosperity: Farm Employment, Immigration, and Poverty in California. *American Journal of Agricultural Economics* 80, no. 5, 1108–1014.

Martinez, Rebecca. 2018. *Marked Women: The Cultural Politics of Cervical Cancer in Venezuela*. Palo Alto, CA: Stanford University Press.

Maskell, James. 2020. *The Community Cure: Transforming Health Outcomes Together*. Austin, TX: Lioncrest Publishing.

Massart, R., M. Freyburger, M. Suderman, J. Paquet, J. El Helou, E. Belanger-Nelson, A. Rachalski, O. C. Koumar, J. Carrier, M. Szuf, and V. Mongrain. 2014. "The Genome-Wide Landscape of DNA Methylation and Hydroxymethylation in Response to Sleep Deprivation Impacts on Synaptic Plasticity Genes." *Translational Psychiatry* 4, e347.

Matthiessen, Christian. 2013. "Applying Systemic Functional Linguistics in Healthcare Contexts." *Text & Talk: An Interdisciplinary Journal of Language, Discourse & Communication Studies* 33, no. 4–5, 437–466.

Mattingly, Cheryl. 2012. "Two Virtue Ethics and Anthropology of Morality." *Anthropological Theory* 12, no. 2, 161–184.

Mattison, Siobhán M., Brooke Scelza, and Tami Blumenfield. 2014. "Paternal Investment and the Positive Effects of Fathers among the Matrilineal Mosuo of Southwest China." *American Anthropologist* 116, no. 3, 591–610.

Maupin, Jonathan N., and Alexandra Brewis. 2014. "Food Insecurity and Body Norms among Rural Guatemalan Schoolchildren." *American Anthropologist* 116, no. 2, 332–337.

Mauss, Marcel. (1934) 2010. "Techniques du Corps." In *Transatlantic Voyages and Sociology*, edited by Cherry Shrecker. Farnham, UK: Ashgate.

Mayer, Emeran. 2016. *The Mind-Gut Connection: How the Hidden Conversation Within Our Bodies Impacts Our Mood, Our Choices, and Our Overall Health*. New York: Harper Wave.

Mays, V., S. Cochran, and N. Barnes. 2007. "Race, Race-Based Discrimination, and Health Outcomes among African Americans." *Annual Review of Psychology* 58, 201–225.

McClintock, Nathan. 2011. "From Industrial Garden to Food Desert: Unearthing the Root Structure of Urban Agriculture in Oakland, California." In *Cultivating Food Justice: Race, Class, and Sustainability*, edited by Alison Hope Alkon and Julian Agyeman. Cambridge, MA: MIT Press.

McElroy, Ann. 2015. *Medical Anthropology in Ecological Perspective*. New York: Routledge.

Meloni, Maurizio. 2014. "Remaking Local Biologies in an Epigenetic Time." *Somatosphere*. http://somatosphere.net/2014/remaking-local-biologies-in-an-epigenetic-time.html/.

Menéndez, Eduardo. 1994. "La enfermedad y la curación. ¿Qué es medicina tradicional?" *Alteridades* 4, no. 7, 72–74.

———. 1996. *De algunos alcoholismos y algunos saberes: Atención primaria y proceso de alcoholización*. México, D.F.: CIESAS.

———. 2003. "Modelos de atención de los padecimientos: De exclusiones teóricas y articulaciones prácticas." *Ciência & Saúde Coletiva* 8, no. 1, 185–207.

———. (2002) 2010. *La parte negada de la cultura: Relativismo, diferencias y racismo*. Rosario, Argentina: Prohistoria Ediciones.

Miller, Daniel. 2020. "How to Conduct an Ethnography during Social Isolation." YouTube, May 3. https://www.youtube.com/watch?v=NSiTrYB-0so.

Miller, Sean. 2013. *Strung Together: The Cultural Currency of String Theory as a Scientific Imaginary*. Ann Arbor: University of Michigan Press.

Mitchell, Richard J., Elizabeth A. Richardson, Niamh K. Shortt, and Jamie R. Pearce. 2015. "Neighborhood Environments and Socioeconomic Inequalities in Mental Well-Being." *American Journal of Preventative Medicine* 49, no. 1, 80–84.

Moffitt, Mike. 2020. "What They Don't Tell You about Surviving Covid-19." *SFGATE*. https://www.sfgate.com/news/editorspicks/article/What-they-don-t-tell-you-about-surviving-15347792.php#.

Mol, Annmarie. 2003. *The Body Multiple: Ontology in Medical Practice*. Durham, NC: Duke University Press.

———. 2009. *Introduction to Syndemics: A Critical Systems Approach to Public and Community Health*. San Francisco: Jossey-Bass.

Molotsky, Irvin. 1987. "US Approves Drug to Prolong Lives of AIDS Patients." *New York Times*, March 21.

Montgomery, Beronda. 2020a. "Planting Equity: Using What We Know to Cultivate Growth as a Plant Biology Community" (Letter to the Editor). *Plant Cell* (September 2020), tpc.00589.2020.

———. 2020b. "Lessons from Microbes: What Can We Learn About Equity from Unculturable Bacteria?" *American Society for Microbiology* 5, no. 5, e01046–20.

Montoya, Michael. 2011. *Making the Mexican Diabetic: Race, Science, and the Genetics of Inequality*. Berkeley: University of California Press.

Moran, A. J., A. Musicus, M. T. Forski Findling, Ian F. Brissette, Ann A. Lowenfels, S. V. Subramanian, and Christina A. Roberto. 2018. "Increases in Sugary Drink Marketing during Supplemental Nutrition Assistance Program Benefit Issuance in New York." *American Journal of Preventative Medicine* 55, no. 1, 55–62.

Morris, Zoë Slote, Steven Wooding, and Jonathan Grant. 2011. "The Answer Is 17 Years, What Is the Question: Understanding Time Lags in Translational Research." *Journal of the Royal Society of Medicine* 104, no. 12, 510–520.

Morris, Devin, Melissa Khurasany, Thien Nguyen, John Kim, Frederick Guilford, Rucha Mehta, Dennis Gray, Beatrice Saviola, and Vishwanath Venketaraman. 2013. "Glutathione and Infection." *Biochimica et Biophysica Acta* 1830, no. 5: 3329–3349.

Murphy, Robert. 1987. *The Body Silent: The Different World of the Disabled*. New York: W. W. Norton.

Myers, Amy. 2017. *The Autoimmune Solution: Prevent and Reverse the Full Spectrum of Inflammatory Symptoms and Diseases*. New York: HarperOne.

———. 2021. *The Thyroid Connection: Why You Feel Tired, Brain-Fogged, and Overweight—And How to Get Your Life Back*. New York: Little, Brown Spark.

Nader, Ralph. 1965. *Unsafe at Any Speed*. New York: Grossman Publishers.

Nading, Alex. 2017. "Can Microbes Give Gifts?" *Medical Anthropology Quarterly Book Forum Blog Series*. http://medanthroquarterly.org/?p=419.

NASA. 2018. "NASA Twins Study Investigators to Release Integrated Paper in 2019." https://www.nasa.gov/feature/nasa-twins-study-investigators-to-release-integrated-paper-in-2019.

National Institutes of Health. 2005. *Progress in Autoimmune Diseases Research.* https://www.niaid.nih.gov/sites/default/files/adccfinal.pdf.

National Library of Medicine. 2022. PubMed.gov. https://pubmed.ncbi.nlm.nih.gov/?term=microbiome&filter=years.1956-2019&timeline=expanded.

Navaro, Yael. 2020. "Methods and Social Reflexivity in the Time of Covid-19." *Wenner-Gren Blog,* June 19. http://blog.wennergren.org/2020/06/the-future-of-anthropological-research-ethics-questions-and-methods-in-the-age-of-covid-19-part-i/.

Neely, Abigail. 2015. "Internal Ecologies and the Limits of Local Biologies: A Political Ecology of Tuberculosis in the Time of AIDS." *Annals of the Association of American Geographers* 105, no. 4, 791–805.

Nestle, Marion. 2006. *What to Eat.* New York: North Point.

———. 2013. *Food Politics: How the Food Industry Influences Nutrition and Health.* Berkeley: University of California Press.

———. 2016. "The Farm Bill Drove Me Insane." Politico. March 17. https://www.politico.com/agenda/story/2016/03/farm-bill-congress-usda-food-policy-000070/.

Niewöhner, Jorg. 2011. "Epigenetics: Embedded Bodies and the Molecularisation of Biography and Milieu." *BioSocieties* 6, no. 3, 279–298.

Niewöhner, Jörg, and Margaret Lock. 2018. "Situating Local Biologies: Anthropological Perspectives on Environment/Human Entanglements." *BioSocieties* 13: 681–697.

Nowakowski, Alexandra C. H. and J. E. Sumerau. 2019. "Reframing Health and Illness: A Collaborative Autoethnography on the Experience of Health and Illness Transformations in the Life Course." *Sociology of Health & Illness* 41, no. 4, 723-739.

O'Conner, A. 2017. "In the Shopping Cart of a Food Stamp Household: Lots of Soda." *New York Times.* January 13.

Olszewski, Adam J., Stacie B. Dusetzina, Charles B. Eaton, Amy J. Davidoff, and Amal N. Trivedi. 2017. "Subsidies for Oral Chemotherapy and Use of Immunomodulatory Drugs Among Medicare Beneficiaries with Myeloma." *Journal of Clinical Oncology* 35, no. 29, 3306–3314.

Otero, Gerardo. 2018. *The Neoliberal Diet: Healthy Profits, Unhealthy People.* Austin: University of Texas Press.

Palamara, Anna Teresa. 1995. "Evidence for Antiviral Activity of Glutathione: In Vitro Inhibition of Herpes Simplex Virus Type 1 Replication." *Antiviral Research* 27, no. 3, 237–253.

Pálsson, Gísli. 2008. "Genomic Anthropology Coming in from the Cold?" *Current Anthropology* 49, no. 4, 545–568.

Park, Lisa Sun-Hee, and David N. Pellow. 2011. *The slums of Aspen: Immigrants vs. the environment in America's Eden.* New York: New York University Press.

Paxson, Heather. 2008. "Post-Pasteurian Cultures: The Microbiopolitics of Raw-Milk Cheese in the United States." *Cultural Anthropology* 23, no. 1, 15–47.

Paxson, Heather, and Stefan Helmreich. 2014. "The Perils and Promises of Microbial Abundance: Novel Natures and Model Ecosystems, from Artisanal Cheese to Alien Seas." *Social Studies of Science* 44, no. 2, 165–193.

Pellow, David N., and Robert J. Brulle. 2005. "Power, Justice and the Environment:

Toward Critical Environmental Justice Studies." In *Power, Justice, and the Environment: A Critical Appraisal of the Environmental Justice Movement*, edited by David N. Pellow and Robert J. Brulle. Cambridge, MA: MIT Press.

Pentecost, Michelle. 2018. "The First Thousand Days: Epigenetics in the Age of Global Health." In *The Palgrave Handbook of Biology and Society*, edited by Maurizio Meloni, John Cromby, Des Fitzgerald, and Stephanie Lloyd. London: Palgrave MacMillan.

Pentecost, Michelle, and Fiona Ross. 2019. "The First Thousand Days: Motherhood, Scientific Knowledge, and Local Histories." *Medical Anthropology* 38, no. 8, 747–761.

Pentecost, Michelle, and Maurizio Meloni. 2020. "'It's Never Too Early': Preconception Care and Postgenomic Models of Life." *Frontiers in Sociology* 5, 21.

Petri, William. 2020. "What Doctors Know About Lingering Symptoms of Coronavirus." *The Conversation*. https://theconversation.com/what-doctors-know-about-lingering-symptoms-of-coronavirus-141029.

Petryna, Adriana. 2003. *Life Exposed: Biological Citizens after Chernobyl*. Princeton, NJ: Princeton University Press.

Pew Research Center. 2021. "Mobile Fact Sheet." https://www.pewresearch.org/internet/fact-sheet/mobile/.

Pollan, Michael. 2006. *The Omnivore's Dilemma: A Natural History of Four Meals*. New York: Penguin.

———. 2008. *In Defense of Food: An Eater's Manifesto*. New York: Penguin.

Prescott, Susan, and Alan C. Logan. 2017. *The Secret Life of Your Microbiome: Why Nature and Biodiversity Are Essential to Health and Happiness*. Gabriola Island, BC: New Society Publishers.

Pullano, Nina. 2019. "Humans Can Reverse Their Biological Age, Shows a 'Curious Case' Study." *Inverse*. https://www.inverse.com/article/59096-humans-reverse-epigenetic-clock.

Qazi, Talal Jamil, Zhenzhen Quan, Asif Mir, and Hong Qing. 2017. "Epigenetics in Alzheimer's Disease: Perspective of DNA Methylation." *Molecular Neurobiology* 55, 1026–1044.

Quesada, James, Laurie K. Hart, and Philippe Bourgois. 2011. "Structural Vulnerability and Health: Latino Migrant Laborers in the United States." *Medical Anthropology* 30, no. 4, 339–362.

Rabinow, Paul. 1996. *Essays on the Anthropology of Reason*. Princeton, NJ: Princeton University Press.

Rabinow, Paul, and Nikolas Rose. 2006. "Biopower Today." *BioSocieties* 1, 195–217.

Ramos-Zayas, Ana Y. 2020. "Preliminary Thoughts on Ethics, Purpose, and Anthropology Beyond Covid-19." Wenner-Gren Blog, June 19. http://blog.wennergren.org/2020/06/thefuture-of-anthropological-research-ethics-questions-andmethodsin-the-age-of-covid-19-part-i/.

Ramsey, Scott, David Blough, Anne Kirchhoff, Karma Kreizenbeck, Catherine Fedorenko, Kyle Snell, Polly Newcomb, William Hollingworth, and Karen Overstreet. 2013. "Washington State Cancer Patients Found to Be at Greater Risk for Bankruptcy than People Without a Cancer Diagnosis." *Health Affairs* 32 (6), 1143-1152.

Rapp, Rayna. 1988. "Chromosomes and Communication: The Discourse of Genetic Counseling." *Medical Anthropology Quarterly* 2, no. 2, 143–157.

———. 2000. *Testing Women, Testing the Fetus: The Social Impact of Amniocentesis in America*. New York: Routledge.

Rappaport, S. M. 2016. "Genetic Factors Are Not the Major Causes of Chronic Diseases." *PLos ONE* 11 (4), e0154387.

Rédei, George. 2008. "Multiplicative Effect." In *Encyclopedia of Genetics, Genomics, Proteomics and Informatics*. Dordrecht, Netherlands: Springer.

Rees, Tobias. 2016. *Plastic Reason: An Anthropology of Brain Science in Embryogenetic Terms*. Berkeley: University of California Press.

Richards, Rose. 2016. "Writing the Othered Self: Autoethnography and the Problem of Objectification in Writing About Illness and Disability." *Qualitative Health Research* 18, no. 12, 1717–1728.

Richardson, Sarah S., Cynthia R. Daniels, Matthew W. Gillman, Janet Golden, Rebecca Kukla, Christopher Kuzawa, and Janet Rich-Edwards. 2014. "Society: Don't Blame the Mothers." *Nature* 512, 131–132.

Robbins, John, and Ocean Robbins. 2013. *Voices of the Food Revolution: You Can Heal Your Body and Your World—with Food!* Newburyport, MA: Conari Press.

Roberts, Dorothy. 2012. *Fatal Invention: How Science, Politics, and Big Business Re-create Race in the Twenty-first Century*. New York: New Press.

Roberts, R. C., C. B. Farmer, and C. K. Walker. 2018. "The Human Brain Microbiome; There Are Bacteria in Our Brains!" Abstract. https://www.abstractsonline.com/pp8/#!/4649/presentation/32057.

Roehr, Bob. 2013. "Spending on Health in the US Is Projected to Reach Almost 20% of GDP by 2020." *British Medical Journal* 347, f5721.

Rogerson, Jennifer. 2020. *Privileges of Birth: Constellations of Care, Myth, and Race in South Africa*. New York: Berghahn Books.

Rose, Nikolas. 1998. "Life, Reason, and History: Reading Georges Canguilhem Today." *Economic Sociology* 27, 154–170.

———. 1999. *Powers of Freedom: Reframing Political Thought*. Cambridge, UK: Cambridge University Press.

———. 2007. *The Politics of Life Itself: Biomedicine, Power, and Subjectivity in the Twenty-First Century*. Princeton, NJ: Princeton University Press.

Sanchez-Alcaraz, Maria, Pierre Kerkhofs, Michal Reichert, Richard Kettmann, and Luc Willems. 2004. "Involvement of Glutathione as a Mechanism of Indirect Protection against Spontaneous Ex Vivo Apoptosis Associated with Bovine Leukemia Virus." *Journal of Virology* 78, no. 12: 6180–6189.

Schulick, Paul, Thomas Newmark, and Richard Sarnat. 2002. *The Life Bridge: The Way to Longevity with Probiotic Nutrients*. Brattleboro, VT: Herbal Free Press.

Schulz, Laura C. 2010. "The Dutch Hunger Winter and the developmental origins of health and disease." *Proceedings of the National Academy of Sciences of the United States of America* 107, no. 39, 16757–16758.

Seligman, Hilary K., Barbara A. Laraia, and Margot B. Kushel. 2010. "Food Insecurity Is Associated with Chronic Disease among Low-Income NHANES Participants." *Journal of Nutrition* 140, no. 2, 304–310.

Serôdio, P. M., M. McKee, and D. Stuckler. 2018. "Coca-Cola: A Model of Transparency in Research Partnerships? A Network Analysis of Coca Cola's Research Funding (2008–2016)." *Public Health and Nutrition* 21, no. 9, 1594–1607.

Servan-Schreiber, David. 2009. *Anticancer: A New Way of Life*. New York: Viking.

Sessa-Hawkins, M. 2017. "Congress Could Cut Soda and Candy from SNAP, but Big Sugar Is Pushing Back." *Civil Eats.* August 28. https://civileats.com/2017/08/28/congress-could-cut-soda-and-candy-from-snap-but-big-sugar-is-pushing-back/.

Sharp, Lesley A. 2019. "Interspecies Engagement in Medical Anthropology." *Medical Anthropology Quarterly* 33, no. 1, 163–167.

Shook, Beth, Katie Nelson, Kelsie Aguilera, and Lara Braff. 2019. *Explorations: An Open Invitation to Biological Anthropology.* Arlington, VA: American Anthropological Assocation.

Shostak, Sara. 2013. *Exposed Science: Genes, the Environment, and the Politics of Population Health.* Berkeley: University of California Press.

Singer, Merrill. 1994. "Aids and the Health Crisis of the U.S. Urban Poor: The Perspective of Critical Medical Anthropology." *Social Science & Medicine* 39, no. 7, 931–948.

———. 2009a. *Introduction to Syndemics: A Critical Systems Approach to Public and Community Health.* Hoboken, NJ: Wiley.

———. 2009b. "Pathogens Gone Wild? Medical Anthropology and the 'Swine Flu' Pandemic." *Medical Anthropology* 28, no. 3, 199–206.

Skinner, Michael K., Carlos Guerrero-Bosagna, M. Haque, Eric Nilsson, Ramji Bhandari, and John R. McCarrey. 2013. "Environmentally Induced Transgenerational Epigenetic Reprogramming of Primordial Germ Cells and the Subsequent Germ Line." PLoS ONE 8(7): e66318.

Sletvold, Jon. 2014. "Embodied Empathy in Psychotherapy: Demonstrated in Supervision." *Body, Movement, and Dance in Psychotherapy* 10, no. 2, 82–93.

Slocum, Rachel. 2006. "Anti-Racist Practice and the Work of Community Food Organizations." *Antipode* 38, 327–349.

———. 2007. "Whiteness, Space, and Alternative Food Practice." *Geoforum* 38, 520–533.

Smelik, Anneke. 2010. *The Scientific Imaginary in Visual Culture. Interfacing Science, Literature, and the Humanities/ACUME* 2, no. 5. Göttingen, Germany: V&R Unipress.

Smith, Allen, and Harry Dawson. 2006. "Glutathione Is Required for Efficient Production of Infectious Picornavirus Virions." *Virology* 353, no. 2, 258–267.

Sobo, E. J. 2020. *Dynamics of Human Bio-cultural Diversity: A Unified Approach,* 2nd ed. New York: Routledge/Taylor & Francis.

Sobo, E., and M. Loustaunau. 2010. *The Cultural Context of Health, Illness and Medicine,* 2nd ed. Santa Barbara: Praeger.

Sontag, Susan. 1978. *Illness as Metaphor.* New York: Farrar, Straus and Giroux.

Sorenson, Thorkild I. A, Gert G. Nielsen, Per Kragh Andersen, Thomas W. Teasdale. 1988. "Genetic and Environmental Influences on Premature Death in Adult Adoptees." *New England Journal of Medicine* 318, no. 12, 727–732.

Spark, Arlene. 2014. "U.S. Agricultural Policies and the U.S Food Industry: Production to Retail." In *Local Food Environments: Food Access in America,* edited by K. B. Morland. Boca Raton, FL: CRC.

Sparks, Mark. 2011. "Building Healthy Public Policy: Don't Believe the Misdirection." *Health Promotion International* 26, vol. 3, 259–262.

Spivak, Gayatri Chakravorty. 1988a. "Can the Subaltern Speak?" In *Marxism and*

*Interpretation of Culture*, edited by Cary Nelson and Lawrence Grossberg. Chicago: University of Illinois Press.

———. 1988b. *In Other Worlds: Essays in Cultural Politics*. New York: Routledge.

Spivak, Gayatri Chakravorty, and Sarah Harasym. 1990. *The Post-Colonial Critic: Interviews, Strategies, Dialogues*. London: Routledge.

Steenhuysen, Julie. 2020. "Scientists Just Beginning to Understand the Many Health Problems Caused by Covid-19." *Reuters*. https://www.reuters.com/article/us-health-coronavirus-effects/scientists-just-beginning-to-understand-the-many-health-problems-caused-by-covid-19-idUSKBN23X1BZ.

Stingone, Jeanette A., Katharine H. McVeigh, and Luz Claudio. 2017. "Early-Life Exposure to Air Pollution and Greater Use of Academic Support Services in Childhood: A Population-Based Cohort Study of Urban Children." *Environmental Health* 16, no. 2, 1–10.

Strathern, Marilyn. 2005. *Kinship, Law, and the Unexpected: Relatives Are Always a Surprise*. Cambridge, UK: Cambridge University Press.

———. 2020. *Relations: An Anthropological Account*. Durham: Duke University Press.

Summerson Carr, E. 2011. *Scripting Addiction: The Politics of Therapeutic Talk and American Sobriety*. Princeton, NJ: Princeton University Press.

Sun, Benjamin B., Joseph C. Maranville, James E. Peters, David Stacey, James R. Staley, James Blackshaw, Stephen Burgess, Tao Jiang, Ellie Paige, Praveen Surendran, Clare Oliver-Williams, Mihir A. Kamat, Bram P. Prins, Sheri K. Wilcox, Erik S. Zimmerman, An Chi, Narinder Bansal, Sarah L. Spain, Angela M. Wood, Nicholas W. Morrell, John R. Bradley, Nebojsa Janjic, David J. Roberts, Willem H. Ouwehand, John A. Todd, Nicole Soranzo, Karsten Suhre, Dirk S. Paul, Caroline S. Fox, Robert M. Plenge, John Danesh, Heiko Runz, and Adam S. Butterworth. 2018. "Genomic Atlas of the Human Plasma Proteome." *Nature* 558, 73–79.

Sureshbabu, Jaya. 2021. "Pediatric Mononucleosis and Epstein-Barr Virus Infection." *Medscape*. https://emedicine.medscape.com/article/963894-overview.

Swistun, Debora Alejandra, and Javier Auyero. 2009. *Flammable: Environmental Suffering in an Argentine Shantytown*. New York: Oxford University Press.

Szasz, Andrew. 2007. *Shopping Our Way to Safety: How We Changed from Protecting the Environment to Protecting Ourselves*. Minneapolis: University of Minnesota Press.

Taylor, Janelle S. 2003. "'The Story Catches You and You Fall Down: Tragedy, Ethnography, and 'Cultural Competence.'" *Medical Anthropology Quarterly* 17, no. 2, 159–181.

Terzic, Andre, and Scott Waldman. 2011. "Chronic Diseases: The Emerging Pandemic." *Clinical and Translational Science* 4, no. 3, 225–226.

Thayer, Z., and A. Non. 2015. "Anthropology Meets Epigenetics: Current and Future Directions." *American Anthropologist* 117, no. 4: doi:10.1111/aman.

US Census Bureau. 2016. American Community Survey: 2014 and 2015 data [Data set]. https://www.census.gov/programs-surveys/acs/news/data-releases/2014/release.html.

US Department of Agriculture. 2016. "Foods Typically Purchased by Supplemental Nutrition Assistance Program (SNAP) Households." https://www.foodpolitics.com/wp-content/uploads/SNAPFoodsTypicallyPurchased_16.pdf.

USDA Economic Research Service. 2021. "Food Security and Nutrition Assistance. https://www.ers.usda.gov/data-products/ag-and-food-statistics-charting-the -essentials/food-security-and-nutrition-assistance/?topicId=c40bd422-99d8-4715 -93fa-f1f7674be78b.

US Environmental Protection Agency. n.d. "Glyphosate." https://www.epa.gov /ingredients-used-pesticide-products/glyphosate.

Vallgårda, Signild. 2015. "Governing Obesity Policies from England, France, Germany, and Scotland." *Social Science and Medicine* 147, 317–323.

Veblen, Thorstein. (1902) 2006. *Conspicuous Consumption.* New York: Penguin.

Vega, Rosalynn. 2018. *No Alternative: Childbirth, Citizenship, and Indigenous Culture in Mexico.* Austin: University of Texas Press.

Verlinde, Evelyn, Nele De Laender, Stéphanie De Maesschalck, Myriam Deveugele, and Sara Willems. 2012. "The Social Gradient in Doctor-Patient Communication." *International Journal for Equity in Health* 11, 12.

Verma Liao, Pamela. 2012. "Half a Century of the Oral Contraceptive Pill: Historical Review and View to the Future." *Canadian Family Physician* 58, no. 12, e757–e760.

Vickerstaff Joneja, Janice M. 2013. *The Health Professional's Guide to Food Allergies and Intolerances.* Chicago: Academy of Nutrition and Dietetics.

Virchow, H. Christian. 2014. "Eosinophilic Esophagitis: Asthma of the Esophagus?" *Digestive Diseases* 32, no. 1–2, 54–60.

Vogel, Sarah A. 2013. *Is It Safe? BPA and the Struggle to Define the Safety of Chemicals.* Berkeley: University of California Press.

Waggoner, Miranda. 2017. *The Zero Trimester: Pre-Pregnancy Care and the Politics of Reproductive Risk.* Berkeley: University of California Press.

Wahlberg, Ayo. 2016. "Exposed Biologies and the Banking of Reproductive Technology in China." Paper delivered at the American Anthropology Association Meetings, Minneapolis, MN.

Walker, Renee E., Christopher R. Keane, and Jessica G. Burke. 2010. "Disparities and Access to Healthy Food in the United States: A Review of Food Deserts Literature." *Health and Place* 16, no. 5, 876–884.

Wallerstein, Immanuel. 1976. *The Modern World-System: Capitalist Agriculture and the Origins of the European World-Economy in the Sixteenth Century.* New York: Academic Press.

Wang, Chao, Yu An, Huanling Yu, Lingli Feng, Quanri Liu, Yanhui Lu, Hui Wang, and Rong Xiao. 2016. "Association between Exposure to the Chinese Famine in Different Stages of Early Life and Decline in Cognitive Functioning in Adulthood." *Frontiers in Behavioral Neuroscience* 10: 146.

Ward, Elizabeth, Ahmedin Jemal, Vilma Cokkinides, Gopal K. Singh, Cheryll Cardinez, Asma Ghafoor, and Michael Thun. 2004. "Cancer Disparities by Race/Ethnicity and Socioeconomic Status." *CA: A Cancer Journal for Clinicians* 54, 78–93.

Waterland, Robert A., and Randy Jirtle. 2003. "Transposable Elements: Targets for Early Nutritional Effects on Epigenetic Gene Regulation." *Molecular Cell Biology* 15: 5293–5300.

Wayne County Health Environment Allergy and Asthma Longitudinal Study. 2015. https://getasthmahelp.org/documents/Johnson-CC-E-Lansing-Michigan-Oct -2015.pdf.

Weinhold, B. 2006. "Epigenetics: The Science of Change." *Environmental Health Perspectives* 114, no. 3, 160–167.

Wiley, Lindsay F., Micah L. Berman, and Doug Blanke. 2013. "Who's Your Nanny? Choice, Paternalism, and Public Health in the Age of Personal Responsibility." *Journal of Law, Medicine, and Ethics* 41, supplement 1, 88–91.

Willen, Sarah S., Michael Knipper, César E. Abadía-Barrero, and Nadav Davidovitch. 2017. "Syndemic Vulnerability and the Right to Health." *Lancet* 389, no. 10072, 964–977.

Wilson, Ara. 2004. *The Intimate Economies of Bangkok: Tomboys, Tycoons, and Avon Ladies in the Global City.* Berkeley: University of California Press.

Wilson, Elizabeth. 2015. *Gut Feminism.* Durham, NC: Duke University Press.

Winders, Bill. 2009a. "The Vanishing Free Market: The Formation and Spread of the British and US Food regimes." *Journal of Agrarian Change* 9, no. 3, 315–344.

———. 2009b. *The Politics of the Food Supply: U.S. Agricultural Policy in the World Economy.* New Haven, CT: Yale University Press.

Wolf-Meyer, Matthew J. 2017. "Multitudes without Politics." *Medical Anthropology Quarterly Book Forum Blog Series.* http://medanthroquarterly.org/?p=406.

World Health Organization. 2020. "Lack of New Antibiotics Threatens Global Efforts to Contain Drug-Resistant Infections." https://www.who.int/news/item/17-01 -2020-lack-of-new-antibiotics-threatens-global-efforts-to-contain-drug-resistant -infections.

World Health Organization and Secretariat of the Convention on Biological Diversity. 2015. "Connecting Global Priorities: Biodiversity and Human Health." https:// www.cbd.int/health/SOK-biodiversity-en.pdf.

Wyatt, S. B., D. R. Williams, R. Calvin, F. C. Henderson, E. R. Walker, and K. Winters. 2003. "Racism and Cardiovascular Disease in African Americans." *American Journal of the Medical Sciences* 325, no. 6, 315–331.

Xin, Xueling, Weijing Wang, Hui Xu, Zongyao Li, and Dongfeng Zhang. 2019. "Exposure to Chinese Famine in Early Life and the Risk of Dyslipidemia in Adulthood." *European Journal of Nutrition* 58, 391–398.

Yehuda, Rachel, Nikolaos P. Daskalakis, Linda M. Bierer, Heather N. Bader, Torsten Klengel, Florian Holsboer, Elisabeth B. Binder. 2016. "Holocaust Exposure Induced Intergenerational Effects on FKBP5 Methylation." *Biological Psychiatry* 80, no. 5, 372–380.

Yeoh, Yun Kit, Tao Zuo, Grace Chung-Yan Lui, Fen Zhang, Qin Liu, Amy YL Li, Arthur CK Chung, Chun Pan Cheung, Eugene Y. K. Tso, Kitty S. C. Fung, Veronica Chan, Lowell Ling, Gavin Joynt, David Shu-Cheong Hui, Kai Ming Chow, Susanna So Shan Ng, Timothy Chun-Man Li, Rita W. Y. Ng, Terry C. F. Yip, Grace Lai-Hung Wong, Francis K. L. Chan, Chun Kwok Wong, Paul K. S. Chan, and Siew C. Ng. 2021. "Microbiota Composition Reflects Disease Severity and Dysfunctional Immune Responses in Patients with COVID-19." *Gut* 0, 1–9.

# INDEX

Photos and illustrations are indicated by italicized page numbers.

functional medicine (*continued*)
35–36; illness denormalized in, 52–57;
individualistic emphasis in, 98; information vetting in, 37; intake process
for, 72–73; living healthy and, 91–93;
mechanisms in, 121–122; meta-
ethnography on, 19–20; modifiable
factors in, 141–142; 'Modifiable
Personal Lifestyle Factors' in, 68;
on non-Westerners, 98; on organs,
93; paradigm shifts in, 9, 20, 28–29;
participatory nature of, 53; person
centeredness in, 19, 33–34, 68; pharmaceuticalization and medicalization
critiqued in, 41–47; preconceptions
and patient care in, 61–63; privilege
in, 69, 142, 244, 264; protocols in,
59–60; "revolutionaries" in, 36–37;
scientific papers for, 57–58; social
inequality and, 99–101; structural
inequality lacking in, 69; structural
myopia in, 149–150; success stories in,
51; translational gap closed by, 57–60;
vaccines in, 38–39; vocabulary in, 54;
writing in three registers about, 19–21
Fung, Jason, 144

Gaia 2.0: farm animals in, 211; Gaia
hypothesis in, 209–210; in nested
ecologies, 207–211
Galland, Leo, 67–68
Gates, Donna, 162–163, 170–171
Gaudet, Tracy, 144
Gawande, Atul, 45
genetic profiles, 105–106, 134; as overwhelming, 109–110; SNPs in, 109
genomics, 115; advances in, 116–117; in
treatment protocols, 116, 121
Gentempo, Patrick, 144, 213
germs. *See* microbes
Glick, Bryan, 134
Global Food Security Act (2009), 242
glutathione S-transferase (GST): as
antioxidant, 107–108; functions of,
108–109
glyphosate, 259; chronic disease from,

213–214; in commodity crops,
234–235; cost of avoiding, 228–229;
in meat, 235; regulation of, 212–213;
ubiquity of, 211–212
GMOs, 212; in commodity crops, 234;
gag order about, 242–243; genetic
colonization in, 240–243; information
warfare on, 240; labeling of, 237, 253;
seed patents in, 240–241; subsidies
for, 234–235
government subsidies: commodity crops
and, 234–236, 253; dietary recommendations and, 235–236; for GMOs,
234–235; for meat and dairy, 235
grassroots movements: in food activism,
259–264; food justice organizations
as, 260–261; regenerative farming in,
261–262
Gratrix, Niki, 127
Gray, John, 180
Green, Lesley, 225–226
green spaces, 217, 223
Greenwood Food Blockade, 241
GST. *See* glutathione S-transferase
gut: addiction and, 179–180; aging and,
177; brain connection with, 172–182;
as command center, 174; as disease
source, 99–100; dysbiosis of, 77, 102,
177, 179, 201, 203–204; emotions
determined by, 178–179; as endocrine
organ, 174; personality shaped by,
178–179; reframing of, 181–182; sensory network in, 172; serotonin from,
175; as unique, 173
Guthman, Julie, 244; on class, 249; on
farmers, 250; on food activism, 263;
on romanticization, 246, 261

Haase, David, 117, 136
Hari, Vani, 259
Harrington, Kevin, 188–189
Hazen, Stanley, 171, 183, 191
health: bioconsumer purchase of, 98;
functional medicine creating, 47–52;
incentives for, 56; optimization of,
49–51; political ecology and, 211–217;

as primordial state, 67; as process, 265–267; resiliency in, 52, 72, 84, 265; social determinants of, 136; wellness-based industry for, 55
healthcare: costs of, 45; as disease care, 49; preparedness in, 56; profit incentives shaping, 92; recovery in, 52–53
health insurance, 49; changing of, 55–56; for disease care, 56; liquid biopsies lacking coverage in, 137; privilege in, 56–57
HealthMeans, 12–13
healthspan, 50
Herbert, Martha, 52–53, 102
Herpes Simplex 1 (HSV-1), 2; misconceptions about, 25; stigma about, 23–24; vulnerability to, 109
Heyman, Andrew: on being wrong, 61–62; on Cartesian split, 39; on diagnosis, 88; on disease management, 43–44; on personalized treatment, 60; on pharmaceuticals, 44; on translational gap, 59
Hislop, Rasheed, 251
histamine intolerance, 11, 155–156
holobiont: definition of, 190–191; microbiome and, 191; in nested ecologies, 192, 220
Hood, Leroy, 116
hookworms, 189
Horvath, Steven, 140
House Agriculture Committee, 236
"Household Food Security in the United States in 2020," 247
HSV-1. *See* Herpes Simplex 1
Human Genome Project, 119, 165
human papillomavirus, 2, 23, 80
hygiene: allergies and, 199–200; as antibios, 199–203; autoimmune diseases and, 200; germ theory and, 199; hypothesis of, 199–200
Hyman, Mark, 36–37; on anthropological approach, 64–65; on chronic disorders, 44; consumption recommendations by, 244; on delayed self-belief, 60; on diet, 205–206, 248;

on farming, 216, 251–252, 261–262; on FMT, 206; on food, 164, 232–234, 241, 249–250, 254, 263–264; as food activist, 237; on government, 237; on gut dysbiosis, 204; on health, 48; on health insurance, 56; on health optimization, 50; on information assimilation, 57; on information warfare, 237–238, 245; on naming disease, 88–89; on pharmaceuticalized medicine, 43–44; on policies, 253, 255, 262; on reductionism in medicine, 93–94; on SNAP, 255–258; on specialists, 87; on subsidies, 235–236; on supratentorial patients, 40–41; on systems biology, 85, 88
hyper self-reflexivity: absence of, 148–149; in anthropology, 26–28; as method, 28; privilege and, 27–28

iatrogenesis, 42, 202
IBS. *See* Irritable Bowel Syndrome
idiopathic, 77
illness: denormalization of, 52–57; in identity, 52; recovery from, 52–53. *See also* disease; functional illness
immune system, 183, 200
infectious diseases: narratives about, 24; stigma about, 22–24
inflammation, 151–152, 169
informational biology, 10, 29, 120; bioconsumers of, 117–119; emergence of, 116; mass marketing of, 117. *See also* genetic profiles
Ingelfinger, Franz J., 66
inter-kingdom communication, 171
Irritable Bowel Syndrome (IBS): antibiotics and, 76; as idiopathic condition, 77; as incurable, 266; serotonin and, 175–176; Terbutaline and, 74
irritable uterus, 73–74
IVF, 80–81

Jacka, Felice, 205
Ji, Sayer, 128; on ancestral diet, 196–197; on bacteriophages, 187; on body

Printed and bound by CPI Group (UK) Ltd, Croydon, CR0 4YY

09/06/2025

14685837-0001